A
Source Book
in
Chinese
Longevity

Livia Kohn

Three Pines Press
P.O. Box 530416
St. Petersburg, FL 33747
www.threepinespress.com

9   8 7 6 5 4 3 2 1

First Edition, 2012
Printed in the United States of America
⊗ This edition is printed on acid-free paper that meets
the American National Standard Institute Z39.48 Standard.
Distributed in the United States by Three Pines Press.

Cover: A talisman for enhancing long life. Picture by the author.

Library of Congress Cataloging-in-Publication Data
Kohn, Livia, 1956-
  A sourcebook in chinese longevity / Livia Kohn. -- 1st ed.
      p. cm.
  Includes bibliographical references and index.
  ISBN 978-1-931483-22-3 (pbk. : alk. paper)
  ISBN 978-1-105-55628-9 (electronic)
  1. Medicine, Chinese. 2. Longevity. 3. Health. 4. Nutrition. 5. Mind and
body. I. Title.
  R601.K65 2012
  613.2--dc23
                          2012007641

Contents

List of Illustrations

Introduction

People today live longer than in any time in history. In the 20th century, the average life expectancy in industrialized societies has almost doubled, increasing from about forty to close to eighty years of age. This is due to widespread efforts in public health—drastic improvements in sanitation and hygiene—coupled with enhanced nutrition, the conquest of infectious diseases through antibiotics and vaccinations, as well as the advances of medical technology that has made joint replacements, organ transplants, and genetic analysis commonplace.

Not only has life itself been extended, but the quality of life continues to improve, so that now centenarians are the fastest growing segment in industrialized populations. As this trend speeds up, more and more people are likely to grow considerably older without suffering the ill effects traditionally associated with aging. Research in gerontology and detailed studies of the aging process are leading to radical changes in our understanding of why and how we grow older, not only extending life expectancy—the culturally determined age people can be expected to reach at a certain time and place in history—but even placing life span—the biologically determined, species-specific limit of life—into question. Many scientists now believe that humans will soon live routinely beyond a hundred years, getting closer to the traditional life span of 120, and may even reach ages above this, pushing biological limits and altering the very nature of the species (e.g. Couzin 2005).

Modern efforts toward longevity (healthy old age) and prolongevity (radical life extension) that may lead eventually to immortality (freedom from death)[1] work in two main thrusts: personal lifestyle modifications and

---

[1] The understanding of human aging as an essentially curable disease in the modern age was proposed first by a group known as "the immortalists" (see Ettinger 1964; Harrington 1977). It is increasingly common among research scientists today (see Benecke 2002; Bova 1998; Hall 2003; Shostak 2002). For a study of the religious implications of these developments, see Maher and Mercer 2009.

advanced medical research. The former, as documented in numerous self-help books, works mainly with diet (especially calorie restriction), supplements (vitamins, growth hormones), exercise (aerobics, weight training, stretches), and stress reduction (relaxation, meditation).[2] The latter, described in more specialized literature, focuses on various forms of bioengineering, such as cloning, genetic modification, xenotransplants, cryonics, and more.[3]

Both are thoroughly rooted in the Western tradition and work with a model that inherits the Platonic, Biblical, and Cartesian understanding of the body as mere flesh, a material entity different from and opposed to the immortal soul, which alone belongs to God. Conceived as threatening and dangerous, full of unruly, ungovernable, and irrational passions, the body in this understanding has to be controlled in its locations, excretions, and reproduction.

Since the Enlightenment and the industrial revolution, moreover, control of body and world has been a central issue: control of the flesh through conquering sexuality and passions; control of the mind through systematic training, education, and political propaganda; control of nature through agriculture and industry, doing away with wilderness and wild life, allowing them to persist only in parks and zoos; control of the outer world by conquest of alien societies and the establishment of colonies; and control of all otherness though the increasing unification of world culture, the McDonaldization of society (see Feher 1989; Foucoult 1973).

In many ways, modern efforts at life extension are a continuation of this dominant trend which, in the late 20th century, merged with consumerism, an attitude of hedonistic enjoyment that proclaimed the body a vehicle of pleasure and rejected all "unnecessary" suffering and decline. The result is a volatile mix of rules and ascetic propositions of body control—manifest in health clubs, diet fads, low-calorie drinks, nonfat foods, vitamin supplements, and generally visions of athletic beauty—combined with the hedonistic pursuit of bodily desires—through nice meals, spa vacations, fancy clothes, electronic gadgets, sexual attractiveness, and so on.

The body in Western society has thus become a battle ground between asceticism and hedonism, control and suppression versus letting go and unashamed display. It has become an ideal, a vision, a project that has to be pur-

---

[2] See, for example, Chopra 1993; Lan et al. 2002; Plasker 2007; Réquéna 2010; Robbins 2006; Roizen and Oz 2007; Sawyer 2007; Weil 2005.

[3] Works of this type include Bailey 2005; Klein and Sethe 2004; Olshansky and Sethe 2001.

sued and made, refashioned by face-lifts, breast augmentations, diets, jogging, weight-lifting, massages, and so on. Yet despite its new image, the body has remained an object, a firm, solid, separate entity that needs to be shaped and molded. In that respect it has not changed despite social and doctrinal transformations. Life extension, as a result, is still dominantly a mechanical undertaking of manipulating different aspects and parts of the body. It is not, as yet, an integrated enterprise that transforms the entire person toward a new dimension of being. Chinese longevity practices, described in terms of "nourishing life" or "nourishing vitality" (*yangsheng* 養生), "nourishing inner nature" (*yangxing* 養性), "longevity" (*shou* 壽), "long life" (*changsheng* 長生), or "not dying" (*busi* 不死), are grounded in a process-oriented, energy-based worldview and have a history of several millennia. They go a long way toward realizing this new dimension and help expand the modern perspective of what can and should be done in the quest for longer, healthier, and happier lives.[4]

The Chinese Body

The body in traditional China is not separate from the cosmos, but forms an integral part of Dao, the underlying power of life and root of creation. There is only one Dao; all beings are part of it. It flows naturally along predisposed channels—in body, nature, society, and the universe. Like water, it is steady, fluid, easy, soft, and weak; it never pushes, fights, or controls. Like a mother, it brings forth and nurtures, cares and raises, supports and moves along: whatever people are and do, they are always part of Dao. One way of describing Dao is as "organic order"—organic in the sense that it is part of the world and not a transcendent other as in Western religion, order because it can be felt in the rhythms of the world, in the manifestation of organized patterns (see Schwartz 1985).

Another way to think of Dao is as two concentric circles, a smaller one in the center and a larger on the periphery. The dense, smaller circle in the center is Dao at the root of creation—tight, concentrated, intense, and ultimately unknowable, ineffable, and beyond conscious or sensory human attainment. The looser, larger circle at the periphery is Dao as it appears in the world, the patterned cycle of life and visible nature. Here Dao is manifest: it

---

[4] A few modern voices on prolongevity come from the Chinese tradition, but tend to also subscribe to a more Western body system. See Liu 1990; Ni 2006.

comes and goes, rises and sets, rains and shines, lightens and darkens. It is, in fact, the ever changing yet ever lasting alteration of natural patterns, life and death, yin and yang (Kohn 2001, 20).

In both forms, moreover, Dao manifests in a vital energy known as *qi* 氣, which can be described as a bioenergetic potency that causes things to live, grow, develop, and decline. The basic force of all existence, *qi is* the world, nature, society, and the human body—all of which are part of a dynamic cosmos that never stops or ends. This also means that there is no division of body, mind, and nature but that these are only different aspects of *qi*-flow, moving at various vibrational speeds and levels—an understanding that closely matches modern quantum physics.[5]

According to the Chinese vision, human life is the accumulation of *qi*, death is its dispersal. People as much as the planet consist first of all of primordial *qi* that connects them to the greater universe and is given to them at birth. They need to sustain it throughout life by drawing postnatal or external *qi* into the body from air and food as well as from other people through sexual, emotional, and social interaction.

But they also lose *qi* through breathing bad air, living in polluted conditions, overburdening or diminishing their bodies with food and drink, getting involved in negative emotions, engaging in excessive sexual or social interactions, and in general suffering from various forms of stress. Although life expectancy or "destiny" is thus a function of primordial *qi*, the way in which people nurture or dissipate it in their use of postnatal *qi* determines ultimately how well and how long they live. Since *qi* as part of Dao is everlasting, there is moreover no fundamental limit to the life one can attain.

As a result, health and long life in the Chinese vision are defined as the smooth alignment with Dao as it manifests in one's personal physical and psychological characteristics and opens paths to full self-realization. It means the presence of a strong vital energy and of a harmonious, active *qi*-flow that moves in a steady alteration of yin and yang, two aspects of the continuous flow of creation: the rising and falling, growing and declining, warming and cooling, beginning and ending, expanding and contracting movements that pervade all life and nature. Yin and yang continuously alternate and change from one into the other. They do so in a steady rhythm of rising and falling, visible in nature in the rising and setting of the sun, the warming and cooling of the seasons, the growth and decline of living beings.

---

[5] See Bentov 1977; Bohm 1951; Gerber 1988; Gribbin 1984; Zukav 1979.

This flow of *qi* in undulating waves is further systematized into a system of the so-called five phases (*wuxing* 五行) which are in turn symbolized by five material objects:

minor yang	major yang	yin-yang	minor yin	major yin
wood	fire	earth	metal	water

These five continue to produce each other in a harmonious cycle in the presented order. *Qi* that flows in this order and in the right amount is known as proper *qi* (*zhengqi* 正氣). In addition to personal health, this is also manifest by harmony in nature, i.e., regular weather patterns and the absence of disasters, and as health in society, the peaceful coexistence among families, clans, villages, and states. This harmony on all levels, the cosmic presence of a steady and pleasant flow of qi, is what the Chinese call the state of Great Peace (*taiping* 太平), venerated by Confucians and Daoists alike.

Qi, on the other hand, that has lost harmonious flow is called wayward (*xieqi* 邪氣). Disorderly and dysfunctional, it creates change that violates the normal order. When it becomes dominant, the *qi*-flow can turn upon itself and deplete the body's resources. Thus, any sick person, decimated forest, or intrusive construction no longer operates as part of a universal system and are not in tune with the basic life force.

Whether proper or wayward, *qi* constitutes all the different systems of the body, which are not classified according to skeletal, muscular, or hormonal, but in terms of yin organs (1) that store *qi* and center the body's functioning, yang organs (2) that move *qi* and take care of digestion and respiration, body fluids that moisturize the body including the lymph and sweat glands, parts that make the body come together, senses that connect it to the outside world, emotions that characterize negative reactions to the world, and virtues that enhance positive attitudes.

phase	organ1	organ2	fluid	body	sense	emotion	virtue
wood	liver	gall	tears	joints	seeing	anger	kindness
fire	heart	small int.	sweat	blood	touch	joy	propriety
earth	spleen	stomach	oral	muscles	taste	worry	honesty
metal	lungs	large int.	nasal	skin	smell	sadness	righteousness
water	kidney	bladder	saliva	bones	hear	fear	wisdom

The same system of the five phases also connects the body to the outside world, to the seasons, directions, colors, and other aspects of nature, creating a complex network of energetic pathways that work closely together and are intimately interconnected.

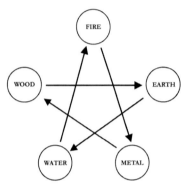

Fig. 1. The five phases

Within the body, moreover, the organs are the key storage and transformation centers of *qi*. They connect to the extremities through a network of energy channels called meridians (*mai* 脈). There are twelve main meridians that run on both sides of the body. They include ten channels centered on the five yin and yang organs, plus two added for symmetry: the Triple Heater (yang), a digestive organ that combines the *qi* from food and from air and transports it to the heart; and the pericardium (yin), supplementing the heart.

There are also eight extraordinary vessels which run only along one line in the body. They are considered primary and more elemental than the twelve meridians, carrying a deeper blueprint of the human being. They include four lines that run along the arms and legs, supporting the basic yin and yang structure of the body, plus two that create a cross inside the torso: the Belt Vessel (*daimai* 帶脈) which encircles the waist horizontally and the Penetrating Vessel (*chongmai* 沖脈) which runs vertically straight through the center from head to pelvic floor. The remaining two are the Governing (*dumai* 督脈; yang) and Conception Vessels (*renmai* 任脈; yin), which run along the back and front of the torso, both originating near the base of the spine and ending around the mouth. They form an essential energy circuit along the torso and are essential in all aspects of life cultivation.

Healing, Longevity, and Immortality

The body being an integrated organism of different forms, levels, and inter-actions of *qi*, healing, longevity, and immortality are also part of the same structure and form a closely knit continuum of practice. Most basic and best known is medical healing, which is usually administered by someone outside the person in the form of acupuncture, herbs, and massages, as well as dietary, exercise, and lifestyle recommendations. This part of the practice serves to replenish *qi* when people have lost their vitality due to bad habits, stress, infections, accidents, and the like.[6]

Having recovered health, many continue in their old ways and eventu-ally get sick again. Some, and especially older people who have undergone repeated cycles of health and decline, realize just how much conscious life-style choices contribute to their well-being. Having attained good health and gained an increased awareness of *qi*-patterns, they may decide to increase their primordial *qi* to the level they had at birth or even above it.

To do so, they follow a variety of preventative medical or longevity techniques—including moderation, diet, exercise, self-massages, breathing, and meditations—to absorb their *qi*-exchange with the environment and cultivate its inner flow (see Kohn 1989). The practice ensures the full realiza-tion of people's natural life expectancy in health and vigor. It often leads to an increase in years, a youthful appearance, and continued strength and en-joyment of life. People enhance and empower the natural patterns of life, consciously following the patterns of yin and yang and creating harmony in themselves and their surroundings.

Immortality, third, raises the practices to a higher and transcendent level. Unlike medical healing and longevity, it means moving beyond the natural cycle and applying the techniques in a reverse manner. To attain it, people have to transform all their *qi* into primordial *qi* and proceed to refine it to subtler levels. This finer *qi* will eventually turn into pure spirit (*shen* 神), with which practitioners increasingly identify to become transcendent spirit people.

The path that leads there involves intensive meditation and trance training as well as more radical forms of diet and other longevity practices. It results in a bypassing of death, so that the end of the body has no impact on the continuation of the spirit person. In addition, practitioners attain super-

---

[6] On Chinese medicine, see Kaptchuk 1983; Kendall 2002; Kohn 2005; Larre et al. 1986; Liu 1988; Porkert 1974; Sivin 1988.

sensory powers and eventually gain residence in otherworldly realms. Unlike medicine and longevity, immortality thus comes with an extensive, vibrant mythology that describes splendid heavens, fabulous creatures, and a host of divine beings.[7]

The very same kinds of practices may be used on all three levels, albeit in different ways and with caution. Certain practices that are useful in healing may be superfluous in the attainment of longevity, while some applicable for immortality may even be harmful when healing is the main focus. Take breathing as an example. When healing or extending life, natural deep breathing is emphasized, with the diaphragm expanding on the inhalation. When moving on to immortality, however, reversed breathing is advised, which means that the diaphragm contracts on the in-breath. Undertaking this kind of reversed breathing too early or at the wrong stage in one's practice can cause complications, from dizziness to disorientation or worse.[8]

This holds also true for sexual practices. In healing, sexual activity with a partner is encouraged in moderation, with both partners reaching regular climaxes. In longevity practice, sexual activity may still be performed with a partner, but ejaculation as a loss of *qi* is avoided and sexual stimulation is used to increase the positive flow of *qi* in the body. In immortality, finally, sexual practices are undertaken internally and without a partner. They serve the creation of an immortal embryo through the refinement of sexual energy into primordial *qi* and cosmic spirit. Going beyond nature, immortality practitioners are not interested in creating harmony and balance, but strive to overcome the natural tendencies of the bodymind and actively lessen or even relinquish earthly existence in favor of cosmic and heavenly states.[9]

Diets are another case in point. Chinese medical diets use ordinary ingredients and recipes, focusing strongly on rice, beans, and vegetables as well as meats, tofu, and other forms of protein. They require the more conscious adaptation to seasonal patterns and the application of warming or cooling foods, spices, herbs, depending on the patient's condition. Eating for long life uses the same principles and is still grain-based, but involves the abstention

---

[7] On the cosmology and mythology of immortality, see Campany 2002; Despeux and Kohn 2003; Miller 2008.

[8] There is as yet no good book on Chinese breathing. For a historical study of the Six Healing Breaths or Sounds, see Despeux 2006.

[9] There are numerous works on Chinese sexual practices, as any Google search will reveal. A good survey of the different kinds and comprehensive translation of texts, most relevant to the longevity tradition, is found in Wile 1992.

from heavy meats and fats as well as from strong substances such as alcohol, garlic, and onions. Practitioners are encouraged to eat lightly and in small portions, matching the seasons and always conscious of their internal *qi.* Contrary to this, immortality practice is to "avoid grain" (*bigu* 辟穀). They eliminate main staples, eat mainly raw food, and increasingly rely on herbal and mineral supplements. Their goal is the refinement of *qi* to a level where food intake is completely replaced by the conscious absorption of *qi* through breath, leading to extended periods of fasting.[10]

The Longevity Tradition

Longevity techniques occupy the middle ground between healing and immortality, medicine and religion. The culmination of healing, they form the ultimate of medical practice; serving as the path to perfect health, they are the foundation of Daoist immortality. Placed between two completely different dimensions yet connected to both, they represent a separate tradition that from its very beginning appears as both preventative and anti-aging medicine and also as a way of personal and spiritual self-cultivation. Only a few dedicated scholars have contributed significantly to its understanding.[11]

As outlined in detail in *Chinese Healing Exercises* (Kohn 2008), longevity practices appear first in manuscripts uncovered at Mawangdui, contained in six of a total of forty-five texts known collectively as the "Chinese medical manuscripts" (trl. Harper 1998). The tomb was closed in 168 BCE, dating the texts to the early Han dynasty (206-6 BCE). Before this time, however, traces of longevity methods appear in inscriptions and philosophical works, such as the "Inward Training" chapter of the *Guanzi,* indicating that awareness of *qi* and methods of its internal circulation and meditational enhancement already formed part of the spiritual and self-cultivation culture of ancient China (see Roth 1999).

Both physicians and philosophers continued to develop the tradition, as documented in the early 3rd century CE in Hua Tuo's Five Animals Frolic as well as in Xi Kang's *Yangsheng lun* (On Nourishing Life). More elaborate

---

[10] On dietary practices of the three levels, see Arthur 2006; Craze and Jay 2001; Lu 1986; Kohn 2010a. For a more comprehensive presentation of various longevity methods, on a popular level and from a medical background, see Reid 1989 and 2003.

[11] See Despeux 1987; 1988; Engelhardt 1987; Kohn 1989; 2006; Sakade 1988; 2007a; Stein 1999.

sources that also show the increasing interaction between the two dimensions appear in the 4th century. In 317, the imperial court of the Jin dynasty fled from the invading Huns and moved south, replacing southern aristocrats in government offices. With time at hand and no careers to pursue, they turned to various other endeavors, including the pursuit of health and spiritual advancement. The result was not only the first comprehensive book on longevity practices but also the founding of the Daoist school of Highest Clarity. Based on a combination of traditional cosmology, early Daoist ritual, and operative alchemy, its followers focused on connecting to the gods and starry palaces above and practiced elaborate visualizations and ecstatic excursions as well as the concoction of elixirs that would instantaneously transport them to the otherworld. In preparation for these endeavors, they applied longevity techniques, using them to strengthen their senses, extend their life expectancy, and clear their energy channels. Longevity practices thus formed an active part of both aristocratic and religious culture.

This in turn led to a proliferation of texts in the course of the Six Dynasties (420-589) that outline a plethora of different methods involving ways of internal *qi* manipulation, physical exercises, and dietary control—contained in the Daoist canon as well as recouped in medical literature. The longevity tradition was finding its unique expression while continuing to straddle both realms of medicine and religion.

The Tang dynasty (618-907) was the heyday of Daoism as well as the longevity tradition. It established the first stable rule after many centuries of division, and much of its culture was dedicated to unification and integration. This was obvious not only in the political realm but also in the world of thought and religion, creating integrated organizational structures and worldview systems. In terms of the longevity tradition, it led to three major systematizations: the texts by the physician and Daoist Sun Simiao, a prolific author especially of medical works who was active in the 7th century and is still revered as a grand master of and God of Medicines; the *Yangxing yanming lu* (Record on Nourishing Inner Nature and Extending Life), a comprehensive collection of all sorts of different methods that also includes a collection of references to longevity methods in previous literature; and the medically based outline of *qi*-absorption methods by the Highest Clarity patriarch Sima Chengzhen, court Daoist of the 8th century and best known for his work on Daoist meditation, "Sitting in Oblivion" (trl. Kohn 2010b).

In the wake of this explosion of techniques, which were also transmitted to Japan and recorded systematically in the *Ishinpō* (Essential Medical Methods; trl. Hsia et al. 1986) of 974, the longevity tradition its active presence in both medical and religious sources, including Daoist texts as well as technical compendia from the Song (960-1260), Ming (1368-1644) and Qing (1644-1911) dynasties.

A major medical source is the *Chifeng sui* (Marrow of the Red Phoenix; trl. Despeux 1988), a collection of longevity methods by Zhou Lüjing, dated to 1578. Reflecting the typical career of a longevity master, Zhou was the son of an aristocratic family, trained for office and married. Then, however, he contracted tuberculosis and could not find help among the medical establishment. Concerned with his health, he made survival his first priority and left the family to reside in a Daoist temple. He got well, but found the world of long life and spiritual cultivation so enticing that he remained a recluse, developing numerous skills, such as sword fighting, paper making, painting, calligraphy, and long life techniques. [12] He collected prescriptions for healing, including herbs, talismans, rituals, exorcisms, and spells, which he wrote up variously (Despeux 1988, 12-13). Integrating many earlier methods, his book consists of three sections: techniques of breathing and guiding *qi*, exercise sequences including the Five Animals Frolic, and meditative exercises based on internal alchemy. It is comprehensive and has remained a key resource for practitioners today.

Within the Daoist tradition, longevity techniques have continued to be initiatory and supplementary, ensuring that practitioners are energetically open for the more advanced spiritual transformations of *qi*. Works on internal alchemy, as a result, mention the methods only in passing, taking them for granted as a prerequisite. However, their take on the human body and its internal powers is different enough to have made an impact on the longevity tradition, especially when it comes to practices specifically geared toward women. Known as women's alchemy, they are recorded from the late 18th century onward, reflecting an increase in women's literacy as well as a greater awareness of the unique features of the female body.

---

[12] Sun Simiao has a similar background story (Sivin 1967; Kohn 2008, 129-31); Jiang Weiqiao 蔣維橋(1872–1955), the author of the *Yinshizi jingzuo fa* 因是子靜坐 法 (Quiet Sitting with Master Yinshi) and major forerunner of qigong in modern China, too, was stricken by tuberculosis and dedicated himself to healing full-time (Kohn 2002; Liu Guizhen 劉貴珍 (1920-1983), the initiator of qigong in the Communist Party, suffered from numerous ailments that medicine could not heal but Daoist-preserved longevity techniques could (Palmer 2007); and Hu Fuchen 胡孚琛 (b. 1945), a Western-trained pharmacologist, came to longevity fasting in the 1990 after being diagnosed with multiple serious diseases (Arthur 2006b, 113).

Today longevity pervades Chinese culture in the form of qigong and taiji quan, practiced widely among the general populace and a mainstay of Daoist cultivation (see Cohen 1997). The exercises described in the literature over the millennia are still actively used, recreated, enhanced, and transformed. They are also increasingly brought into a Western scientific context, notably in energy medicine and psychology (see Feinstein et al. 2005; Gallo 2004; Oschman 2000; Shealy 2011; Carlson and Kohn 2012). However, to date there are only few translations of relevant texts, preventing the proper appreciation of the tradition.[13]

This volume hopes to remedy this lack. It presents translations of numerous sources on longevity practice from a variety of periods, including comprehensive guidelines on lifestyle moderation as well as the major compendia of the Tang. It offers materials on specific practices, such as diets, exercise, self-massages, breathing, and the guiding of *qi*, in each case selecting the most representative and most widely cited works. It does not repeat translations already available, such as of the Han-dynasty manuscripts (Harper 1998) and texts on sexual (Ishihara and Levy 1970) and women's practices (Wile 1992). It does, however, cover the main periods of the longevity tradition, beginning with the 4th century BCE, when the earliest materials appear, and systematically moves through Chinese history, all the way to late Qing period and its development of special techniques for women.

Opening the traditional Chinese texts, their worldview, body vision, and concrete methods, to a wider Western audience, the book hopes to contribute not only to the better understanding of Chinese culture but also to aid the contemporary search for a way to enable more people to live longer and healthier lives.

---

[13] Translations in French and German include Despeux 1988; Engelhardt 1987; Stein 1999. In English there are only four: Harper 1998 translates the manuscripts found in the Mawangdui tomb of the Han dynasty; Hsia et al. 1986 has the longevity chapters of the Japanese collection *Ishinpō* (dat. 984); Huang and Wurmbrand 1987 offers a collection of texts on breathing from the Daoist canon, albeit with no annotation; and Berk 1986 presents an illustrated Qing-dynasty work on healing exercises.

Chapter One

Nourishing Body and Self

The earliest records on how best to enhance vitality by nourishing body and self come from the late Warring States through early Han, dating from the 4th to the 2nd centuries BCE. They divide clearly into two groups, transmitted philosophical texts connected to certain "masters" (*zi* 子) and excavated technical manuscripts containing "methods" (*fang* 方). Philosophical texts are mainly pre-Han and only hint at concrete practices, yet their later commentaries attach new explanations and practice instructions to their verses. Excavated manuscripts tend to come from Han tombs, but there are also earlier finds that outline practices. The overall tendency is, as Donald Harper points out, that while pre-Han texts present "a theoretical exposition on the physiology of the sage, the excavated texts are meant to teach how to do it—whether it be breath cultivation, exercise, sexual cultivation, or dietetics" (1998, 125). These two kinds of sources are thus representative for the two-fold thrust of the tradition: theoretical and practical, spiritual and physical.

As the two kinds of sources go back to different historical periods, their fundamentally distinct nature also signals a shift in overall accessibility and spread of the methods. "One is inclined to think of Warring States cultivation practice as an arcane matter with few actual practitioners," Donald Harper notes. In contrast, early Han sources "paint a rather different picture of the popularity of macrobiotic hygiene among the elite in the 3rd and 2nd centuries BCE," the literature being widely available and consisting almost entirely of practice instructions (Harper 1998, 126).

At the same time, the two kinds of sources already point to the integration of the two dimensions, the ultimate goal combining physical perfection with spiritual transcendence. They agree that harmony of spirit and peace of mind have a profound effect on the body, while physical control and a mod-

erate lifestyle open the self to spiritual cultivation. Thus the medical manuscript *Shiwen* 十問 (Ten Questions) says about "fullness of life": "Above it
spans Heaven and below it spreads over Earth. Who succeeds in attaining it
becomes a spirit and as such can release his bodily form" (Harper 1998, 398).

This attitude is also fundamental in the philosophical text *Zhuangzi* 莊
子 (Book of Master Zhuang), whose materials were compiled in the mid-3rd
century BCE and in part go back to the 4th.[1] Rather impatient with purely
physical cultivation, Zhuangzi ridicules those who merely "huff and puff,
exhale and inhale, blow out the old and draw in the new, do the 'bear-hang'
and the 'bird-stretch'" as "Pengzu's oldsters" (ch. 15; Graham 1986, 265). On
the other hand, the text contains several sets of meditation instructions important in the later tradition, such as "sitting in oblivion" (*zuowang* 坐忘)
and "mind-fasting" (*xinzhai* 心齋) (see Kohn 2010b; Saso 2010; Santee 2008).
While emphasizing the centrality of *qi*—rather than using the mind or senses
to perceive, practitioners should attune themselves to the subtler level of
energy perception—the text's key focus is on mental disengagement and
spiritual cultivation, noting the connection to the body only in some passages.

An early text that also provides meditation instructions but focuses
more strongly on the mind-body connection in terms of *qi* is the "Neiye" 內
業 (Inward Training) chapter of the *Guanzi* 管子 (Works of Master Guan; trl.
Roth 1999). According to this, adepts refine their *qi* through physical control
and moderation in lifestyle and diet, withdrawal from sensory stimulation,
and sitting in meditation. They pursue the fourfold alignment of body, limbs,
breath, and mind. First they take a proper upright posture and align their
limbs, then breathe deeply and consciously, regulating the breath and creating a sense of quietude within. From there they practice single-minded focus
for the attainment of a tranquil mind, also described as the "cultivated," "stable," "excellent", and "well-ordered" mind. This well-ordered mind then creates an open space within, a lodging place where *qi* can come to stay and
flow about freely.

Once filled with the potency of *qi*, adepts achieve complete balance in
body and mind. They reach a level of simplicity that allows them to let go of
things and be free from sensory overloads. Finding a state of serenity and
repose in detachment from emotions that resembles the state of clarity and
stillness proposed in the *Daode jing* 道德經 (Book of the Way and Its Power),

---

[1] The original text with the pioneering translation by James Legge can be found
at http://ctext.org/Zhuangzi. Other prominent translations include Watson 1968a;
Graham 1981; 1986; Mair 1994; Kohn 2011. For a complete list, see Mair 2010, 228-32.

they walk through life in harmony with all, free from danger and harm. At peace within and in alignment with the world, they attain a level of physical health that keeps them fit and active well into old age. Reaching beyond ordinary life, they gain a sense of cosmic freedom that allows them to "hold up the Great Circle [of the heavens] and tread firmly over the Great Square [of the earth]" (Roth 1999, 112-13).

Another combination physical practices and spiritual attainment appears in the Han-dynasty commentary to the *Daode jing* attributed to Heshang gong 河上公, the Master on the River. A Daoist sage of some renown, he is said to have lived near the Yellow River under Emperor Wen (r. 179-156 BCE), studying the *Daode jing.* The emperor was a great devotee of Laozi and his teachings. He had the text recited at court, but had difficulties understanding certain passages. He learns about Heshang gong and summons him to court, but the master refuses. Impatient, the emperor goes to see him, scolding him for his lack of respect. Instead of groveling before the ruler, the master rises in levitation to hover between Heaven and Earth, thus making it clear that he is beyond all civil authority. Deeply awed, the emperor apologizes and begs to receive his teachings, upon which Heshang gong hands over the manuscript of his commentary.[2]

Now contained in the Daoist Canon under the title *Heshang gong zhangju* 河上公章句 (Verses and Sayings of the Master on the River, DZ 682),[3] it focuses mainly on the link between personal cultivation and the perfection of rulership. It explains the rather abstract philosophical verses of the *Daode jing* in terms of *qi* control through breathing, dietetics, and the visualization of psychological agents or "spirits" in the five central organs of the body, thus linking longevity and transcendence (see Sakade 2007b).

As far as concrete methods go, the earliest practice instructions on specifically physical techniques appear in an inscription on a dodecagonal jade block that dates from the 4th century B.C.E. and is entitled *Xingqi* 行氣 (Guiding *Qi*). The original function of the block remains uncertain (see Chen 1982),

---

[2] The Heshang gong legend is detailed in the *Laozi daode jing xujue* 道德經序訣 (Introductory Explanation to the Perfect Scripture of the Dao and Its Inherent Potency) which dates from the about the 5th century CE and survives in several Dunhuang manuscripts (S. 75, P. 2370). For a detailed study of the figure and the text, see Chan 1991.

[3] Numbers in the Daoist Canon refer to the extensive annotated catalog by Schipper and Verellen (2004). A full translation of the commentary appears in Erkes 1958; sections on inner cultivation are also rendered in Needham 1983, 130-35.

but its forty-five characters describe a fundamental *qi* practice that reappears in the first section of the *Shiwen* (Harper 1998, 386-87), forms an important part of longevity practice throughout the middle ages, and is still central to internal alchemy and qigong today under the name Microcosmic Orbit (*xiao zhoutian* 小周天; see Chia and Chia 1993). [4]

To perform the practice, people inhale deeply, allow the breath to enter both the chest and the mouth, and in the latter mix it with saliva, another potent form of *qi* in the body. Moving their tongue around their mouth, they gather the saliva and gain a sense of fullness, then swallow, allowing the *qi* to sink down. They feel it moving deep into their abdomen, where they let it settle in the central area of gravity, known in Chinese medicine as the Ocean of *Qi* (*qihai* 氣海) and in Daoism as the cinnabar or elixir field (*dantian* 丹田). There the *qi* rests and becomes stable, growing stronger as it accumulates. Eventually it does not remain in the lower abdomen but begins to spread through the body or, as the text says, it "sprouts." Once this is felt, adepts can consciously guide it upwards, in close coordination with deep breathing pushing it down to the pelvic floor and then moving it up along the spine. The goal of the practice is to open the body to *qi* while harmonizing its flow, and thus ensuring inner focus and physical health.

More extensive and detailed *qi* practices are outlined in six medical manuscripts unearthed at Mawangdui 馬王堆 (168 BCE). Two texts deal almost solely with sexual cultivation, discussing the best times and frequency of sexual intercourse as well as herbal remedies for impotence and weakness. They are the *He yinyang* 和陰陽 (Harmonizing Yin and Yang) and the *Tianxia zhidao tan* 天下至道談 (The Perfect Dao in the World). Two texts focus on breathing, dietetics, and herbal drugs: the *Yangsheng fang* 養生方 (Recipes for Nourishing Life;) and the *Shiwen*. Two further works focus on breathing and exercises. The *Quegu shiqi* 卻穀食氣 (Eliminating Grains and Eating *Qi*) covers ways of fasting by means of controlled breathing, repeatedly contrasting "those who ingest *qi*" with "those who ingest grain," while the *Daoyintu* 導引圖 (Exercise Chart) presents forty-four color illustrations of human figures performing healing exercises.[5]

---

[4] The original of the block is reprinted in Li 1993, 320-23. Discussions appear in Engelhardt 1996, 19; Harper 1998, 126; Wilhelm 1948.

[5] All these texts are translated with extensive annotation and detailed explanations in Harper 1998. Those on sexual practices also appear in Wile 1992, 77-83. They are not included in this anthology.

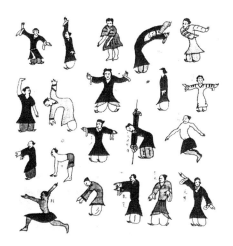

Fig. 2. The "Exercise Chart" from Mawangdui

Another set of early cultivation texts was unearthed at Zhangjiashan 張家山 and dated to 186 BCE: the *Maishu* 脈書 (Channel Book), a compilation of several texts with lists of ailments and descriptions of eleven *qi*-conduits (Harper 1998, 31-33; Ikai 1995, 29); and the *Yinshu* 引書 (Stretch Book), a short text presents seasonal health regimens, a series of about a hundred exercises in three sections, and a brief discussion on the etiology of disease and ways of prevention. The *Yinshu* is the earliest text to outline specific exercises and their medical application in great detail; it also prescribes certain breaths to use for the balancing of *qi*, curing of diseases, and extension of life. Unlike the earlier texts but very much like the Mawangdui manuscripts, it is very clearly a medical work, representing the physical dimension of Chinese longevity.[6]

---

[6] The original text of the *Yinshu* is reprinted in modern characters Wenwu 1990, 84-85; Li 1993, 340; Ikai 2004, 27-28. The first section also translated in Harper 1998, 110-11; other parts appear in Harper 1998, 132-33. The various exercises are translated and discussed in Engelhardt 1996; Kohn 2008, 41-61.

Translation

Everlasting Life [7]

The Yellow Emperor retired, left the world, set up a solitary hut, spread a plain mat, and went on retreat for three months. After that he went to see Guangchengzi, the Master of Wide Accomplishments. He found him lying down with his head to the south. In abject submission, the Yellow Emperor approached him on his knees, knocked his head to ground twice, and asked: "I have heard that you have attained utmost Dao. May I ask what self-cultivation I should practice to reach extended longevity?"

The Master got up quickly: "What a great question! Come and I will tell you all about utmost Dao. Its innermost essence is serene and obscure; its highest ultimate is murky and silent.

"Practice being unseeing and unhearing, guard your spirit in stillness, and your body will automatically right itself.

"Practice clarity and stillness, never labor your body, never agitate your essence, and you can reach long life.

"With your eyes unseeing, your ears unhearing, and your mind unknowing, your spirit will keep your body whole, and it will live forever. Protect your inner being, close off outside contacts: much knowledge leads to defeat.

"I will take you to the Heights of Great Radiance, the source of Utmost Yang. I will guide you through the Gate of Serene Obscurity, the source of Utmost Yin. This is where Heaven and Earth are administered, where yin and yang are being kept.

"Protect your physical self, and things will naturally be vigorous. I constantly guard the One and rest in its deepest harmony. I have cultivated myself for 1,200 years, and my body has yet to decay."

Deeply impressed, the Yellow Emperor again knocked his head to ground: "You really are like Heaven!"

"Come and I will tell you," the Master said. "That thing I have been talking about is limitless, yet people all think it has a limit. It is immeasurable, yet people all think its can be measured.

---

[7] From *Zhuangzi* 11. The rendition here follows Kohn 2011, 129-31.

"Attaining Dao will make you a sovereign above and a king below. Losing Dao, you may see the light above but you'll remain mere dust below— like all the flourishing creatures that arise from dust and return to dust.

"For this reason, I leave all that behind, go through the gate to the limitless, and frolic in the fields of infinity. I join my light with that of the sun and moon, extend my life span to that of Heaven and Earth. Things come near me—I remain with chaos. Things move away from me—I stay in oblivion. All others may well die—I alone survive!"

Inward Training [8]

People's vitality always comes from being straight and upright. It is always lost due to joy, anger, worry, and resentment. To stop anger, nothing beats poetry; to stop worry, nothing beats music. To choose the right music, the best way is by propriety; to maintain propriety, the best way to through respect; to cultivate respect, the best way is in stillness.

Being still within and respectful without, you can recover your true inner nature; by resting in your inner nature, you find great stability.

Eating the right way. Fill up greatly and your *qi* suffers, causing the body to decline; restrict your intake greatly and your bones dry up, causing the blood to clot. The median between filling and restricting is called "harmony complete." Here vital essence lodges and awareness springs forth.

If ever you lose the right measure of hunger and satiation, make a plan: when full, exercise vigorously; when hungry, empty your thoughts [of food]; when feeling old and tired, let go of worries.

If you don't exercise vigorously when full, your *qi* cannot flow to your four limbs. If you don't empty your thoughts when hungry, you won't be able to stop when you next eat. If you don't let go of worries when you feel old and tired, your inner resources will quickly be depleted.

Expand your mind and let it run free; open you *qi* and let it be wide. Keep your body still and don't move; guard the One and release all vexations.

Look upon profit without attraction, look upon potential harm without fear. At ease with others, you can be benevolent to all. Happy alone, you can delight in yourself.

This is what we call letting the *qi* circulate freely: in intention and action always modeling Heaven.

---

[8] From the *Neiye* chapter of the *Guanzi*, sects. 22-25.

People's vitality always comes from inner joy. The moment you worry, you lose your core thread; the moment you get angry, you lose your stabilizing ends. As long as you are given to worry, sadness, joy, or anger, Dao has no place to stay!

Thus immediately still all cravings and desires; straighten out all foolish [assumptions] and upsetting [thoughts]. Never pull, never push—good fortune arrives of itself, Dao naturally comes to roost.

Yes, make your lists and plans, but know this: Keep still and you will succeed, get nervous and you will fail.

Controlling *Qi* [9]

Image Complete

Nourish the spirits and you will not die. [*The spirit of the valley does not die.*]

"Valley" means "nourish." If one can nourish the spirits, one does not die. The "spirits" are the spirits of the five organs: the spirit soul in the liver, the material soul in the lungs, the spirit in the heart, the intention in the spleen, and the essence in the kidneys. If the five organs are exhausted or harmed, the five spirits will leave and one dies.

This is called the mysterious and the female. [*It is called the mysterious female.*]

This means that the Dao of no-death lies in the mysterious and the female. The mysterious is heaven; in the human body it is the nose. The female is earth; in the human body it is the mouth.

Heaven feeds people with the five *qi*, which enter the organs through the nose and settle in the heart. The five *qi* are pure and subtle; they cause people to have sentience and spirituality, intelligence and perception, sound and voice, as well as the five kinds of inner nature. They are represented in the spirit soul, which is male and leaves and enters the human body through the nose in order to interact with heaven. Therefore, the nose is the mysterious.

---

[9] From *Heshang gong zhangju*, chs. 6, 50, and 10. Chapters 6 and 50 also appear in *Yangxing yanming lu* 1.1b-2b. The translation of the original verses reflects the commentary's interpretation. The standard rendition is added in brackets. For a searchable online text of the *Daode jing*, see http://ctext.org/dao-de-jing.

Earth feeds people with the five flavors, which enter the organs through the mouth and settle in the stomach. The five flavors are turbid and heavy; they cause people to have body and skeleton, bones and flesh, blood and pulses, and the six kinds of emotional passions. They are represented in the material soul, which is female and leaves and enters the human body through the mouth in order to interact with earth. Therefore the mouth is the female.

The gates of the mysterious and the female are called the root of Heaven and Earth.

"Root" means "prime." This means that the gates of the nose and the mouth are whereby the primordial *qi* that pervades Heaven and Earth comes and goes.

It goes on forever. [It is an endless flow of inexhaustible qi.]

Breathe through nose and mouth softly or hard. In either case, do so without interruption and very subtly, hardly knowing whether the breath is coming or going, is there or not there.

Use it and never be strained. [Use it, and it will never be exhausted.]

In using the breath you should be open and relaxed, never rushing or straining.

Honoring Life

Coming into life,

This means that as emotions and passions issue from the five inner organs, the spirit soul is stable and the material soul still. Then there is life.

We enter into death.

This means that as emotions and passions enter into chest and intention, essence scatters and spirit is confused. Then there is death.

Following life: there are ten and three; following death, there are ten and three.

This passage speaks about the different aspects of life and death. Each of them has thirteen. To wit, there are nine orifices and four passes. They are alive when the eyes do not see wantonly, the ears do not hear wantonly, the nose does not smell wantonly, the mouth does not speak wantonly, the hands do not point wantonly, the feet do not walk wantonly, and when essence does not move wantonly. They die when the opposite occurs.

Alive, yet moving toward death: there are also ten and three.

People wish to pursue life and activity, yet they act contrary to that and move toward death in thirteen ways.

Why is that? It is because they pursue the intensity of life.

The reason why people move toward death is that they pursue life's activities and great intensity. Thereby they get farther away from Dao and go against heaven, acting wantonly in all they do.

Now, I have heard that someone who is good at supporting life when walking on dry land will not encounter rhinos or tigers, when joining the army will not be exposed to shields and weapons. At such a person rhinocenroces do not butt their horns, tigers do not point their claws, soldiers do not thrust their knives. Why is this? It is because there is no death in him.

It is because he does not violate any of the thirteen points above that there is no death in such a person.

Can You?

Sustaining qi and the material soul, and thereby embracing the One, can you prevent it from leaving? [*Can you balance your life force and embrace the One without separation?*]

"*Qi* and material soul" are the same as "spirit and material souls." People sustain the two kinds of souls and thereby obtain life. They should love and nurture them, realizing that joy and hatred cause the spirit soul to vanish while haste and alarm make the material soul leave. The spirit soul resides in the liver, the material soul in the lungs. Indulging in wine and sweet delicacies harms the liver and lungs. Instead people should keep the spirit soul tranquil so that their will can be set on the Dao, and they will be free from trouble. They should maintain the material soul in a state of peace so that they attain long life and can extend their years.

The second part says: if one can embrace the One and cause it to remain in the body, one will live forever. The one is the first product of Dao and virtue or inherent potency, the essential energy of Great Harmony. Therefore it is called the One. The One pervades everything in the world. Heaven attains it to become clear; Earth attains it to become solid; princes and kings attain it to become upright and just. Entering people, it forms their mind; emerging from people, it forms their activities; spreading through people, it forms their inherent potency [virtue]. All this is simply called the One. What it ultimately means in practice is that one makes the will one and not two.

Concentrating on the breath and attaining softness, can you be like an infant? [*Can you control your breath, quietly, like a baby?*]

Concentrating firmly on essence and breath without letting it be disturbed, your whole physical being will adapt to it and become soft and pliant. On the inside be without yearnings and worries, on the outside without ambitions and affairs: then the spirits will not leave.

Purifying and cleansing your mysterious perception, can you be without error? [*Can you clarify your dark vision without blemish?*]

You should purify your mind and make it clean and pure. With the mind resting in mysterious union, perception can know everything. Therefore the text speaks of mysterious perception.

Then you will be free from lasciviousness and wrongdoing.

Nurturing the people, governing the country, can you be without action? Regulating the body means nourishing *qi* and breath; this will make the body whole. Governing the country means nurturing the people; this will put the land at peace.

Regulating the body means inhaling and exhaling essence and breath without allowing the ears to hear it. Governing the country means spreading inherent potency [virtue] and compassion without letting the people know it.

As the Gate of Heaven opens and shuts, can you be like the female? [*Can you open and close the Gate of Heaven without clinging to earth?*]

The Gate of Heaven is the constellation Purple Tenuity in the North Culmen. It opens and shuts, begins and ends in accordance with the five phases. In regulating the body, the Gate of Heaven is the nostrils. To open it, breathe hard; to shut it, breathe softly.

In regulating the body, you should be like the female, quiet and tranquil, soft and weak. In governing the country, you should be in accordance with the world's transformations and never take the lead.

Brightly penetrating the four quarters, can you be without knowledge? [*Can you brighten the four directions without knowledge?*]

This means that Dao is as bright as the sun and the moon, penetrates all directions, and fills the world even beyond its eight ultimate poles. Therefore it is said: "Look for it and do not see it; listen for it and do not hear it" [*Daode jing* 14]. Manifest everywhere in the ten directions, it is radiant and shines brilliantly. Yet nobody knows how Dao fills the world.

It generates and nurtures them. [*Give birth and cultivate.*]
Dao gives birth to the myriad beings and nurtures them.

It generates but does not possess. [*Give birth and do not possess.*]
Dao gives birth to the myriad beings but it does not take possession of them.

It acts but does not depend on them. [*Act without dependence.*]
Dao acts widely everywhere but never depends on or expects any reward.

It raises them but does not control them. [*Excel but do not rule.*]
Dao raises and nurtures the myriad beings but it does not control them or hold them back, thereby turning them into mere tools.

This is called mysterious potency.
This means that Dao and its inherent potency in their mysterious union cannot be seen, yet they wish to make people know Dao.

Guiding *Qi* [10]

To guide the *qi*, allow it to enter deeply [by inhaling] and collect it [in the mouth]. As it collects, it will expand. Once expanded, it will sink down. When it sinks down, it comes to rest. After it has come to rest, it becomes stable.

When the *qi* is stable, it begins to sprout. From sprouting, it begins to grow. As it grows, it can be pulled back upwards. When it is pulled upwards, it reaches the crown of the head.

It then touches above at the crown of the head and below at the base of the spine. Practice this and attain long life. Go against this and die.

---

[10] From the Dodecagonal Jade Block.

The Stretch Book [11]

Spring: generate; summer: grow; fall: collect; winter: store—such is the way of Pengzu.

Spring days. After rising in the morning, pass water, wash and rinse, clean and click the teeth. Loosen the hair, stroll to the lower end of the hall to meet the purest of dew and receive the essence of Heaven, and drink one cup of water. These are the means to increase long life. Enter the chamber [for sex] between evening and late midnight [1 a.m.]. More would harm the *qi*.

Summer days. Wash the hair frequently, but bathe rarely. Do not rise late and eat many greens. After rising in the morning and passing water, wash and rinse the mouth, then clean the teeth. Loosen the hair, walk to the lower end of the hall and after a while drink a cup of water. Enter the chamber between evening and midnight. More would harm the *qi*.

Fall days. Bathe and wash the hair frequently. As regards food and drink, let hunger or satiation be whatever the body desires. Enter the chamber however often the body finds it beneficial and comfortable—this is the way to greatest benefit.

Winter days. Bathe and wash the hair frequently. The hands should be cold and the feet warm; the face cold and the body warm. Rise from sleep late; while lying down, stretch out straight. Enter the chamber between evening and early midnight [11 p.m.]. More would harm the *qi*.

1. Lifting one shin across the opposite thigh, moving it up and down thirty times is called Crossing Thighs.

2. Extending the shin, then pointing and flexing the toes thirty times is called Measuring Worm.

3. Placing the feet parallel, then rocking back and forth thirty times is called Shifting Toes.

4. Extending the shin, straightening the heel and rocking thirty times is called The Parapet.

5. Stretching the toes, then raising and rocking them thirty times is called Stretch Move.

6. Bending the shins, alternating right and left, forward and back thirty times is called Forward Push.

---

[11] From *Yinshu*.

7. Rubbing the shin with the opposite foot, moving along its front and back thirty times is called [unnamed].

8. Extending the feet straight forward thirty times is called Stretching Yang.

9. Rubbing the backs of the feet thirty times on each side is called [unnamed].

10. Hamstring Stretch: interlace the fingers [lit. "join the hands"] at the back and bend forward.

11. Upward Gaze: interlace the fingers at the back, then look up and turn the head.

12. Bend and Gaze: interlace the fingers at the back and bend forward, then turn the head to look at your heels.

13. Side and Back: interlace the fingers at the back, then lean sideways and turn [the head] toward the [opposite] shoulder.

14. Duck in Water: interlace the fingers at the back and move the head back and forth.

15. Rotating Stretch: interlace the fingers, raise the arms, and twist backward.

16. Upright Swivel: interlace the fingers at the back, contract the neck, and turn the head.

17. Snapping Yin: place one foot forward [with bent knee], interlace the fingers, bend forward, and hook them around [the knee].

18. Reverse Rotation: interlace the fingers, bend forward, and look up, moving the arms from side to side.

19. Dragon Flourish: step one leg forward with bent knee while stretching the other leg back, then interlace the fingers, place them on the knee, and look up.

20. Lower Back Stretch: step one leg forward with bent knee while stretching the other leg back, then interlace the fingers, twist, and revolve backwards.

21. Snake Wriggle: interlace the fingers at the back, click the teeth and swivel the head around.

22. Twisting the Tail Bone: with both hands [text missing].

23. Great Spread: place both hands on the floor with vigor, then step the feet back and forth between them.

24. [Forward Hold]: spread the legs wide and bend to hold the left foot with the right hand; alternate right and left.

25. Limbs Dropping: place the hands on the hips, then twist one arm forward toward the feet and bend.

26. Gibbon Hold: hold the left foot with the right hand and twist the left hand back as you bend to the right and left.

27. Triple [Stretch]: raise both arms high and [while bending] extend them forward, then out to the sides.

28. Hanging Forward: bend forward, raise both hands and look up as if looking for something.

29. Arm Punch: propel both arms forward as if hitting someone.

30. Pointing Back: interlace the fingers, raise them overhead and bend back as far as possible.

31. [Reaching] Below: step one leg forward with bent knee while stretching the other leg back, then lift one arm and stretch it with vigor.

32. Tiger Stretch: place one foot forward, raise one arm and bend.

33. Yin Stretch: interlace the fingers with palms facing out and lift them, then bend forward as far as you can.

34. Yang Stretch: interlace the fingers, stretch the arms forward, and look up as far as you can.

35. Double Deer: raise both arms, push up, then bend forward as far as you can.

36. Tiger Crouch: with arms parallel, rotate the shoulders up and back, alternating on the right and left.

37. Leaping Toad: with arms parallel, swing them to the right and left, up and down.

38. Cart Cover: with arms parallel, swing them outward to the right and left, then lower them straight down and swing them back and forth.

39. Nose to Belly: bend forward and lift both arms to the right and left.

40. Calculating Wolf: place the hands beneath their respective armpits and rotate the chest.

41. Warrior Pointing: with the left foot forward, use the left hand to point the fingers forward, stretching the arm.

42. To relieve inner tension: Sit in dignified kneel with the tailbone supported. With the left hand stroke the neck and with the right hand stroke the left hand. Now, bend forward as far as you can, then very slowly let go as you exhale with *xu*. Sit up straight and look up. Repeat five times, then change sides in the handhold, for a total of ten repetitions.

43. To relieve neck pain and difficulties in turning the neck: Lie down flat, stretch the hands and feet [*next five characters illegible*]. Then lift the head from front to back as far as you can. Very slowly come back to a straight position and rest. Repeat ten times. Afterwards cover the mouth and hold the breath. Wait until you sweat and you will feel better.

44. To relieve fatigue at the onset of a disease, when you note that your mind wanders restlessly and your body aches all over: practice Eight Meridians Stretch and quickly exhale with *hu* and *xu*, thereby releasing yang. Also, soak the face with cold water for the time it takes to eat a bowl of rice, then discard the water. Take a bamboo cloth in both hands and rub it over your face, moving it up and down. All the while continue to exhale *hu*, *hu*. Repeat ten times.

45. To relieve the onset of an intestinal ailment: The first sign is swelling. When you notice the swelling, place your intention on the lower abdomen and exhale with *chui*. Repeat a hundred times.

46. Grasp a pole with the right hand, face the wall, hold the breath, and place the left foot forward and up against the wall. Rest when you get tired. Similarly, take the pole in the left hand and step forward with the right foot against the wall. Again stop when tired. This makes the *qi* flow down from the head.

47. To relieve tense muscles: Stand with legs hip-width apart and hold both thighs. Then bend the left leg while stretching the right thigh back, reaching the knee to the floor. Once done, [change legs and] bend the right leg while stretching the left leg back and reaching that knee to the floor. Repeat three times.

48. Get a piece of wood that can be easily carved, about a fist in circumference and four feet long. Cover its ends [with cloth] and hang it about four feet above the floor with a new rope. Sit on the piece of wood, hold the rope with both hands and kick out with your feet. Do a thousand repetitions each in the morning, at noon, in the evening, and at midnight, and within ten days you will be fine.

49. To relieve ankle pain: Put your weight on [lit. "stand on"] the inner ankle of the right foot and stretch the right inner calf. Then put your weight on the outer ankle and stretch the right outer calf. After this, put your weight on the inner ankle of the left foot and stretch the left inner calf. Then put your weight on the outer ankle and stretch the left outer calf. Repeat this three times on each side.

50. If the right knee hurts, hold on to a staff with the left hand, then turn the right foot in and out a thousand times. If the left knee hurts, hold on to a staff with the right hand, then turn the left foot in and out a thousand times. Next, grab the left toes with the left hand and pull them backwards ten times, while the right hand still holds the staff. Then grab the right toes with the right hand and pull them back ten times while holding the staff with the left hand. . . .

Holding the Breath is good for stretching the muscles.
Hall Dropping is good for balancing the meridians.
Snake Wriggle is good for enhancing the brain.
Duck in Water is good for opening the neck.
Flushing Flesh along the meridians is good for all from heel to head.
Side and Back is good for the ears.
Upward Gaze is good for the eyes.
Opening the Mouth and looking up is good for the nose.
Spitting without Emitting is good for the mouth.
Rubbing the Heart and lifting the head is good for the throat.
Upright Swivel is good for the base of the neck.
Tiger Turn is good for the neck.
Triple Stretch is good for the shoulder muscles.
Limbs Dropping is good for the armpits.
Bird Stretch is good for the shoulder joints.
Turn and Shake is good for abdomen and belly.
Turn and Twist is good for the sides.
Bear Amble is good for the lower back.
Repeated Hold is good for the hips.
Step of Yu is good for the thighs.
Forward Loosening is good for the knees.
Turn and Push is good for feet and heels.
Shifting Toes is good for the *qi* of the feet.
Stomping Heels is good for the chest.
All these should be done with three repetitions.

Chapter Two

Moderation and Self-Control

In the early middle ages, during the Three Kingdoms (220-265), Western and Eastern Jin dynasties (265-419), documents on nourishing life come dominantly from aristocrats who, either by choice or because they were deprived of official careers due to political circumstances, had time on their hands to think and write about lifestyle and self-cultivation. Their primary concern is the balancing of *qi* through various measures that involve time, space, nature, and human interaction. Their advice ranges from the very general—structure of the body and nature of mind and life—to the highly particular. Applying common household knowledge of Chinese medicine, they provide specific guidelines for dressing, sleeping, bathing, eating, sexual relations, mental attitudes, social behavior, and more, always indicating which organs will suffer. Under their impact and reflecting their key concerns, longevity literature mushrooms into a massive hodgepodge of suggestions, combining deep insights with detailed instructions, petty limitations, and abstruse taboos.

The first and best known among longevity writers of this period is Xi Kang 稽康 (223-262), born into a clan of officials under the Wei Kingdom (in modern Anhui) and married to a princess of its royal Cao family around 245. When the Sima clan of the future Jin rulers took over the government in 249, he was made redundant and retired to his country estate where he headed a group of similarly placed men known as the "Seven Sages of the Bamboo Grove" (Nienhauser 1986, 410-11).

They pursued various leisure activities, engaged in spirited philosophical debates, dabbled in longevity practices, and wrote beautiful poems and intellectual essays. Although they held a firm belief in immortality and sought contact with the higher spheres, their practice was less religious than escapist (see Balasz 1948; Holzman 1956). It involved consuming wine in large quantities and taking narcotic and psychedelic drugs, notably the notorious Cold Food Powder (*hanshi san* 寒食散), which caused great visions and made the body feel very hot. This in turn inspired the "sages" to remove their clothing and jump into the cooling waters of nearby ponds and rivers, giving them a reputation of wild eccentricity and reckless abandon (Wagner 1973).

Their main contribution to the longevity tradition centers on Xi Kang's essay, *Yangsheng lun* 養生論 (On Nourishing Life). In this work, he professes a strong belief in immortality yet claims that not everyone can attain it because it requires a special gift that manifests itself in the presence of an extraordinary *qi*. Yet even without this special *qi*, by practicing various longevity techniques and controlling all excesses one can extend one's life to several hundred years.

His position was criticized severely by his fellow sage Xiang Xiu 向秀 in the *Nan Yangsheng lun* 難養生論 (Criticizing "On Nourishing Life"). A hedonist, he proposes to experience life as intensely as possible, to pursue all the happiness that can be afforded by the senses. For him, realization means to appreciate and savor all the feelings of being alive. He criticizes the efforts of longevity-seekers who deny themselves all sensual gratification in order to prolong a merely physical existence. He asks: What good is a life I cannot enjoy? His attitude differs from the classic ideals of perfection, which claimed that the only life worth enjoying was the purified and tranquil sojourn on earth in as much alignment and contact with Dao, gods, and the virtue of Heaven and Earth, bringing a more hedonistic and ecstatic dimension of fullness of life into the foreground.[1]

Another aristocrat who turned away from politics to engage in life-extension was the would-be alchemist and scholar Ge Hong 葛洪 (283-343), who called himself Baopuzi 抱朴子 (Master Who Embraces Simplicity). Born into the southern aristocracy, he grew up in a small town near Jiankang 建康 (modern Nanjing). Rather than being motivated by a lack of opportunities, he was inspired by a family interest for otherworldly pursuits and became a disciple of the hermit and alchemist Zheng Yin 鄭隱 at the age of fourteen, studying with him for five years. After serving in the imperial administration in various minor capacities, he resigned his position to study longevity and immortality full time (Pregadio 2000, 167). He wandered around the country

[1] Complete translations and detailed discussions of these works cam be found in Henricks 1983; Holzman 1957. They are not translated here.

in search of ancient manuscripts and learned masters, then came home to write down his findings.

In his autobiography—the first of its kind in Chinese literature (see Wells 2009)—he describes how he eschewed official positions and even avoided social interaction with his peers because his one aim in life was to become immortal, i.e., reach a state of perfect health and extended longevity that would allow the concoction of an alchemical elixir and ascension to the heavens (Ware 1966, 6-21). The foundation of this state were the longevity techniques— exercises, breathing, dietetics, and meditations—followed by the great alchemical endeavor, which alone could lead to ultimate immortality (Pregadio 2006, 125).

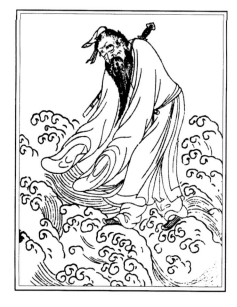

Fig. 3. Ge Hong

His most important work is the *Baopuzi neipian* 抱朴子內篇 (Inner Chapters of the Master Who Embraces Simplicity, DZ 1185; trl. Ware 1966), which was first completed in 317, the very year when Central Asian invaders forced the Chinese court to take refuge in the south, leading to the change from the Western to the Eastern Jin dynasty. A twenty-chapter compendium on the techniques and practices of the immortals, it provides an overview of the various esoteric practices prevalent at the time, including much material on longevity practices (Robinet 1997, 78-113).

Two short texts that focus on this aspect of Ge Hong's work survive in the Daoist Canon. One, the *Baopuzi yangsheng lun* 抱朴子養生論 (Baopuzi on Nourishing Life, DZ 842), is associated specifically with him; the other, the *Pengzu shesheng yangxing lun* 彭祖攝生養性論 (Pengzu on Preserving Life and Nourishing Inner Nature, DZ 840), connects to the immortal Pengzu often called the "Chinese Methuselah" since he supposedly lived for 800 years.[2] They prescribe moderation in all things, physical, emotional, and

---

[2] He has a biography in the *Liexian zhuan* 列仙傳 (Immortals' Biographies, DZ 294), see Kaltenmark 1953, 60) as well as in Ge Hong's *Shenxian zhuan* 神仙傳 (Biog-

mental, emphasizing control of the senses and balance of food and clothing in accordance with the seasons. Their list of twelve things to do "little" is cited widely in longevity materials throughout the middle ages and their emphasis on spirit and *qi* is essential in the literature. The two dimensions of longevity—spiritual and medical—are thoroughly merged at this time, and there are increasingly detailed instructions on daily living, food consumption, and mental attitudes.

Another important document of the same period is the *Yangsheng yaoji* 養生要集 (Long Life Compendium) by the aristocrat and official Zhang Zhan 張湛 (fl. 370). He is best known as the first and most important commentator to the Daoist philosophical text *Liezi* 列子 (Book of Master Lie; trl. Graham 1960), which supports a similar view of the body as the *Yangsheng yaoji* (see Sakade 1986, 10; Kohn 2009).[3] Zhang Zhan, also called Chudu 處度, does not have a biography in the dynastic histories despite the fact that he wrote several philosophical commentaries in the Profound Learning (Xuanxue 玄學) tradition of Daoism, authored two compendia on longevity practices, served as imperial secretary under the Eastern Jin, and was born into a family of senior officials under the Western Jin (Despeux 1989, 228). Rather, information about him is anecdotal, some found in the story collection *Shishuo xinyu* 世說新語 (A New Account of Tales of the World; trl. Mather 1976), some in the biographies of contemporary officials and later descendants.

According to these sources, Zhang Zhan was philosophically minded and a follower of Dark Learning thinkers such as the *Zhuangzi* commentator Guo Xiang 郭象 (d. 312), whom he frequently cites in his *Liezi* commentary. He also had medical knowledge and was eager to improve the *qi* in his residence by planting various kinds of pine trees. The *Jinshu* 晉書 (History of the Jin Dynasty) biography of Fan Ning 范寧 further mentions that he was susceptible to eyestrain, for which he took a longevity recipe consisting of six ingredients: read less, think less, focus inward, scan outward, sleep late, and go to bed early. He was to mix these ingredients with *qi* and take them to

---

raphies of Spirit Immortals, JHL 89) (Campany 2002, 194-204). The abbreviation JHL stands for *Daozang jinghua lu*. The numbering refers to Komjathy 2002.

[3] The first mention of authorship of the commentary is in the bibliographic section of the *Suishu* 隋書 (History of the Sui Dynasty) of the 7th century (Despeux 1989, 228). Zhang Zhan is a common name, and it is also remotely possible that the author was an official in northern China, known as Zhang Ziran 張自然 (Zhu 1986, 102).

heart for seven days. This would enhance his vision and extend his life (Stein 1999, 101).

An imperial official and well-educated thinker with time on his hands, Zhang Zhan engaged in wide reading and practiced long life techniques. Like other aristocratic authors on the subject, he had the material cushion necessary to indulge his interest in medical learning and was well connected to the literati. The practices he mentions were probably well known and widely used at the time, and he may well have put together the *Yangsheng yaoji* to help his fellow aristocrats stay healthy and live moderately despite their riches and newly found leisure, thus using long life practices predominantly for this-worldly advancement.

The *Yangsheng yaoji* has not survived as an independent text, being lost probably after the rebellion of An Lushan 安錄山 in 755 (Barrett 1980, 172). It survives in fragments, notably in Tang medical and longevity works, recently collated and translated by Stephan Stein (1999). The earliest among its sources is the *Zhubing yuanhou lun* 諸病源候論 (Origins and Symptoms of Medical Disorders), a medical compendium in 50 *juan*. Compiled by a committee under the guidance of the court physician Chao Yuanfang 巢元方, it was presented to Emperor Yang of the Sui in 610 (see Despeux and Obringer 1997). Its selections tend to emphasize the more medical dimensions of longevity practice.

Another important source is the *Yangxing yanming lu* 養性延命錄 (Record on Nourishing Inner Nature and Extending Life, DZ 838), a Daoist collection of meditative, breathing, and physical practices in two *juan*, ascribed alternatively to the Highest Clarity master, alchemist, and naturalist Tao Hongjing 陶弘景 (456-536) and to the master physician and Daoist Sun Simiao 孫思邈 (581-682). It includes many passages close to Sun's other works and goes back to at least the mid-seventh century (see Mugitani 1987; Despeux in Schipper and Verellen 2004, 345) (see ch. 7 below).

The most extensive source of *Yangsheng yaoji* citations is the *Ishinpō* 醫心方 (Essential Medical Methods; trl. Hsia et al. 1986), an extensive Japanese medical collection by the court physician Tamba no Yasuyori 丹波康頼 (912-995), presented to the emperor in 984 (Sakade 1989, 3-9). It consists of thirty chapters and cites 204 largely Chinese sources that were partially lost in China itself and thus only survive here. Chapter 28, for example, provides the foundation of much information we now have on medieval Chinese sexual cultivation (see Ishihara and Levy 1970; Wile 1992), while chapter 26 discusses the theory of life extension and 27 presents a thorough outline of various longevity practices. Passages from the *Yangsheng yaoji* appear here as well as in several other chapters, notably such as ch. 29 on nutrition and ch. 30 on medical substances (Stein 1999, 122).

As outlined in the *Yangxing yanming lu*, the text has ten sections:

1. Endowed with Spirit 稟神
2. Caring for *Qi* 愛氣
3. Nourishing the Body 養形
4. Guiding and Stretching 導引
5. Speaking and Talking 言語

6. Eating and Drinking 飲食
7. The Bedchamber 房室
8. Rejecting Habits 反俗
9. Medicinal Supplements 服藥
10. Various Taboos 雜忌

The text thus begins with an outline of practices that support the spirit and *qi*, focusing on establishing a moderate lifestyle and harmonious balance of worldly activities and personal cultivation as well as setting up a daily routine of *qi*-absorption. It then moves on to more mundane matters of sleep, baths, and hair care to continue with recommendations for exercises, the proper use of speech, and dietary and herbal suggestions, including monthly taboos and food combinations. Sexual practices tend to focus on temporal and physical constraints, while "Various Taboos" involve warnings against doing things in excess. It is not clear what "Rejecting Habits"(*fansu* 反俗) means and there are no fragments under this heading.

Translation

Nourishing Life [1]

[1a] The Master Who Embraces Simplicity said:

The human body resembles a country. The role of the belly and stomach is like that of the central palace. The position of the limbs and skeleton is like that of the outer regions. The arrangement of bones and joints is like that of the hundred officials. The arrangement of the connective tissue is like the four imperial highways. The spirit is like the ruler. The blood is like the ministers. The *qi* is like the people. Thus the accomplished person governs himself just as an enlightened ruler governs his country.

---

[1] *Baopuzi yangsheng lun*. Some parts of this also appear in *Baopuzi* 13 and 18.

Loving the people is a prime way to stabilize the country. Loving the *qi* is a key method to make the body whole. If the people are distressed, the country will perish. If the *qi* declines, the body fails. Thus, all accomplished people and superior gentlemen take medicines before the onset of illness and do not pursue a cure after it has been defeated. Know therefore: Life is hard to preserve and easy to disperse. *Qi* is hard to keep pure and easy to get turbid. If you can always seize opportunities and manage to control your lusts and desires, you can preserve and maintain inner nature and destiny. [1b]

To be good at nourishing life, first of all eliminate the six harms [of the senses and emotions]. Then you can extend your years to a hundred. What to do?

     1. Let go of fame and profit!
     2. Limit sights and sounds!
     3. Disregard goods and wealth!
     4. Lessen smells and tastes!
     5. Eliminate lies and falsehood!
     6. Avoid all hate and envy!

Without eliminating the six harms, how can longevity cultivation be pursued?

Now, if you have not seen the benefit of the practice yet, even though your heart is attuned to the wondrous Dao, your mouth recites perfect scriptures, you suck and chew on bright florescence, and you inhale and exhale the luminants and heavenly signs, you still cannot supplement your life's shortcomings. Thus be very careful not to throw away the practice at the root and forget its branches. Be deeply aware of this!

To preserve harmony and complete perfection: think little, reflect little, laugh little, speak little, enjoy little, anger little, delight little, grieve little, like little, dislike little, engage little, deal little.

If you think much, the spirit disperses.
If you reflect much, the heart is labored.
If you laugh much, the organs and viscera soar [get excited].
If you speak much, the Ocean of *Qi* is empty and vacant.
If you enjoy much, the gall bladder and bladder take in outside wind.
If you anger much, the connective tissue pushes the blood around. [2a]
If you delight much, spirit and heart is wayward and unsettled.
If you grieve much, hair and whiskers dry and wither.
If you like much, will and *qi* is one-sided and overloaded.
If you dislike much, essence and power race off and soar away.

If you engage much, muscles and meridians tense and get nervous.
If you deal much, wisdom and worry are confused.

These attack life more than axes and spears; they diminish destiny worse than wolves and wolverines.

Also, do not sit for long, walk for long, watch for long, or listen for long. Do not force yourself to eat unless hungry; do not push yourself to drink unless thirsty. If you force yourself to eat without being hungry, your spleen will be labored; if you push to drink without being thirsty, your stomach will become swollen. The body should always be exercised; food should always be minimal. Yet even in exercise do not go to extremes; in minimizing food do not go to emaciation.

On winter mornings do not empty your mind; on summer nights do not eat your fill. Rise early but not before cock crow; rise late but not after sunrise. Keep your mind pure so that perfected spirits maintain their position; keep your *qi* stable so that deviant entities leave your body.

If you practice cheating and treachery, the spirit grieves; if you practice competition and strife, it is harmed. [2b] If you despise and insult people, your destiny is reduced; if you kill and harm living beings, your longevity suffers. Thus, if you perform even one good deed, the spirit souls rejoice; if you perform even one bad deed, the material souls are glad. [Note: The material souls like death; the spirit souls love life.]

Always reside in openness and generosity and preserve deep inner serenity. Then body and self will be calm and at peace, disasters and harm will not dare to come close. Your name will be entered in the registers of life while your record will be expunged from the ledgers of death. The entire principle of nourishing life rests on this.

As for refining reverted cinnabar to nourish the brain, transforming the golden fluid to maintain the spirit: this is the wondrous Dao of the highest perfected. These methods cannot be pursued and cultivated while still eating grain and taking blood [meat]. Among ten thousand people, only very few can attain it. Pay due attention!

Lord Lao said: "As for actualizing this Dao of mine: the highest practitioners will completely cultivate it and extend their years and life; medium practitioners will half cultivate it and be free from sickness and disasters; lesser practitioners will occasionally cultivate it and avoid untimely death; the ignorant, finally, will lose it utterly and forfeit their inner nature!" (*Daode jing* 41). This is just it.

Preserving Life and Nourishing Inner Nature [2]

[1a] When spirit is strong, you live long. When *qi* is strong, you easily perish. Soft and weak, in awe of greatness—that means the spirit is strong. Burning with anger, the will proud—that means the *qi* is strong.

When ordinary people see that they do not have the determination to attain a certain goal and think about it compulsively, their will is injured. When they see that they do not have the strength to overcome a certain obstacle and push against it violently, their body is injured. Constantly sad without end, the spirit souls are harmed. Accumulating laments without end, the material souls disperse. [1b]

Indulging in excessive joy and anger, spirit leaves its residence.
Hating and loving without constancy, spirit exits the body.
Being full of anxieties and desires, spirit is troubled.
Worrying and panicking, spirit is defeated.

Talking and laughing for a long time, the inner organs and viscera suffer.
Sitting and standing for a long time, the muscles and bones suffer.
Sleeping and resting losing track of time, the liver suffers.
Moving and panting to fatigue and exhaustion, the spleen suffers.

Holding the bow and pulling the string, the muscles suffer.
Floating high and wading low, the kidneys suffer.
Getting drunk and throwing up, the lungs suffer.
Eating to fullness and sleeping on the side, the *qi* suffers.

Galloping like a horse and running around wildly, the stomach suffers.
Shouting and cursing with vile language, the gall bladder suffers.
Failing to keep yin and yang in proper exchange, ulcers develop.
Failing to balance bedchamber activities, fatigue and exhaustion result.

People in every generation hope to live for a long time, but even a long life does not normally go beyond 30,000 days [82 years]. If you cannot be even one day without lessening or harming one aspect [of yourself]—if you

---

[2] *Pengzu shesheng yangxing lun.* The second half of the text is identical with *Baopuzi* 13.8ab.

cannot have even one day of cultivation and supplementation [of *qi*]—the spirit will not stay and the body will not be healthy. Is this not deplorable? [2a]

For this reason, the method of nourishing life involves not spitting far and not walking hastily. Let the ears not listen to excess; let the eyes not look around extensively. Do not sit until tired; do not sleep beyond your needs. Wait until it is cold before you put on more clothes; wait until it is hot before you take them off. Do not get too hungry, because hunger harms the *qi*, and when you eat beware of overindulging. Do not get too thirsty before you drink and do not drink too deeply at a time. If you overeat, your bowels will be blocked and obstructed to the point of illness; if you drink too deeply, phlegm will accumulate into lumps.

Also, do not allow any outside *qi* or wind to impact your body too much, but do not try too hard to evade it either. Avoid breaking a sweat; avoid running around madly when intoxicated; and never walk fast after eating your fill. Do not talk too much and do not enter severe cold. Do not eat lots of fatty meats and fancy foods and do not expose your head after washing your hair.

In winter, do not desire being very warm; in summer, do not strive to be very cool. If you are very warm in winter, in spring you will suffer from violent attacks. If you are very cool in summer, in fall you will suffer from recurring fevers. Do not sleep out in the open, exposed to sun and moon; and never allow yourself to approach the dirty leftovers of others, even if very hungry.

Do not toss and turn while sleeping; do not expose your head soon after a meal. When hot, avoid drinking ice-cold water; when cold, avoid getting close to the burning stove. [2b] After a bath, do not get out into a fierce wind; after breaking a sweat, do not immediately take off your clothes.

To combat heat, do not jump into cold water and immerse your whole body; to urinate or defecate, avoid facing the sun and moon or straight north and south. Never expose your body to the stars and planets; never try to push away natural events like frost and fog, storm and wind. All these will cause harm to the inner organs and viscera, create defeat for the spirit and spirit souls.

Make sure to eat selectively of the five flavors. Too much sour food [wood] harms the spleen [earth]; too much bitter [fire] harms the lungs [metal]; too much pungent [metal] harms the liver [wood]; too much sweet [earth] harms the kidneys [water]; and too much salty [water] harms the heart [fire]. All these follow the system of the five phases as they invisibly underlie the four limbs. Following this, you can understand and penetrate the patterns.

A person of strong will and high valor will be careful about all of this! Also, if you happen to violate one, take care not to diminish them all, because the effect accumulates over long periods of time and creates defeat and decay.

Remember: the heart is the ultimate master of the five organs and the *qi* is the supervisor of the hundred bones. Using them with proper movement to create harmony is the horse; following along in mysterious serenity is the cart. When the limbs and joints are troubled and exhausted, do healing exercises. [3a]

If you do not practice the arts of long life or follow the Dao of harmony, your *qi* will decline more and more, and your body will wither before your eyes. Exercise your perfect body, maintain our serene thinking. Listen to this Dao and way of nourishing life, and be very careful about it.

Thus the perfected are serene day in and day out and never come even close to being rushed or hectic. The ignorant, on the other hand, are loose and unsettled in intention. They diminish their bodies and defeat their spirits and spirit souls, harming even their material souls. Deplorable indeed!

Life's Essentials [3]

1. Endowed with Spirit

For the eyes, avoid seeing irregular sights; for the ears, avoid listening to ugly and distressing sounds; for the nose, avoid smelling offensive, stinking odors; for the mouth, avoid tasting harsh, poisonous flavors; for the mind, avoid all planning, scheming, and cheating. All these put the spirit to shame and reduce longevity.

There is no point sitting around and sighing deeply, all day and night whistling for good things to come. Yes, while still immersed in ordinary life it is impossible to be completely free from desires or let go of affairs, but you can make a constant effort to balance your mind, control your thoughts, calm

---

[3] Representative selections from several chapters of the *Yangsheng yaoji*, avoiding passages identical with those in the *Yangxing yanming lu*, which is translated in full below (ch. 7). Those found in the *Ishinpō* are also available in Hsia et al. 1986. Most passages translated here are from the *Zhubing yuanhou lun*, reprinted in Stein 1999, 285-92 and translated in Stein 1999, 233-46. I abbreviate it *Zhubing*.

your body, and reduce possessions. Begin simply by removing all that disturbs your spirit and harms your inner nature: this is the key practice to realize full endowment with spirit. (50; *Ishinpō* 23)

2. Caring for Qi

Master Luo states: People are in *qi* like fish are in water. If the water is polluted, fish die; if the *qi* is turbid, people get sick. Turbidity, moreover, does not only refer to the natural *qi* being dark or cloudy. It also occurs when thoughts and worries trouble the mind, when gain and loss keep alternating in your life, and when you get stuck in continuous push-pull—all these we call "turbid." (71; *Ishinpō* 23)

The three months of spring are the time of unfolding and alignment. Heaven and Earth join to generate new life and the myriad beings flourish. Go to bed late and rise early, then walk vigorously around the yard, loosen your hair, and relax the body—thus you allow the power of spring to arise. Nurture life and abstain from killing, give freely and avoid taking, reward generously and avoid punishing. In this manner you match the *qi* of spring. This is the way of nourishing life. Going against it, you harm your liver and are likely to suffer from a cold disorder in the summer, reducing your chances at long life.

The three months of summer are the time of luxurious, even excessive growth. The energies of Heaven and Earth mingle, and the myriad beings flourish and ripen. Go to bed late and rise early, avoid all resentment during the day, and make sure not to let anger enter your mind. Allow your florescence to flourish in its full expression and let the *qi* spread widely, as if all you love was outside. In this manner you match the *qi* of summer. This is the way of nurturing longevity. Going against it, you harm your heart and are likely to suffer from fevers in the fall.

The three months of fall are the time of maturation and regulation. The *qi* of Heaven is stormy, that of Earth is bright. Go to bed early and rise early, matching the daily rhythm of the chickens. Make sure your mind is calm and peaceful to alleviate the disturbing influences of fall. Contain your spirit and *qi*, so you can regulate the *qi* of fall. Avoid directing your mind toward outward affairs and keep the *qi* of your lungs clear. In this manner you match the *qi* of fall. This is the way of nurturing the harvest. Going against it, you harm your lungs and are likely to suffer from obstructions and colds in the winter.

The three months of winter are the time of closing and storing. Water freezes, and the Earth develops cracks. Avoid disturbing your inner yang. Go to bed early and rise late, waiting until the sun has risen. Keep your mind contained within, as if you were harboring selfish intentions and had already achieved all you want. Avoid the cold and keep yourself warm. Make sure nothing leaks out through your skin, lest your *qi* is reduced. In this manner you match the *qi* of winter. This is the way of nurturing preservation. Going against it, you harm your kidneys and are likely to suffer from reduced virility in the spring. (35-40; *Zhubing* 15)

3. Nourishing the Body [4]

Getting drunk and falling asleep in a position where you are exposed to wind causes sudden loss of voice. (1)

If you see a straight wall about ten yards long, don't lie down to sleep in the direction it is running. This will expose you to wind that can cause seizures and feelings of heaviness. (15)

Eating to satiation and going to sleep on your back, if done habitually, makes you prone to *qi* ailments and head wind. (7)

After eating, don't immediately lie down to sleep. Over a prolonged period this can cause *qi* ailments and hip pain. (26)

After breaking a sweat, don't sleep without covers or take a cold bath. This can cause chills, hot and cold flashes, as well as wind-based eczema. (19)

When you go to bed at night, make sure to cover your ears, not leaving even a small opening. If wind enters the ears, the mouth can be affected. (2)

Don't sleep with your mouth open, since this leads to extreme thirst and sallow complexion. (30)

During sleep, don't let your feet hang down from a raised platform. This will soon lead to excessive water in the kidneys. (51)

After waking, don't drink cold water and go back to sleep. This causes water stagnation. (46)

4. Guiding and Stretching

Every morning, ingest the Jade Spring and click the teeth. This strengthens the body, lightens the complexion, eliminates parasites, and stabilizes the teeth. The Jade Spring is the saliva in the mouth. Before getting up in the morning, rinse the entire mouth with saliva. Allow it to fill up, then swallow

---

[4] Passages on sleeping as found in fragments from the *Zhubing yuanhou lun*.

it. Click your teeth twenty-seven times. Repeat this process three times, then stop. This is called "refining essence." (23; *Zhubing* 3)

The *Yuanyang jing* [Scripture of Primordial Yang] has: Always pull the *qi* in through the nose, hold it in the mouth and mix it with saliva, swishing it around the tongue and teeth, then swallow it. Doing this a thousand times in the course of a day and night is excellent.

Also make sure to eat and drink little. If you eat a lot, the *qi*-flow goes awry and the hundred arteries are clogged. Once they are clogged, the *qi* cannot flow, and no *qi*-flow causes disease. (76; *Ishinpō* 23)

Always practice after midnight, during the hours of rising *qi*. Hold the breath in for a certain period while counting mentally. Make sure there are no pauses in the count, lest you give rise to error and confusion. Or you can count with your fingers. If you make it to a thousnd, you're getting close to immortality. Exhale. Always make sure to take in much and expel little. Breathe in through the nose and out through the mouth. (82; *Ishinpō* 23)

5. Speaking and Talking

Always strive to regulate the breath and nourish the spirit. Hold the breath in as long as possible, then let it out as subtly as you can. Also, avoid excessive talking or loud yelling. They cause the spirit to be labored and diminished. (20; *Zhubing* 3)

Excessive laughter causes the kidneys to twist and leads to pain in the hips (28; *Zhubing* 4)

People should talk and laugh sparingly and never raise their voice. Raising the voice comes when you argue about theories and principles, debate about right and wrong, get involved in shouting matches, or use rude and abusive language.

Whenever you are faced with a situation like this, immediately empty your mind and lower your *qi*, avoiding any form of conflict. Excessive talking and laughter injure the lungs, harm the kidneys, and cause agitation in essence and spirit. (98; *Ishinpō* 27)

6. Eating and Drinking

Prohibition: Do not eat too much—the hundred arteries will be clogged.
Prohibition: Do not eat too little—the gall bladder will be agitated.
Prohibition: Do not eat too hot—it harms the five energies.
Prohibition: Do not eat too cold—it causes congestive ailments.
Prohibition: Do not eat raw—it hurts the stomach.

Prohibition: Do not get intoxicated—it harms vital *qi.* (115; *Ishinpō* 27)

Eating meat that has been dried in the sun rather than over a fire leads to pain and agitation. (45; *Zhubing* 20)

Eating poultry together with seal meat leads to chronic infections (56; *Zhubing* 24)

Blackened chicken eaten together with carp can cause abscesses. (95; *Zhubing* 33)

Eating sweet yogurt and vinegar together may cause blood in the urine. (59; *Zhubing* 27)

If any of the six domestic animals dies suddenly during an epidemic or after getting sick during the summer, don't eat their brain. This causes abscesses in the digestive tract. (100; *Zhubing* 33)

In the 6th month do not eat the five kinds of fruit after they have already dropped to the ground and been chewed on by ants, grasshoppers, or beetles. This leads to the nine kinds of ulcers. (104; *Zhubing* 34)

Sitting around after a meal and not going for a walk or doing something else active is not only useless for the body but can cause congestion of *qi* and digestive issues. It can also lead to paralysis in the arms and legs as well as cause dark yellow spots in the face. (71; *Zhubing* 27)

7. The Bedchamber

Essence is stored in the Jade Chamber [elixir field]. Excessive sexual intercourse leads to a loss of essence. This in turn causes depression, fear, and accelerated heart beat. (7; *Zhubing* 1)

The husband should not sleep with his head pointing north, since this agitates the spirit and the spirit soul, which may lead to depression and forgetfulness (88; *Zhubing* 31)

Engaging in sexual intercourse when intoxicated can lead to aggressive infections (109; *Zhubing* 35)

If you suffer from sadness or anger and cry frequently, you will be likely to fail in establishing the proper harmony for the union of yin and yang. This can cause irregular menstruation: sometimes heavy, sometimes scant. It can also lead to internal heat and pathological thirst. The complexion becomes sullen, the muscles dry out, and the body feels heavy. (115; *Zhubing* 35)

If husband and wife have an argument and the husband forces the wife to submit to his sexual advances without having first resolved their issues, this can cause a closing of the uterus and a pathogenic accumulation of *qi.*

This in turn may lead to a wax-like vaginal discharge of a yellow or white coloring. (117; *Zhubing* 38)

Engaging in yin-yang before menstruation has ceased causes essence and *qi* to flow inward. This may cause irregular menstruation and on the inside give rise to *qi* accumulations, which in turn may lead to infertility. (119; *Zhubing* 39)

9. Medicinal Supplements

In taking medicinal supplements, pick those that are beneficial for your inner nature and carefully examine whether their warming and cooling tendencies are appropriate for you. There is no point taking an herb just because you notice that someone else is benefiting from it. When you first take medicinal supplements, begin with herbs, then move on to roots, and finally to minerals. In all cases balance the various supplements with each other. As we say, "Subtle and gross each take their turn." And, "Move from the gross to the subtle." (2; *Ishinpō* 1)

On the 1ˢᵗ day of the 1ˢᵗ month, pick herbs of the five fragrances and boil them into a decoction. Wash your hair with this to prevent graying. (65; *Zhubing* 27)

10. Various Taboos

If someone moans or shouts while having a nightmare, and you call him loudly, he is likely to die soon. It is much better to wake him with a soft, calm voice. Also, do this from a distance and don't get too close to the person, lest he lose his spirit or material soul. (53; *Zhubing* 23)

Do not look upon a decaying corpse on an empty stomach. Its putrid *qi* will enter your spleen, causing your tongue to show white and yellow discoloration and creating a nasty taste in your mouth. (84; *Zhubing* 30)

If you have been crying heavily due to a case of mourning, don't eat immediately after you stop. This will, over a period of time, lead to *qi* ailments. (34; *Zhubing* 13)

If there are old wells or ditches in your area, don't fill them in, lest this causes people to go deaf and blind. (73; *Zhubing* 28)

Chapter Three

Chants, Visualizations, and Self-Massages

The longevity tradition first actively connected with Daoism in the 4th century, in a transcendent self-cultivation movement called Highest Clarity (Shangqing 上清),whose followers used stretches and self-massages to ready themselves for contact with the divine, then entered visualizations to connect to the gods and invoked them with sacred chants. Their organization and practices integrate the magical and alchemical traditions but in terms of Daoism they follow upon the earliest organized Daoist school of Orthodox Unity (Zhengyi 正一), also known as the Celestial Masters (Tianshi 天師). [1] Centered in Sichuan, they surrendered to Cao Cao 曹操 in 215, and soon after were made to leave the area, moving across country and settling in different parts of China. In each new location, they mingled with local cults and influenced the development of new forms of religion.

The Highest Clarity movement was one result of this mixture. It began with the popular practice to establish communication with one's ancestors with the help of a spirit-medium, mainly to find causes for unexplained illness and misfortune, but also to learn of their destiny in the otherworld and to obtain advice on current affairs. In the 360s, two brothers of the aristocratic Xu family who lived in a village near Maoshan 茅山 southeast of Jiankang hired the medium Yang Xi 楊羲 (330–386?) to establish contact with a deceased wife. She appeared and told them about her status in the otherworld, explained the overall organization of the heavens, and introduced the

---

[1] On the Celestial Masters, their organization, worldview, and practices, see Hendrischke 2000; Kleeman 1998; Kobayashi 1992; Stein 1963; Tsuchiya 2002.

medium to various other spirit figures. In a series of revelations, which continued well over a decade, these divine guides provided the medium with a detailed description of the organization and population of the otherworld, and especially of the top heaven of Highest Clarity. They also revealed specific methods of personal transformation, meditations, visualizations, and alchemical concoctions, including longevity practices—thus not only bringing the longevity tradition into Daoism but also expanding its repertoire with various Daoist methods.

The gods' instructions resulted in an extensive corpus of texts that was carefully transmitted for about fifty years while local aristocrats continued to follow the practices it prescribed. In the 5th century they were scattered throughout the country while Buddhism and other Daoist schools, notably that of Numinous Treasure (Lingbao 靈寶), rose to the foreground. Around the year 500, the ritual master and alchemist Tao Hongjing reassembled the corpus in his masterful work *Zhen'gao* 真誥 (Declarations of the Perfected, DZ 1016) and propelled the school to the leading position in medieval Daoism.[2]

Revealing deities included various figures prominent in the Highest Clarity pantheon, pure cosmic powers of Dao as well as human beings turned perfected immortals. High among them is the Queen Mother of the West (Xiwang mu 西王母), who represents the cosmic power of yin and governs the paradise of Mount Kunlun in the west, where she grows the peaches of immortality and maintains the registers of the immortals. Her major attendants, who accompany her on her revelatory jaunts to earth include Lady Wang (Wang Furen 王夫人) as well as the Mysterious Woman of the Nine Heavens (Jiutian xuannü 九天玄女), a powerful goddess who "ruled war, sexuality, and everlasting life" (Cahill 2006, 70).

The Queen Mother's yang counterpart is the Lord King of the East (Dongwang gong 東王公) who in Highest Clarity appears as the Green Lad (Qingtong 青童), ruler over the paradise realm of Fangzhu 方諸 in the east and strongly associated with longevity practices that harness the regenerative forces of spring and newly rising yang. He manages particularly the registers of earth immortals, beings that have reached perfection but continue to live

---

[2] On the history and texts of Highest Clarity, see Bokenkamp 2007; Miller 2008; Robinet 1984; 2000; Strickmann 1978; 1981.

on earth for many centuries and serves as a manager in the office of the Ruler of Destiny (Siming 司命), another major revelatory deity.[3]

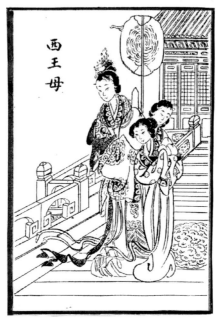

Fig. 4. The Queen Mother of the West

The Ruler of Destiny is more of a divine official than a particular deity. Already mentioned in a bronze inscription of the 6th century BCE, he is in charge of the section in the otherworldly administration that keeps records of human deeds and metes out punishments, aka the Department of Destiny. He appears prominently in a manuscript unearthed at Fangmatan, which describes the resurrection of a man named Dan in 297 BCE. Having killed another, he committed suicide and was buried after three days of public exposure, only to reappear, alive but not quite hale, after three years.

His resurrection was effected through the workings of an otherworld bureaucracy, to whom a surviving friend petitioned on the grounds that Dan had been taken before his allotted time had run out. Accordingly, "he made a

---

[3] For details on Xiwangmu, see Cahill 1993; 2006; Despeux and Kohn 2003; Yoshikawa in Pregadio 2008, 1119-20. One of her most celebrated revelations, according to Shangqing legend, was to Emperor Wu of the Han. See Schipper 1965; Smith 1992. For more on the Azure Lad, see Kroll 1985; Smith in Pregadio 2008, 803.

declaration to the senior scribe of the Ruler of Destiny, who then had a white dog dig up the pit to let Dan out." Reporting on his experiences in the other-world, the wronged man explains that "the dead do not want many clothes" and people "sacrificing at tombs should not spit" (Harper 1994, 14).[4] Under the Han, the Ruler of Destiny came to be associated with a star in the con-stellation Literary Glory (Wenchang 文昌), located above the Northern Dip-per (Beidou 北斗), another major deity in charge of the destiny of both the world at large and of individual people.

His underlings include the Three Deathbringers or Three Corpses (*san-shi* 三尸), a mixture of demons and parasites residing in the head, chest, and abdomen. Assisted by the Nine Worms (*jiuchong* 九蟲), they benefit from their host's death and incite the individual to engage in excessive emotions and commit bad deeds. They ascend to Heaven on every *gengshen* day, the 57th day of the sixty-day cycle, to report the person's violations to their su-pervisor who not only records everything in the ledgers of life and death but also orders the Deathbringers to make the person sick and cause misfortune.[5] To attain long life, it is absolutely essential that one gains control over the Deathbringers and replaces them with the Three Ones, deities of pure Dao that open celestial connections and preserve integrity.

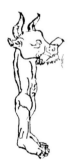 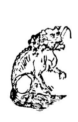 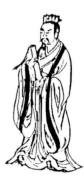

Fig. 5. The Three Deathbringers

Among humans who attained immortality and rose to high rank in Highest Clarity, the most important is the former leader of the Celestial Mas-

---

[4] Similar reports have recurred over the ages and are still current today. See Teiser 1988, 1994; Pas 1989.

[5] For Siming, see Yamada in Pregadio 2008, 914-15. On underworld officers in Warring States stories, see Harper 1994. The Three Deathbringers are described first in Ge Hong's *Baopuzi* (Ware 1966, 115-16). For a study, see Kohn 1995a.

ters, Wei Huacun 魏華存 (251–334), known also as the Lady of the Southern Peak (Nanyue furen 南嶽夫人). One of the first to connect to the medium, she revealed numerous texts and provided detailed practice information; she has been vigorously venerated ever since.

Another prominent figure is Lord Pei 裴君 who allegedly lived under the Han and originally followed Buddhism. On his wanderings he once met a Daoist master who transmitted alchemical recipes to him. After taking the elixir, he went on an ecstatic excursion around the polar mountains where he met various divinities who gave him food of the immortals and sacred books, enabling him to journey to Highest Clarity where he took up an official position. Methods associated with him include a technique to make various immortals and planetary spirits descend into the adept's body; a way to expel the Three Deathbringers; and a method of ingesting solar and lunar energies to enhance vitality and attain long life.[6]

These various methods are typical of Highest Clarity followers, who used longevity techniques less to transform the body than to develop and enhance their relation to various deities, both outside in the greater universe and deep within the body. To activate this divine connection, they used physical moves and various forms of *qi*-manipulation to enhance vitality and the keenness of their senses as part of their daily routine, especially after getting up in the morning. In addition, they integrated religious and ritual activities, such as specific guided visualizations of divine manifestations as well as talismans and incantations—sacred strips of paper covered with celestial script in red ink that tallied with the divine powers of the otherworld and lengthy chants that invoked specific deities and expressed the seeker's immortality aspirations.

A key text that outlines these techniques is the *Xiwang mu baoshen qiju jing* 西王母寶神起居經 (The Queen Mother of the West's Scripture on Treasuring the Spirit in Daily Living, DZ 1319), fully translated here. Dating from the 5th century, it consists of materials from the original revelations and in content closely echoes the *Zhen'gao* (chs. 9, 10) as well as Tao Hongjing's *Dengzhen yinjue* 登真隱訣 (Secret Instructions on the Ascent to the Perfected, DZ 421) (Robinet 1984, 2:359-62). It also refers to various other Highest Clarity scriptures, mostly associated with the Queen Mother and often now known otherwise.

---

[6] On Wei Huacun, see Schafer 1977; Valussi in Pregadio 2008, 1131-32. For her role on the Southern Peak and its development, see Robson 2009. For more on Lord Pei, see Robinet 1984, 2:375-84; 2000, 115.

One of the better known texts is the *Dadong zhenjing* 大洞真經 (Perfect Scripture of Great Pervasion, DZ 6) in thirty-nine sections, the most fundamental of all Highest Clarity texts. Transmitted by the highest deity of the pantheon to the Queen Mother before the creation of the world, each section centes on a celestial divinity, providing a description and visualization instructions for specific body gods. Its recitation, accompanied by a complete liturgy, formed another core practice of the school.[7]

Other texts used here include fundamental works on exorcism and alchemical elixirs, such as the *Xiaomo jing* 消魔經 (Scripture on Dissolving Demonic Influences, DZ 1344), which contains spells for commanding demons (Robinet 1984, 2:179-86); the *Taisu danjing* 太素丹經 (Elixir Scripture of Great Simplicity, DZ 1359), which in content predates the Highest Clarity revelations and describes methods for escaping imminent physical dangers; as well as the *Taiji jing* 太極經 (Scripture of the Great Ultimate), possibly connected to a text associated with the Perfected of Great Ultimate that spelled out how to concoct and use the elixir of nine cycles (see Pregadio 2000, 174). Other works the text refers to have not survived independently.`

In terms of methods, Highest Clarity most strongly impacted the longevity tradition in its vision of the body as a miniature version of the universe, constituting its own inner landscape inhabited by numerous body gods. Deities in the body as mentioned in the text include the Three Primes (Sanyuan 三元), originally rulers of the Celestial Masters pantheon; the Great One in the abdomen who represents the center of the cosmos; the deities of the head and hair known as Niwan 泥丸 and Xuanhua 玄華; as well as the spirit and material souls (*hun* 魂, *po* 魄), now grown to three and seven in number and given specific names and tasks (see Robinet 1993, 100).

The different parts of the body, moreover, especially those activated in self-massages and visualizations, now have new, colorful, and vibrant names, including Jade Pond (mouth), Spirit Terrace (heart), Cassia Bridge (lungs), Heavenly Perfection (corner of eyes), Mountain Spring (nostrils), Flowery Court (third eye), and so forth. The body, from being merely a vehicle of health and long life, in its Daoist dimension has thus become the residence and playground of the gods—just as enhancing vitality has transformed into a stepping stone to immortality.

---

[7] For more on this text, see Robinet 1984: 1:A2; 1993, 97-119; 2000, 201; in Pregadio 2008, 295-97.

Translation

Treasuring the Spirit in Daily Living [8]

[1a] When you wake up at dawn after a good night's sleep and are about to rise, always once more close your eyes completely, click your teeth nine times, and swallow the saliva three times. Once done with this, curl your tongue back toward the throat, then shake your head and move your neck seven times. With both hands rub the sides of your nostrils to the right and left, up and down for several sets of ten. Once done, chant softly:

> Highest Emperor of the Nine Heavens,
> [in my] Three Primes preserve infancy.
> Highest Connected Florescence,
> [in my] Jade Chamber bring forth essence.
> Let my seven gates [orifices] summon the gods,
> My nine chambers [organs] receive brilliance.
> Allow my ears to be keen, and my eyes to be bright,
> So I can penetrate perfection and reach utmost numen.

> Oh, Holy Peaks of Heaven,
> Harmonize my *qi* to perfect evenness.
> Proud Maid of Cloudy Rectitude,
> Eye Lad of Radiance and Brilliance,
> Your mysterious windows shining forth,
> Hundred pavilions crisp and cold,
> Protect and harmonize my Highest Prime
> And let me wander to the Golden Court.

> My five organs brilliant and florescent,
> My ears and eyes always alive,
> My Spirit Terrace dense and strong,
> My Cassia Bridge never bent,
> Let my seven material souls be fresh and pure,
> My three spirit souls yellow and at peace,
> The Highest Lord reaches out his hand

---

8 *Xiwangmu baoshen qiju jing.*

To journey along with me. [1b]
The Five Elders merge together,
Wuying supplements my defensive *qi*.
The myriad misfortunes dissolve,
Whatever I desire comes to pass.
Sun and moon guard my gates,
My heart matches luminants and stars.
Whatever the immortal sovereign's orders,
The myriad spirits respectfully obey.

Upon waking up from sleep, once you have done the massage, always chant this chant without fail. Even when the Dao of perfection is complete, still continue this practice.

The *Xiwang mu baoshen jing* centers on the above method. It helps people make their ears keen and eyes bright, strongly aware and vastly clear. Their nostrils harmonized to perfect balance, they no longer produce discharge or foulness. The four ministers and eight subordinates [firmly in place], their faces have a youthful appearance. They control the spirit souls and order the material souls, exorcising and dispelling the myriad demons.

This, then, is the wondrous way in which the perfected rise and rest. The reason why we speak of "rise and rest" is that the practice should always be undertaken at all times of rise and rest.

Also, with both hands rub the face and eyes, creating a low heat and always using a set number of strokes. The Old Mother [Amu] says: "When people get older, the wrinkles in their faces always start from beneath the eyes. [2a] When people's bodies decline, the decrease in *qi* always begins with the two nostrils." These two areas are accordingly the gates to all wrinkles and decline, the passages and fords of *qi* and vigor. For this reason, at all times of rise and rest always practice this method. Doing so, you can avoid wrinkles and decline and have strong *qi* and vigor to maintain perfect health and harmony.

The *Xiwang mu baosheng wusi yujing* (Queen Mother's Jade Scripture on Treasuring Life and Being Free from Death) says: With your hands spread over the sides of the Flowery Court, roll [the fingers] and extend harmony to Heavenly Perfection. Moving upward, enter with spirit into the Luscious Chamber [third eye], where the Jade Valley [nose] meets the Heavenly Mountains [forehead]. Further inward, the [Mountain] Spring is mysterious to behold. The myriad demons naturally find destruction, and you live forever without dying, your jade registers filed among those of emperors and lords. All this from harmonizing Heavenly Perfection and rubbing the dark Mountain Spring.

"Heavenly Perfection" is located between the eyebrows at the two corners of the inner eyebrows. Heavenly Perfection is one millimeter beneath them. This is the upper chamber to attract the numinous spirits. [2b]

"Mountain Spring" is beneath the nose and above the human center. Originally located sideways beneath the nostrils, it is the small opening into the Inner Valley [nose]. It is the gate that blocks and destroys the myriad demons.

"Flowery Court" is beneath the two eyebrows, the central area beneath the point where the eyebrows face each other. This is the ford and bridge of penetrating vision.

In the morning before rising and in the evening before lying down, close the eyes completely and curl the tongue back toward the throat. Swallow the saliva three times, then quickly with your hands rub the three places just listed nine times each. Rub them continuously and do not lift the hands. Doing this will always make people live long and be free from death, make the numinous forces descend and the vision perspicacious, as well as block and destroy the way of the myriad demons. When done with the hand rubbing, chant:

The Highest Sovereign of Emptiness opens and spreads the Jade Court:
Golden chambers clear and resplendent, turquoise terraces shimmering green.
I cultivate the threefold way, destroy all demons, and give rise to numen;
I am free from death and equally free from life. [3a]
I live long in eternal spontaneity, reverse aging and return to youth.
My spirit and material souls receiving purity,
My five spirits [of the organs] are restful and at peace.
I return in a flying carriage to go north and visit Jade Clarity,
Ascend to Great Nonbeing, and journey with the sun.
Becoming a perfected, I merge in mystery with emperors and lords.
Whatever the Three Primes now order
The myriad spirits respectfully obey.

In the old days, in the times of Lord Zhuang of Chu, there was a city mayor called Song Yuanfu. He had a kind heart and often in person went out to sweep the city streets. After a long time, one day a beggar entered the city.

Throughout the year, every morning he would beg while singing loudly. His song was:

The Heavenly Court gives rise to the Golden Flower,
The Inner Source blocks off all things dark and bad.
The Jade Valley joins the mysterious leaders,
The Jasper *Qi* supports the celestial network.
Heavenly Perfection stands right above the sun,
Flying Buds emit numinous powders.
At clear dawn rub the Heavenly Horse,
Then ride the spirit back to the home of mystery,
Where immortals enter the inner chamber.

He also had a song on how to destroy and remove the hundred demons and one that he posted on the city gates. Although confronted with all this information, the people of Chu city did not understand, but Yuanfu in his intention had some awakening and wondered if the beggar was not in fact an immortal. However, he did not understand the song or other pointers. [3b]

So he kowtowed to him and humbly asked for an explanation. For a long time, the beggar did not respond, but eventually he said: "I am indeed a perfected. My song consists of verses from the Queen Mother of the West, who resides on Mt. Kunlun, on how to treasure life and be free from death. Who follows them will not die."

Then he gave Yuanfu the key methods. He practiced them for twenty years and then ascended to Heaven in broad daylight to become an immortal minister in the Mystery Prefecture. There he discovered that the beggar was in fact Master Redpine, the Perfected of the Southern Peak. He had divided his form and spread out his shadow, entered the world of dust and grime and wandered all over to invite an auspicious meeting with a potential perfected.

The Perfected of Clarity and Emptiness, Lord Pei, revealed the *Shenbao jing* (Scripture on Treasuring Spirit). To pursue Dao, it is of utmost importance that one first makes the eyes bright and the ears keen. The ears and eyes are the key stages and ladders in the pursuit of perfection; they are the gateway to pervasive numen. All success and failure are established through them, all life and death are examined with their help. Today I offer this scripture to show all of you how this can be achieved.

First, to eliminate demons: Rub the ears many times on the right and left, even uncountable times. This is called "Supervising the City Wall." You will have your name entered into the r of emperors.

Similarly rub the nose many times on the right and left, but only for a certain number. This is called "Infusing the Central Peak." You will have your name entered into the register of emperors. NOTE: These two items were revealed by Lady Li at midnight on the 12th day of the 9th month.

The Dao said: Every day rub the small hollow outside the eyebrows three times. Also, using your palms and fingers rub underneath the eyes and above the cheek bones, after which you massage the ears thirty times.

Next, massage all the way up to the forehead, three sets of nine repetitions each. For this, begin at the center of the eyebrows, then move up all the way to the hairline. While swallowing the saliva, rub as many times as possible along the sides of the mouth. [4b] This daily practice will allow your eyes to get brighter and improve your vision. After one year you can write at night and discern people's secrets.

The small hollow outside the eyebrows is Upper Prime. It is also the Prefecture of the Six Harmonies, which presides over birth and transformation as well as over the brilliance of the eyes. It is important that you protect the gods of the eyes—this is the primary method of the perfected undertaken whether sitting or standing. It is also described in the *Changju neijing* (Inner Scripture of the Perfected on Constant Presence]. If you want to write at night, practice constant presence. It will also give you the ability to see sideways to the four extremes and into the eight far reaches.

Underneath the eyes and above the cheeks is Open Brightness. It protects the inner chambers and leads the person back to the perfect Dao of infancy. To activate it, hold the ears with the hands and perform the practice of increasing radiance. Thereby the blood and joints will be straightened and all wrinkles and discoloration will be prevented. The eyes will shine with mysterious brilliance, and you will harmonize essence and be filled with spirit. [5a]

To stay young and live long, you have to start with eyes and ears. All aging begins with the area to the right and left of the eyes. To prevent this, with both hands hold the forehead while visualizing an infant in your eyes, shining with the doubled radiance of the sun and the moon and filling your Upper Prime with tremendous joy. Do this for three sets of nine repetitions, which make one cycle. After completing this, speak in audience with the Three Primes and ask them to stabilize your health and enhance your hair.

Next, hold the four sides of the head with your hands, stroke the hair but not roughly, as if you were grooming and combing it. This will make the blood flow in the head and have it spread smoothly everywhere, preventing any congestion or wind-induced problems. After this, rub the four corners of the eyes for two sets of nine repetitions and notice how you begin to see the light more brightly. This activates the gods of the eyes. Over a long time, you will be able to see the hundred numinous forces.

The *Shijingzi jing* (Scripture of Master Stone Radiance) says: Always use your hands to rub the areas around the mouth and nose to activate the subtle *qi* at the four corners of the eyes. Soon you will feel moisture developing in the hands. Spread this over your face and eyes. It will make you smell nice.

The *Taishang santian guan yujing* (Highest Jade Scripture of the Three Heavenly Passes) says: Always rub the sides of the nose and the corners of the eyes, holding the breath to create greater openness in *qi*-flow. Stop abruptly and exhale, then begin again. [5b] NOTE: The above two practices were revealed by Lady Wei of the Southern Peak.

The *Danzi zishu sanwu xunxing jing* (Scripture on Appropriate Practice in Cinnabar Characters and Purple Script) says: Sit and close your eyes, internally envision the five organs, intestines, and stomach. Do this for a long time, and you will attain discernment and brightness.

The *Taisu danjing jing* (Scripture of Great Simplicity on Cinnabar Radiance) says: Rub both hands together to generate *qi* and heat, then rub your face with them. This opens the body and makes people look radiant and glossy. It prevents wrinkles and discolorations. Over five years you will gain a complexion like a young girl.

It also says: Rub both hands together to generate heat, then rub your face and eyes. [6a] Guide the hands to stroke the hair like grooming or combing it, also crossing the arms and using the hands on opposite sides. This will prevent the hair from getting white.

The chapter on "Essential Radiance Massage" in the *Dadong zhenjing* (Perfect Scripture of Great Pervasion) says: When you get up in the morning, always calm your breath and sit up straight, then interlace the fingers and massage the nape of your neck. Next, lift the face and look up, press the hands against the neck while moving the head back. Do this three or four times, then stop. This will cause essence to be in harmony, the blood to flow well, and prevent the entering of wind or bad *qi*. Over a long time it will keep you free from disease and death.

Next: bend and straighten the body; extend the hands to the four extremes [up, down, right, left]; bend backward and stretch out the sides; shake out the hundred joints. Do each of these three times.

Also, when first getting up, take a cloth and rub the forehead, the four sides of the head, and the area behind the ears. Let all these places get warm

and moist. Then stroke the hair like grooming it and, finally, massage the
face and eyes. [6b]This makes people's eyes bright and prevents wayward *qi*
from arising. Also, the body will never be dirty or defiled. At the end of the
practice, swallow the saliva thirty times to guide your internal fluids. NOTE:
The previous item comes from the *Dadong jingjing jing* (Scripture of the Essential Luminants of Great Pervasion).

The *Xiwang mu fantai anmo yujing* (Queen Mother's Jade Scripture on
Massages for Returning to the Womb) says: In the Dao of nourishing life, the
cultivation of eyes and ears is foremost. If you keep seeing mixed things, your
eyes will darken; if you keep listening to things widely, your ears will close
up. These are diseases that come from the inside of the body and are not un-
wanted guests brought in from without.

People say how hard it is to hear of Dao. But is not hard to hear of Dao,
it is only hard to practice it. No, it is not hard to practice Dao; it is only hard
to follow through with it.

If the eyes and ears are disturbed and confused, your imagination cannot let go of difficulties and problems, then, even if your feet step into an
immortals' pavilion and your hands take hold of a dragon's porch, it will do
no good.

Rather, always practice the massage of returning to the womb on yang
days. The first of the month is a yang day; the second is a yin day. [7a] On
every such yang day, in the morning and evening, before you go to sleep at
night and when you first wake up in the morning, quickly close your eyes,
face your birth direction, then rub the hands together to generate some heat.
Using the palms, rub the eyes to the right and left, as well as the ears under
their opening. Brush the hands back to the center of the next. Repeat this
nine times. Now, visualize a cloudy vapor in the eyes in three colors: purple,
red, and yellow. Each sinks down and enters the ears. After some time, chant:

> Oh, Eye Lads of the Three Clouds,
> Perfected Lords of Both Eyes:
> Be radiant and light in bringing forth essence,
> Open and pervasive as imperial gods.
> Oh, Great Mystery of Cloudy Righteousness,
> Jade Numen of the Expanded Chapters:
> Preserve and enhance my two towers [ears],
> Open and spread my nine gates [orifices].
> Let my hundred joints respond and echo
> And my various fluids return to the Niwan Palace.

Allow my body to ascend to the jade palaces above
And let me rank among the highest perfected.

Finish chanting and swallow the saliva three times. This concludes it. You may now open your eyes.

Practice like this on every yang day in the morning. There is no need to also do it in the evening. If you continue to do this for three years, your ears will be keen and your eyes bright. [7b] Also, groom your hair facing your birth direction and chant:

To the Great Emperors spreading numen,
Five Elders reverting spirit,
The gods Niwan and Xuanhua:
Preserve my essence and let me live long.
As my left holds the shadow of the moon
And my right pulls the root of the sun,
May the Six Harmonies become clear and pure
And the hundred deities deliver their grace.

Doing this regularly will keep the head free from all aches and ailments.

The *Taiji jing* (Scripture of the Great Ultimate) says: To groom the hair, face the Jade Pond. Begin your care and softly recite:

The gods Niwan and Xuanhua:
Preserve my essence and let me live long.
As my left holds the shadow of the moon
And my right pulls the root of the sun,
May the Six Harmonies become clear and pure
And the hundred deities deliver their grace.

After this, swallow the saliva three times. If you do this always, your hair will not fall out but grow anew every day. But frequently change the hold and direction of the comb, because moving in different ways will help prevent pain. You can also have a servant comb your hair for you, but have him or her change pressure and direction every so often. This prevents blood stagnation and will strengthen the roots. [8a] NOTE: The above two items were revealed by Jiuhua.

In sitting and sleeping always have your nostrils face your birth direction. Do this also when eating and drinking. If you cannot face your birth direction, use the northeast or northwest. They are also good, because they are the gates and passages of the spirit and material souls.

Also, when rising from sleep, always begin by rocking the body to the right and left and by rotating the neck, twelve times each. After this, sit up straight and raise both hands to support heaven. Hold this for a while, then use your palms to massage your cheeks up to the ears. Do this for some time and chant:

As I roll forwards and point backwards,
Let me become the honored guest of the Heavenly Emperor.
As I rub my left ear and right cheek,
Let me life long and reach great transcendence.
As I raise my head and swallow my *qi*,
Let the Great One reach its ultimate.
As I bend into a hanging moon or dragon form,
Let the Ruler of Destiny climb in his carriage. [8b]
As I drink and ingest the embryonic prime,
Let the Double Towers of Kunlun appear.
As I bend and drop to both knees,
Let the perfected join my will.

Conclude this chant, then inhale deeply and hold the breath. Visualize red *qi* in your navel the size of an egg. Allow it to emerge from the navel and enter into your nostrils. Repeat this three times. Doing this concludes the sequence of self-massages. It allows people's hundred passes to be open and flourishing and helps them live long without getting sick.

You can also visualize a purple *qi* in the center. To do so every day, close your eyes and lie down to rest your body and calm your breath. Lie as if asleep, so that other people won't even know you're not sleeping. Then in inner vision reach out to the four directions. Let your eyes and ears penetrate beyond ten thousand miles. If you do this for a long time, you can even see yourself as far out as ten thousand miles. If done powerfully, using essence and mind, you can even see as far as a million miles. As you do this, you hear the music of gold and jade in your ears together with the soft rustling of leafy bamboo. It is wondrous indeed.

As for the four directions, listen carefully to these words. First work with one direction, until you see and hear it clearly within. [9a] When you first start out, there will be no subtlety, but it gradually gets better and you will come to enter wondrous scenes.

The *Dadong zhenjing* (Perfect Scripture of Great Pervasion) contains a section on the Superior Method of the Great Chant to Expel Pathologies by the Highest Internal Lad. It says:

Every time you pass through a dangerous mountain road or go near a demon shrine, when you have doubts or concerns in your mind or worry about subtle taboos and divine decrees, first curl back your tongue and swallow the saliva three times. Then with the third finger of your left hand press beneath the nose, between the Human Center point and the high area inside the nostrils. Do this thirty-six times. Then with your hands quickly rub the nose any number of times. The high area inside the nostrils is called Spirit Pond. It is also known as Root of Pathologies and Spirit Soul Terrace. After you are done rubbing, click the teeth seven times. Then, with the center of your hands cover your nose, reaching up to the eyes, and chant: [9b]

The Vermilion Bird traverses Heaven.
The Spirit Powers expand within.
My Mountain Spring is completely full.
My Demon Well is emptied and demolished.
All Pathogenic Roots are subdued and contained.

My Spirit Terrace shines forth brightly.
My Jasper Chamber is ringing clearly.
My Jade Perfection is lofty elevated.
My guardians are present in the Hall of Light.
My hands radiate with purple mist.
My head is surrounded by auroral gleam.

Thus I hold and recite the *Cavern Scripture*
In all its thirty-nine sections.
It contains demon dispellers,
Dragons, tigers, and murderous soldiers
That punish and control savage hounds,
Stampeding cattle, cutting knives,
Devouring floods, toppling mountains
Celestial apes, divine birds,
Poisonous six-headed serpents, and even
Fire-spitting, demon-swallowing monsters.

Oh, lightning hogs, thunder fathers:
I hold the stars both flowing and crossing:
Xiao and Ke, swift and brilliant,
Adverse winds, blowing across.
Great birds of prey, swooping like a net,
All are at my side,
Spitting fire as far as 100,000 feet,
And eliminating all that is inauspicious.

The host of sprites reveal the way
To seal and protect all mountains and villages.
The hundred gods, the thousand numinous forces
Fold their hands and kowtow to me.
Noble officials raise lanterns
And burn incense for me.
Wherever I am, wherever I go,
The myriad gods worship and adore me.

Conclude this, then click our teeth three times, open your eyes, and release the hands from the nose, left hand first. [10a]

As you use your hands to rub Mountain Spring, your Demon Well is closed. As you rub Spirit Pond, your Pathogenic Roots are dispersed. As your rub Spirit Terrace, various jade perfected come to guard your passes. Thus the Numinous Root is stimulated, and heavenly beasts come to stand guard for you. The thousand sprites are shaken and submissive, and none dare to invade your *qi*. This is the principle of nature. It all happens quite effectively.

Mountain Spring beneath the nostrils is the energetic control center of the entire body, the pervasive administration of perfection and pathology. Those not perfected give rise to pathogenic *qi* at this point. Those already perfected use it to control the myriad pathologies. Depending on how you rub and massage this area, good or bad fortune will arrive.

The Hall of Light is another center that controls the system of the entire body. It has charge over life and death and serves as the primordial chamber of the seven material souls and also as the numinous residence of the three spirit souls. Visualizing the gods in there makes you perceptive and activates inner vision. Abolishing this practice, on the other hand, leads to stiffness and decay. Be careful and there will be no regrets. NOTE: The above four items are from the "Section on Highest Dao" in the *Dadong zhenjing*. [10b]

The Perfected of Great Numen says: Wind-induced disorders arise because of the darkness and dampness of hills and tombs. They block the three springs, and in response the earth officials send in water-*qi* to flush things out. Thus people come to suffer from wind-induced arthritis. If serious, it may cripple the entire body, but even if light it may still hamper half the body and render the hands and feet immobile.

If you often dream of passing through old houses in the northeast or northwest or see a numinous bed in those directions, you need to adjust the *qi* of your ancestors' tombs. The northeast of a tomb is the direction that cuts off destiny; the northwest is the area of ninefold danger. They are both inauspicious and likely to give rise to posthumous complaints or supernatural lawsuits. If you dream of a deceased person standing in such a place, this is even worse and you need to be more careful. As you wake from the dream, immediately click the teeth three times and chant:

Oh, Great Prime and Highest Mystery,
Ninefold Capital in Purple Heaven:
Regulate my spirit souls and protect my destiny.

Oh, Highest Pure Perfected,
Who have given me the superior methods,
And the teachings of Great Mystery.

Let me live long, have eternal vision,
And my body fly to be like the immortals.
Let my ancestral tombs be forever at peace. [11a]
And all demon complaints be blocked.
Let my souls be joyful and in harmony
And all pathogenic *qi* be gone from me.
Keep wandering sprites and minxes
From coming close to my spirit.

Let the Northern Emperor sit in judgment
And make the *qi* enter the deep abyss.
Let me attain registration with the Highest Sovereign
And my name be inscribed among the celestial rulers.

Repeat this twice, then click the teeth three times and you will no longer dream of tombs or dead ancestors. Such is the power of this secret chant.

You can also use this to fulfill you a wish you have in your heart or if you have other kinds of bad dreams. The practice will eliminate all demonic *qi* and dissolve all pathological influences.

If you cannot raise your hands or arms, it is because deep wind and poisonous *qi* have invaded the meridians and are now creating blockages that create arthritis in the bones. This condition can be helped with needles and moxa. But you can also use the chant of the Northern Emperor. Repeat it a hundred times and the condition will be cured.

First take one hand, and rub the ailing area very slowly. Continue for a long time. Eventually lie down, turn your eyes to inner vision, swallow the saliva three times, click the teeth three times, and from the depth of your heart chant:

[11b] Oh, Highest Lord, let my
Four mysteries, five effluences [phases], and six courtyards,
three spirit souls and seven material souls,
Heavenly Pass, Earth Essence, and Spirit Prefecture,
protective *qi*, heavenly womb, highest radiance,
four limbs, hundred body gods,
nine nodes, and myriad numinous forces
All receive registers and jade stars,
So they communicate easily with the heavenly jade city.

May jade maidens protect my body, jade lads guard my life.
Forever matching the two luminants,
May I fly up as an immortal to Highest Clarity.
May I be as old as the sun and the moon,
And share the same years as they.
Striding in transcendence to rise up to the immortals,
May I attain complete Great Peace.

If ever flowing winds create disease,
That infiltrate like demons or five dragons;
If baleful stars harness their *qi*,
Dark energies twist and revolve around each other;
If they ever usurp my four limbs

Cause me excess and deficiency—
Oh, Highest Lord, let your celestial Ding powers
Dragons and tigers shine forth in their majesty
And behead all demons and inauspicious forces,
Making sure all adverse winds and pathologies are thoroughly destroyed.

Should I be tested by hardship and litigation,
Let the hundred poisons hide and vanish
And let me once again be permanent,
Radiating as brightly as the sun and the moon
Should I be tested by encountering dangers,
Let all northern demons be smitten in destruction.
This I bring to radiant attention above,
Submitting this noble petition to the authorities of the Dipper. [12a]

The *Taishang mingting sanhua jing* (Highest Engraved Scripture on Spreading Efflorescence) in its first chapter has the following massage method:
Always during the hours of living *qi* swallow the saliva for two sets of seven. Then direct your attention to the ailing area in the body and chant:

Mystery on the left, mystery on the right—
My three spirit [souls] join perfection.
Yellow on the left, yellow on the right—
My six efflorescences match each other.
All wind *qi* and bad ailments
Submit to the four directions.
While Jade Liquor flows smoothly
Up and down, pervading all.
Within I extend fire and water,
Without I keep away all that is inauspicious.
Thus I live long and attain spirit immortality,
My body always at ease and strong.

After you finish this, then again swallow the saliva for two sets of seven. If you do this regularly, you will be completely free from all ailments. It also helps if you quickly rub the affected areas 31 times. NOTE: The above was revealed by Lady Wang of Right Radiance, resident of the Palace of the Roaming Cloud Forest on the 22nd day of the 10th month.

The *Xiaomo shangling jing* (Highest Numinous Scripture on Dissolving Demonic Influences) says: [12b]

If the body is not well in a certain area, first curl back the tongue to
block the throat, then swallow the saliva a number of times until all unwell
feelings right themselves. Also, be aware of any feelings of openness in the
body. NOTE: This is from the "Section on Highest Numen" in the *Xiaomo
jing.*

If you have trouble dreaming and waking, or if your material souls tend
to collect pathogenic *qi* and impinge on the heart and mind, you want to
worship the gods with proper devotion. Every time you have a nightmare, in
the morning face north and petition the Highest Lord of the Great Dao by
telling him the circumstances. After doing this four or five times, all should
be well. NOTE: This was transmitted orally by the Azure Lad.

Also, if you feel awful after waking up from a nightmare either day or
night, turn your pillow over several times, then chant:

Oh, jade maidens of Great Harmony,
Attend perfection and guard my spirit souls.
Oh, golden lads of the Six Palaces,
Come and protect my Gate of Destiny.
Transform all nastiness into goodness
And submit a letter to the Three Primes above
To make me live forever,
Stride on the luminants and ride around on the clouds.

[13a] After you finish this, swallow the saliva nine times and click the
teeth seven times. You are now ready to sleep again. If you do this four or
five times, everything should be well. You have turned your nightmares into
auspicious signs. NOTE: This was revealed by Lady Wang of Right Radiance
on the 3rd day of the 11th month.

Now, the mysterious emblem and numinous pivot reach far, observing
everything that approaches. Concentrate your mind, making it smooth and
empty, so your wave-like spirit can taste the flowing waves. Inhale and exhale with Great Harmony, so your body and *qi* become majestic and serene.
Then your jasper shakings emit a gentle sound, a myriad reeds issue a mysterious summons.

Now, *qi* is the vessel of spirit brightness, the ancestor of purity and
coarseness. In the atmosphere, it makes the sky pure; in people, it makes the

body live forever. Life itself never goes through destruction or increase, but flows along between adjustment and control.

If you desire to ingest the six *qi*, always face the sunrise during the period of *yin* or *chou* [1-5 a.m.]. To match the times of heaven's beginning, you must also face the appropriate direction for that time. It is when the great morning cuts its first light, cinnabar yang gives birth to initial radiance, the numinous luminants begin to shine forth, and vermilion essence brings forth its first brightness. [13b]

Then begin by visualizing the sun in the Niwan center, about the size of a chicken egg. Once you have this,

exhale once, visualizing the *qi* black in color: this is corpse *qi*;

exhale twice, visualizing the *qi* white in color: this is old *qi*;

exhale three times, visualizing the *qi* azure in color: this is death *qi*.

Think of these colors and continue to exhale in the pattern for a prolonged period. Once you have expelled all three colors, you have covered all six breaths.

After you finish this, inhale very slowly, taking in yellow *qi* four times. Visualize this *qi* as arising from the sun in your Niwan center and allow it to descend four times for inhalation. After this, swallow the saliva three times. Repeat the entire procedure three times.

Next, visualize the sun *qi* again in the Niwan center, let it reach down to the ears and emerge through them. It then assembles before your mouth, about nine inches before your face. Make it subtly clearer to the eyes, so you can see it well. Then, using the sun, take in red *qi* seven times. Stop. Swallow the saliva three times. Next, get up and shake your four limbs, bending and stretching the body. This will make the joints and arteries harmonious. To conclude, visualize the saliva to be swallowed as green *qi*. [14a]

At night, you can also work with this by visualizing the moon in the Niwan center, just as you did with the sun during the day. If you decide to visualize the moon, begin at midnight on the 1st of the month and work until the 15th. From the 16th to the 30th, the moon *qi* is declining and the heavenly womb contracts. Do not visualize the moon at that time.

This method is most wondrous. Those who do it become immortals. The reason why we inhale and exhale embryonic prime, rinse and breathe with bright perfection, and at the right times summon the five *qi* is that thereby we get the spirit souls to return and the material souls that block our dwellings to go back to the Niwan center. Thus we can live long. Various other methods will not give the same results. NOTE: The above is a formula of the Queen Mother of the West.

In 375, in the night of the 4th day of the 7th month, the Ruler of Destiny, Lord of the Eastern Minister, descended with seven retainers. [14b] As they entered the house, they were seen to hold flowery banners, called numinous banners of tenfold elimination. One of them carried a bag ornamented with metal rings. Three others were holding white ivory caskets that contained sacred writings. Yet another of the group came with a fire bell of flaming gold. All retainers were clad in vermilion robes.

The Ruler of Destiny was very impressive, but only little more so than the retainers. He wore an embroidered skirt of green brocade under a purple feather cape, and his head was covered with a hibiscus headdress. As he entered, his retainers stepped forward and set up a Throne of Destiny for him. He sat down and we talked for a long time.

On the 6th day of the 7th month, the Ruler of Destiny descended again. This time he explained the sacred writings:

"You need to pattern yourself on the mystery, match the cosmic emblems, clear and still. Unaltered by the seasons, follow them or be in the lead, and the host of dark influences appropriately cease. Raise your wings and perch on cosmic impulses. Elevate your taste to match the wondrous abyss. Rest in the hills, steep and majestic—in solitude play with the jade-like scriptures. Treasuring your spirit and your life, let go of all ordinary wishes and desires.

"Create pure harmony with all that's clear and numinous. Ascend in your radiance into the cosmic void; unfold your brightness in all of the five paths [of rebirth]. Sensuality ceases as you change along with the waves [of life]. All you desire is to join with softness. In emptiness and oneness merged with the Great Thoroughfare, you see or hear no more. [15a]

"Moving far off, you match wondrous perfection; inherently strong, you rise to mysterious awakening. Bright potency fills you on the inside, numinous patterns stand firm on your outside. In the end you can harness the clouds, ride on them to reach the Great Empyrean. Your name will be entered in the cinnabar registers of the Ruler of Destiny.

"On the other hand, if your emotions are scattered and you hold a myriad different thoughts, your life is no longer stable. Your qi falls into the waves and grime [of the common world] and your heart no longer contains perfection. This thoroughly labors your body and spirit, enmeshing them in a wild forest, certainly causing you to make mistakes in your studies. Remember: this Dao is obscure and easy to seek; this Dao is abstruse and hard to attain.

"So, every month, at midnight of the 5th day, visualize the sun in your heart, allowing it to enter through your mouth. Let it shine throughout the heart until the entire heart is completely suffused in the radiance of the sun. Next, become aware of the warmth and glowing light of the heart. Continue for a long time, then chant:

Great Brightness nourishes my essence
With purifying my cinnabar heart
Radiance and light join together
Gods and perfected come into my body.

When you finish this, swallow the saliva nine times." NOTE: On the 15th, 25th, and 29th days proceed according to the same method. [15b]

This makes people open to the light and hear with acuity. Their hundred joints are released and free, their face brings forth a jade-like radiance, and their entire body is suffused with golden fluid. Practice this for five years, and the Great One will send a carriage to take you to the Great Empyrean. If you are doing it only to extend your life, there is no need to do it for as many days. NOTE: This comes from the "Esoteric Techniques of the Red Lady of the Southern Peak" in the *Xiaomo jing.*

Also, during meals do not speak of the affairs of the dead and do not expose the foodstuffs to the elements. Either action will attract pathogenic *qi.*

Also, if you frequently take baths and the beginning of the cycle with the *jiazi* day is approaching, do not rush to take your bath but wait until the sun or moon begin to rise. This makes people connect to the numinous and avoid contracting various afflictions during their baths. If you cannot avoid this, make sure to properly purify all smells of decay so that the *qi* of perfection can enter again. NOTE: These two items were revealed by Lady Wei.

The *Taishang jiubian shihua yixin jing* (Highest Scripture of Ninefold Change and Tenfold Transformation toward the New) says:

If you step into defiled or other unwholesome places, [16a] immediately immerse yourself in a bath and release your body to eliminate their influence. The best way is to use ten pounds of bamboo leaves combined with four pounds of the white flesh of peeled peaches and heat them in a cauldron filled with twelve pecks of pure water. Just before the mixture comes to a boil, let it cool to warm and use it to wash your body. The myriad obstructions will be eliminated.

Once you are free from obstructions, to get rid of spleen dampness, sores, ulcers, and similar ailments, make a similar concoction from white bamboo core and the white flesh of peaches. It will eliminate all pathogenic *qi* and extirpate all pollution. For this reason, we use these two recipes to dissolve all [energetic] dregs and staleness in the body. When celestials descend to wander about the world, they inevitably use this before they return to purify themselves. None of similar methods known in the world, such as drinking talisman water, chanting and swishing, and external containment, come even close to the power of this technique. To make bathing even more powerful and efficacious, do not merely use this concoction to wash yourself. In addition also use the plain fluid of corpse purification in your bath. This is truly esoteric and wondrous. NOTE: We were instructed to use the above by Lady Wang of the Mysterious Mound and Feathery Palace of Purple Tenuity. [16b]

At day break, face the ruling direction, hold the talisman written in red and get ready to swallow it, then chant:

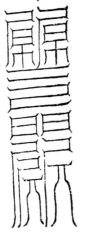

The five spirits open my heart
So I can hear clearly the music of the mystery.
The three spirit souls collect my essence,
Which always protects my cinnabar heart.
Let me not forget anything
And my five organs seek afar.

Fig. 6. The talisman written in red

Bow deeply, take the talisman, swallow the saliva five times, and click the teeth five times. Do not let anybody watch you do this. If you cannot do it at day break, use the moon rise. Every month you can do this on the 1st, 15th, and 27th days. Repeat three times every month for a year and you will have deep experiences.

The *Taixu zhenren koujue* (The Oral Formula of the Perfected of Great Emptiness) says:

On the *yimao* day in spring, the *bingwu* day in summer, [17a] the *gengshen* day in fall, and the *renzi* day in winter, as you get ready for bed, pound cinnabar, realgar, and yellow ochre, three parts each, into a fine dust, then wrap it into cotton and make it into the shape of two small dates. Put these into your ears for sleep. This will dissolve the Three Deathbringers and purify the seven material souls. But don't let anyone know about it.

Next morning, during daylight take a bath in an eastward flowing river. After that, straighten your mat, don loose clothing and create great cleanliness. Sweep the floor near your bed and your entire dwelling, making it all lovely. Set up your pillow, lie down, close your eyes, and make your hands into fists. Now enter into a spirit state. Stay there for a while, then chant:

The Dao of Heaven has its constancy.
It changes and alters the old to the new.
On the auspicious days of the Great Emperor,
It matches perfection to take a bath.
The three *qi* dissolve the Deathbringers;
The vermilion and yellow pacify the spirit souls;
The treasures refine the seven material souls;
They are very close to me. [17b]

This is the supreme method for dissolving defilements, getting rid of the Deathbringers and generally renewing the body. Do it once in every season.

The Perfected of Great Emptiness said: At sunrise, when the sun is thirty to forty feet above the horizon, sit up straight, face the sun, and visualize the three spirit souls joining with the sun's radiance and entering your heat. Keep the radiance in, hold your breath to the count of three, then swallow the saliva three times and quietly chant:

The sun spreads its brightness,
Sending out rays in purple and green.
They come and enter my body,
To illuminate my five limbs.
They eliminate all demonic ploys
And make my heart upright and steady.
On the inside they enhance the nine *qi*;
On the outside, they pervade my womb destiny.
This I fly to Highest Clarity as an immortal
My name firmly planted in the jade registers.

Conclude this chant, then rub your eyes twice seven times and click your teeth twice seven times. This methods makes your three spirit souls concentrate brightness and your cinnabar heart be open and upright. It also helps to contain and subdue the myriad pathologies and prevents the various mental ploys. It is the essential way to perfection. Practice it constantly! [18a]

At the times of fivefold accomplishment, advance quickly to the sun so you sneeze. If you cannot sneeze, use a soft item [like a feather], face the sun, and tickle your nose. This is another way to achieve a sneeze. Once you sneeze, chant:

Radiance of Heaven, come closer to me,
Let my sixfold womb open to the world above.
May my three spirit souls protect my spirit;
My seven material souls never perish.
Connected to the sun, I sneeze loudly
Thus merging with it into a single body.
I fly to Jade Clarity as an immortal
And take up the position of a perfected lord.

Conclude this, and then rub your eyes twice seven times. In this manner your inner essence communicates with the radiance of the sun above and your three spirit souls bring forth brightness within. This makes your heart open to spirit and frees the hundred essences to flow easily through your interior palaces. However, if it is not the time of fivefold accomplishment, you must not practice this.

Also, at the times of fivefold accomplishment, face north and bow five times. Deeply from your heart, call three times upon the sovereign lords of highest perfection and their divine spouses, using their proper names. Once done with this, click your teeth five times.

After this, spread your kerchief and kneel upright, and respectfully announce:

Five Stars, Sun and Moon,
Highest Sovereigns, Lofty Perfected, and Lords of the Dao,
Emperors of the Thirty-two Heavens [18b]
Highest Lord of Jade Clarity,
Highest Sovereign of Highest Clarity,
Highest Emperors of the Great Dao—
All sage lords come and line up before me.

From my ancestors of seven generations down to my father and mother
And to myself in this body,
All thousands of sins and myriads of transgressions,
Handed down all the way from many generations before,
I pray, be released and dissolved.

"May the Three Officials file a proper report to the Heavenly Emperors that cause our long list of sins to be eradicated and all black marks against us to be eliminated. I pray to be endowed with the perfection of the Five Stars so I can join them to rise up to the flowery planets, ascend to Highest Clarity, and easily pass through the celestial Jade Gates."

1/6 noon, 2/1 afternoon, 3/7 midnight, 4/9 breakfast, 5/15 midnight, 6/3 noon, 7/7 midnight, 8/4 noon, 9/2 dawn, 10/1 dawn, 11/6 midnight, 12/2 midnight. [19a] NOTE: These are the times of fivefold accomplishment.

How to Ingest Solar and Lunar Essences:: On the 1st day of the new moon, as the sun reaches twenty feet above the horizon, relax and look into the distance, directly at the sun. Make your hands into fists and perform the Pace of Yu three times while facing east. Open your mouth to take in the solar essence, swallowing it twice seven times for a total of fourteen swallowings. You may be able to repeat this twice in the same day. If then you enter the home of someone who suffers from fever, his disease will stop: it cannot stay. Also, if you practice this persistently in a state of inner lightness, you will reach old age and have a very long life.

On the 3rd day of the month, as the moon rises in the *geng* quadrant, make both hands into fists and face the moon in the southwest. Perform the Pace of Yu three times, then open your mouth and drink lunar essence twice seven times, for a total of fourteen swallowings. Doing so, for the rest of your years you will be free from all sickness and disease. Also, if you enter a house where someone has just died, your sun-moon radiance will dispel all pollution.

These two ways of eating solar and drinking lunar essences reliably dissolve all the myriad ailments!

Chapter Four

Matching, Guiding, and Eating *Qi*

In the wake of the Highest Clarity revelations, medieval sources show that the longevity tradition expanded to enhance practitioners' connection to cosmic patterns while developing techniques already documented in early sources. Several texts from the 5th to 7th centuries outline specific methods, specializing in unique areas of longevity practice, such as working with *qi*, healing exercises, and dietetics.

This chapter concerns the first, translating the *Shenxian shiqi jin'gui miaolu* 神仙食氣金櫃妙錄 (Wondrous Record of the Golden Casket on the Spirit Immortals' Practice of Eating *Qi*, DZ 836), listed in the *Suishu* 隋書 (History of the Sui Dynasty) as consisting of 9 sections and 23 *juan* (34.1048). In contents it predates this period (Loon 1984, 130; Lévi in Schipper and Verellen 2004, 355). The text is ascribed to Master Jingli 京里 or Jinghei 京黑 who supposedly lived in the 4th century and is also listed as the author of the *Daoyin jing* 導引經(Scripture on Healing Exercises, DZ 818), an extensive presentation of various physical practices (see ch. 5 below). He is further associated with the *Shenxian fu'er danshi xing yaofa* 神仙服餌丹石行藥法 (Spirit Immortals' Essential Methods Regarding Dietetics and Mineralogy, DZ 420), a collection of alchemical recipes and general examination of mineral and vegetal substances that seems to predate the Tang (Pregadio in Schipper and Verellen 2004, 100). Its *Yuanyang jing* 元陽經 citation matches a passage in the *Yangsheng yaoji* (*Ishinpō* 27.18a).; its list of 33 healing exercises also appears in the *Daoyin jing*, and its exhortation on "awe and care" features in one of Sun Simiao's works (see ch. 7 below).

The text contains a plethora of methods that work with *qi* in a variety of ways. It repeatedly emphasizes the connection of personal cultivation to the greater universe, insisting that practitioners arrange their regimen to match the cosmic flow of *qi* in terms of day and night, solar and lunar phases, and the overall pattern of the Chinese calendar. It strongly submits to the general rule, expressed in practically all Daoist and longevity texts since the middle ages, that the universe like the human body is a living and breathing entity (Maspero 1981, 500).

Creating the patterns of the circadian rhythm which govern human wake and sleep cycles, the cosmos has an inhalation or living breath (*shengqi* 生氣), which is dominant from midnight to noon, and an exhalation or dead breath (*siqi* 死氣), which controls the period between noon and midnight. For example, the *Baopuzi* says: "The circulating of *qi* should be undertaken at an hour when the *qi* is alive and not when it is dead" (Ware 1966, 139). Similarly the *Jin'gui lu* notes that one should "always practice after midnight [and before noon] in the period of living *qi*. . . . The time after noon and before midnight is called the period of dead *qi*. Do not practice then" (8a). Most exercises thus occur in the wee hours after midnight and around dawn, enhancing the quality of *qi* in the body through the rising energies of nature—a tendency that has continued to the present day, when most practitioners of qigong and taiji quan come to the parks in the early morning.

In addition, the text also specifies specific numbers of repetitions at different times of day, the largest being at midnight when the *qi* begins to rise. This method goes back to Highest Clarity and is documented in more detail in the *Taishang yangsheng taixi qi jing* 太上養生胎息氣經 (Great Scripture on Nourishing Life Through Embryo Respiration and *Qi*, DZ 819) (see Despeux 2006, 55; Jackowicz 2006, 85).

Another Highest Clarity impact appears in the practice of using talismans associated with specific yin and yang days and the invocations of jade maidens in charge of certain weeks within the Chinese calendar. The calendar designates years on the basis of Jupiter, which revolves around the sun once in twelve years, assigning a specific zodiac animal (e.g., rat, ox, hare) as well as a so-called cyclical character or "branch" (e.g., *zi, chou, yin*) to each year. It describes days in terms of a ten-day week, using another set of nominal characters, known as "stems" (e.g., *jia, yi, bing*). Combining the ten stems with the twelve branches in all possible permutations, the Chinese further developed a set of sixty combinations, which they used to count years, months, days, and hours. Odd numbered items are yang in nature, even numbered ones are yin. For example:

1 = *jiazi* (1-rat)	10 = *guiyou* (10-rooster)
2 = *yichou* (2-ox)	11 = *jiaxu* (1-dog)
3 = *bingyin* (3-tiger)	12 = *yihai* (2-pig)
4 = *dingmao* (4-hare)	13 = *bingzi* (3-rat)
5 = *mouchen* (5-dragon)	14 = *dingchou* (4-ox)
6 = *yisi* (6-snake)	etc., until
7 = *gengwu* (7-horse)	59 = *renxu* (9-dog)
8 = *xinwei* (8-sheep)	60 = *guihai* (10-pig)
9 = *renshen* (9-monkey)	61 = *jiazi* (1-rat) = 1

Each ten-day period, moreover, is under the supervision of a specific jade maiden, allowing practitioners to adapt their activities to the subtle flow of *qi* in the greater cosmos.

Beyond this, the *Jin'gui lu* shows the adaptation of Highest Clarity cosmology into the longevity tradition, not only by merging the goals of long life and immortality but also by including body gods, palaces, and nomenclature from the *Huangting jing* 黃庭經 (Yellow Court Scripture, DZ 331, 332), a 4th-century text on visualization of body gods and interior cultivation that today appears in an Outer (*wai* 外) and Inner (*nei* 內) scripture. The work is closely associated with Highest Clarity but in its older (outer) form preceding the revelations.[1]

Thus it emphasizes the importance of the three elixir fields (*dantian* 丹田) in the body: the upper one in the head, called the Niwan Palace 泥丸宮; the middle one in the solar plexus or heart area, also known as the Scarlet Palace (Jianggong 絳宮); and the lower one in the abdomen, also described as the Primordial Pass (Yuanguan 元關) and the Ocean of *Qi* (Qihai 氣海). In all three, celestial rulers reside, the so-called Three Ones (Sanyi 三一), whose visualization will ensure a successful celestial connection, matching a practice described in the Highest Clarity scripture *Jinque dijun sanyuan zhenyi jing* 金闕帝君三元真一經 (Scripture of the Three Primordial Perfect Ones by Lord Goldtower, DZ 253; trl. Andersen 1980; Kohn 1993, 204-14). It also uses a nomenclature for body parts that derives from the *Huangting jing*, such as

---

[1] On the nature and date of the text, see Robinet in Pregadio 2008, 511-14; Schipper in Schipper and Verellen 2004, 96-97, 184-85. For partial translations and studies, see Baldrian-Hussein 2004; Homann 1971; Kohn 1993, 181-88; Kroll 1996; Robinet 1993, 55-96; Saso 1995. For a searchable online version, see http://www.xiulian.com/XMZHF/013htj.htm.

Yellow Court for the spleen, Jade Pond for the mouth, and Numinous Root for the tongue.

Within this setting, the text then details a number of ways of working with *qi*: swallowing (*yan* 嚥), eating (*shi* 食), visualizing (*cun* 存), holding (*bi* 閉), guiding (*xing* 行), absorbing (*fu* 服), pulling and stretching (*daoyin* 導引), as well as overall moderation. It describes the main branches of the longevity system in terms of sexual, dietary, and *qi*-guiding practices—noting that the former two have innumerable variations and "involve a lot of toil and trouble." Only the latter is worthwhile, in all its variations.

Much of what the text describes consists of breathing techniques combined with visualizations. It guides adepts to breathe softly and deeply, then swallow the breath mixed with saliva, so they can fast with ease for three to seven days. The stomach is kept active by body fluids rather than outside materials. If they practice this frequently and do not get dizzy during this time, they can extend the period for as long as three weeks, finding all the while that "*qi* and vigor increase daily." Aided by talisman water (*fushui* 符水), the ashes of a divine writ dissolved in water, and by chants to secure the support of the gods, they learn to ingest *qi* instead of eating solid food.

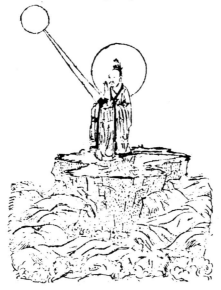

Fig. 7. Ingesting solar energies

A variant of this practice is ingesting yellow *qi*, the energy of the spleen-stomach area associated with the Yellow Court, the lower elixir field, and the central deity of the Daoist universe. This involves more visualization and a more active connection to the deities, not unlike the ingestion of solar and lunar energies that forms a key aspect of Highest Clarity practice and is also described in the text.

In addition, adepts practice holding the breath. In Western terms, about eighty heart beats make one minute, so a count of 120 would mean holding the breath for about ninety seconds and a count of 300 about three or four minutes. A key method to establishing control over the breathing patterns of the body and thus the autonomic nervous system, holding the breath increases diaphragmatic flexibility and enhances breath capacity. It also strengthens inner stillness and calmness of mind, since for the time of holding, the vibrational frequencies in the body stabilize and no mental input takes place. It is important, however, to increase the holding times slowly and carefully, since overlong holding will trigger a sympathetic nervous response and can lead to a renewed creation of stress.

Another technique is guiding the *qi*, a meditative way of deep, relaxed breathing that also involves exhaling with the warming or cooling breaths, letting go of all tensions and emotions, and allowing the *qi* to flow freely throughout the body. This may also lead to the more advanced *qi*-absorption which, rather than merely replacing ordinary nourishment with *qi*, serves to completely internalize *qi*-circulation and ultimately leads to embryo respiration (*taixi* 胎息). "Instead of being supported by a mother's body, he or she is now nourished in the womb of the universe, the body corrected to be only cosmic *qi*. . . . The practitioner in his or her body has returned to the stage of the primordial egg, from which the comic giant Pangu transformed and created the world. Primordial union has been reestablished, and the practitioner partakes of the unlimited supply of original, primordial, ever-circulating *qi*" (Jackowicz 2006, 82-83).

All this, moreover, is predicated on a moderate, controlled, and simple life-style, where one observes the "Twelve Littles" and abstains from getting involved in the world and stays away from gain and fame, indulgence and luxury. It also means developing an overall attitude of awe and care, an inherent amazement at the wonders of the world, a deep-seated adoration of Dao, combined with concern for other beings and strong self-respect.

Translation

Ingesting *Qi*[2]

[1a] **To Ingest Yin-Yang Talismans While Summoning the Six Jia Jade Maidens:** If you want to cultivate long life and study immortality, begin by learning to ingest *qi*, cut out grains, preserve essence, and maintain the spirit. These methods provide gradual progress and come with specific stages. You cannot move suddenly or jump over grades. In your ascent, if you rush you will only create lack of attainment and reversal of progress. Thus rely carefully on the following instructions without neglecting or ignoring any of them.

As for cutting out grains, remain aware of the five spirits [of the organs], reject all false imaginings, and make it your main concern to properly take the spirit immortals' talisman for cutting out grains. To prepare its ingestion, every day in the early morning sit facing east. In your left hand hold the talisman, in your right hand hold a cup of water. Silently recite: [1b]

I, so-and so, love and relish the Dao of perfection,
Ingest and ingest the *qi* of central harmony.
Oh, Jade Maiden of Great Mystery of the *jiazi* day,
Chengyi, come and serve me.
Wherever I, so-and-so, practice this diet method [lit. "kitchen"],
May the method work perfectly as chosen.
May it prevent me from feeling hungry and thirsty,
And let even armies big or small, people few or many
Be satisfied completely.

After this, take the talisman with water. Begin the practice on a *jiazi* day and continue it for sixty days, always using the same chant, except on the days following change the name of the day and with it the name of the responsible jade maiden. Always include her full name when you call on her, but do not change anything else in the chant. Dao has two patterns: yin and yang. Follow the instructions accordingly. [2a] This talisman serves from *jiazi* to *bingyin*. Change it appropriately as the day comes, matching all thirty

---

[2] *Shenxian shiqi jin'gui miaolu* (DZ 836).

yang days of the cycle. This talisman serves from *yichou* to *dingmao*. Change it appropriately as the day comes, matching all thirty yin days of the cycle.

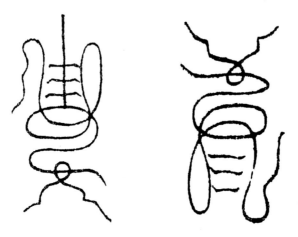

Fig. 8. The two talismans

Yang talismans match days that contain [the stems] *jia*, *bing*, *mou*, *geng*, and *ren* as well as [the branches] *zi*, *yin*, *chen*, *wu*, *shen*, and *xu*. Yin talismans match days that contain [the stems] *yi*, *ding*, *si*, *xin*, and *gui* as well as [the branches] *chou*, *mao*, *si*, *wei*, *you*, and *hai*. Write yang talismans in vermilion ink, and use black ink for yin ones. [2b]

The Jade Maiden of *jiazi* is called Great Mystery, personal name Chengyi.
The Jade Maiden of *jiaxu* is called Yellow Simplicity, personal name Feiqian.
The Jade Maiden of *jiashen* is called Great Simplicity, personal name Zhenshi.
The Jade Maiden of *jiawu* is called Purple Palace, personal name Yunling.
The Jade Maiden of *jiachen* is called Worship Essence, personal name Lingsu.
The Jade Maiden of *jiayin* is called Green Center, personal name Huijing.

NOTE: Each jade maiden is in charge of one 10-day week. As specified in the *Scripture*, sit up straight, hold on to the appropriate divine talisman and some water, chant the incantation, and take it. The jade maiden will protect people you specify in your mind and hold in your thoughts.

This method is not only good for your personal self-cultivation, but you can also use it on behalf of others, helping them cut out grains, nor is it limited to five or even ten people. It works perfectly in all cases, but you have to have a pure, clear mind. Mentally line them all up straight before yourself and have them face the sun with proper seriousness, then bow to the master and follow the talisman method. [3a] Thus they can all learn to live without eating and gradually come to realize the power of inherent potency. Every day take a talisman, from the six *jia* to the six *gui*, matching them appropriately and thus giving rise to essence and spirit.

The *Scripture* also says: Who has more than he needs to serve the world truly has Dao. A commentary notes: If you practice this to enhance your elixir fields, just using the way of guiding *qi* and concentrating essence will help your realization.

To Ingest *Qi* During the Twelve Hours, by Xi Jian of the Central Peak: Practice at first light: 7 x 7 times; at sunrise: 6 x 6 times; at daybreak: 5 x 5 times; in mid-morning: 4 x 4 times; at noon: 9 x 9 times; in mid-afternoon: 8 x 8 times; at last light: 7 x 7 times; at sunset: 6 x 6 times; at dusk: 5 x 5 times; [3b] in mid-evening: 4 x 4 times; at midnight: 9 x 9 times; at cock crow: 8 x 8 times.

The *Huangting jing* (Yellow Court Scripture) says: "The clear fluid in the Jade Pond waters the Numinous Root. All can practice this; all can live long." [3]

This refers to eating and drinking spontaneously. Spontaneous indicates the Jade Pond, which is the saliva in the mouth. Breathe as prescribed and swallow it accordingly, and you will never be hungry. To begin, first avoid grain for three days or seven days. This is a small completion. Take care not to get dizzy in your head or eyes. Then continue for twenty-one days and thus complete your training. Your *qi* and vigor will increase daily. Then, if you want to eat you can eat; if you don't want to eat you can just breathe. Avoiding grain by following yin and yang, you will never run out of essence of lose your *qi.* Then it is fine, too, if you eat some grain.

To Ingest *Qi* to Eliminate Grain: Begin by inhaling with a closed mouth. After taking in *qi,* swallow it. Do this 360 times and you will never diminish. [4a] The more you do this, the better. If you can do it a thousand times in one day, you can start to reduce your food intake, and after ten days you can give up food completely. After that, *qi* will always come in and not leave again. And if you maintain the intention that the *qi* be always full, you will find no need to eat for three days and yet feel satisfied in your stomach.

Should you be hungry or feel the urge to urinate, take nine ripe dates and take them one at a time in the morning and evening to release the urge.

---

[3] This appears in *Huangting waijing jing*, l. 6-7.

However, if you don't think of eating, you will not have such urges. But if you use the dates, always keep the pit in your mouth for a while to accumulate more *qi*. This will also improve the saliva and other bodily fluids.

The Way of the Perfected to Ingest Yellow *Qi* : To ingest yellow *qi*, always think of the spleen being full. Be aware of the yellow *qi* in your stomach, rich and abundant. Also find that there is a spirit being present, three inches tall in a yellow robe and standing tall like a statue. With each hand he leads yet another figure, also clad in yellow. [4b] When you see them clearly, silently call to the central figure: "Perfected of the Yellow Court, having arisen in me, become myself!" Then use the sweet spring and pure liquor [of saliva] to enhance your inner elixir and numinous fungus. Imagine all you might want to eat and drink and have it come before you. Practice swallowing it always at cock crow and dusk. Should you ever get hungry, face the sun and do this, and the hunger will go away.

To Guide *Qi*: When you first guide *qi*, it will be shallow and uneven, but it gets easier and better over time. Lie down flat on your back, make your hands into fists, keep your feet about four or five inches apart and your shoulders about four or five inches from the pillow. Now breathe softly for four sets of ninety repetitions, i.e., 360 times. Like a soft robe, all your bones and joints begin to dissolve. This may be hard to do the first thirty times, but it gets easier, even automatic. You can feel the *qi* like a cloudy vapor flowing into the body, pervading the meridians and arteries, moving all around rich and moist, lubricating and enhancing skin, organs, and intestines. [5a] With this, old diseases disperse without stopping, and you reach a state of full health.

NOTE: Making your fists means curling your hands like an infant.

When you first guide *qi*, calm and rest the body, then harmonize the breath. There must be no conflict between breathing and intention, because without internal harmony there can be no progress. Harmonize the breath, then practice constantly without stopping. Little effort means small success. Big effort leads to great accomplishments.

When the *qi* arrives fully, the body is calm. When the body is calm, the nasal breath is in harmony. When the breath is in harmony, the pure *qi* arrives. When the pure *qi* arrives, the body feels hot. When the body feels hot, sweat begins to flow. When sweat flows without outer incitement, spirit is at peace. When spirit is at peace, Dao manifests spontaneously.

To nourish the *qi* in the desire to keep it forever, also make sure to eliminate all greed, anger, sadness, and worry. When you eliminate these, the *qi* will not be confused. When the *qi* is not confused, proper *qi* will arrive.

When proper *qi* arrives, there will be a sweet fragrance in the mouth. When the mouth is fragrant, there is lots of saliva. [5b] When there is lots of saliva, your nostril breathing will be subtle and long. When the breath is subtle and long, the five organs are at peace. When the five organs are at peace, their *qi* flows in its proper course. Then all diseases will retreat and vanish. All food and drink will be sweet and savory. The three kinds of *qi* in perfect alignment, the body is light and strong; you reach high old age and can live forever.

To guide the *qi*, inhale through the nose and exhale through the mouth. Breathe in slowly and subtly: this is what we call a long breath. There is only one way to inhale, but there are six ways to exhale. The inhalation is called *xi*, the six exhalations are called *chui, hu, xi, he, xu,* and *si.* Normal people just use one way each to inhale and exhale, they do not know the other ways. But if you want to practice the long breath, you need to use the different ways of exhalation.

For example, when you are cold, use *chui.* When you are warm, use *hu.* To cure diseases, similarly use *chui* to expel cold and *hu* to expel heat, *xi* to expel wind or pain, *he* to expel vexations and lower the *qi*, *xu* to disperse blockages, and *si* to dissolve extremes. [6a] When ordinary people find themselves in extremes, they make heavy use of *xu* and *si*, but Daoists tend to avoid these because they prevent the long breath. All this can be found in the scriptures of the immortals.

Essence is the greatest treasure of Dao. When shared with another person, it gives new life. When kept in the body, it gives life to oneself. Giving life to oneself, one can transcend the world and have one's name entered among the ranks of the immortals. Giving new life to another, on the other hand, one pursues fame and merit in this world. Pursuing fame and merit, one places oneself last. Placing oneself last, one falls among ordinary people and is reduced to playing a minor role in the game of life. How much worse is it to foolishly share one's essence, wasting it not even knowing how much one is losing, thereby forsaking long life and falling into untimely death? Heaven and Earth have yin and yang. Yin and yang should be valued by people. Value them and find harmony with Dao. To do so, first of all be careful about what you do with your essence.

Lord Lao said: Essence is the flowing spring of blood and pulse, the numinous spirit power that protects the bones. If essence goes, the bones wither; when the bones wither, you die. Thus you have to treasure essence. Think of your body as a country: the heart is the ruler, essence is the minister, *qi* is the people. *Qi* transforms into essence, essence transforms into spirit, and spirit creates the immortal embryo. [6b] The immortal embryo grows into a perfected and then turns into the [god] Red Child who represents Perfect Oneness.

Heaven has the three luminants: sun, moon, stars. People have the three treasures: spirit, *qi*, essence. They also have three elixir fields: the upper is the Niwan Palace, located in the head between eyebrows; the middle is the Scarlet Palace, found in the heart; the lower lies beneath the navel. Always think of the Red Child in the three elixir fields. The immortal embryo is the quintessential Dao. Thus we say: Guard the One and the myriad affairs are done. This is just it!

Lord Lao said: From morning to night, always practice without stopping: thus you reach long life. Between the eyebrows, go in one inch and come to the Hall of Light. Two inches, and you find the Grotto Chamber. Three inches, and there is the upper elixir field, called Upper Prime, with its perfected being known as Red Child, aka Primordial Ancestor and also known as Imperial Master.

The heart is the Scarlet Palace. It contains the middle elixir field, called Middle Prime, with its perfected being known as the Perfected, aka Child Cinnabar and also known as Upright Radiance. [7a] The area three inches beneath the navel is the lower elixir field, called Lower Prime, with its perfected being known as the Infant, aka Primordial Yang and also known as Deep Mystery. These three represent the luminants in the body. Whether guiding *qi* or holding it, always actively visualize and think of them.

Formulas on Guiding *Qi*: To pursue immortality, there are three major methods: 1. preserving essence; 2. guiding *qi*; and 3. taking special foodstuffs. Each of the three has shallow and deep ways. Without meeting a perfected and without undergoing some hardship and toil, one cannot know any of them in any depth. Thus, the art of preserving essence comes with several hundred variants; the technique of taking special foodstuffs has thousands of specifics. They all involve a lot of toil and trouble.

Guiding *qi*, on the other hand, is straightforward: it can cure the hundred diseases, eliminate all kinds of infections, protect against snakes and wild beasts, prevent boils and ulcers, float in water, avoid hunger and thirst, and extend the years. [7b] Its most quintessential form is embryo respiration. To practice this, you no longer use the mouth and nose, but learn to breathe like the embryo in the womb, then attain Dao.

The Way of Guiding *Qi*: To practice this method, first you have to be in a secluded chamber, with doors closed and curtains drawn, and with a relaxing bed, warm and secure. The pillow should be 2.5 inches high and support your neck so your head is level with your body. Lie down flat on your back, close your eyes, and hold your breath. Allow it to stop in your chest and keep it so quiet that a down feather held before your nostrils will not move. Count to 300. Your ears will no longer hear; your eyes will no longer see; there will be no thoughts in your mind. Then exhale very slowly.

If you eat raw and cold food, the five strong vegetables, meat and fish, and tend to be given to joy and anger, sadness and rage and yet try to guide *qi* like this, the practice will not have any benefit. Unless you first discontinue common emotional and social habits, the practice will on the contrary increase the ailments of your *qi* as it battles and goes against the highest course.

If you cannot yet hold the breath, learn to do so gradually. Begin by holding it to the count of 3, then 5, 7, and 9. Rest and slowly exhale. If you can make it to 12, you have completed a small cycle. [8a] If you can make it to 120, you have completed a big cycle. This is the key to healing the body. Always practice after midnight [and before noon] in the time of living *qi*. Count silently in your mind so that you cannot hear it with your own ears.

In this *qi*-practice, the time after noon and before midnight is called the period of dead *qi*. Do not practice then, except during the *you* hour [5-7 pm], as the sun at this point is still bright and the *qi* is clear and pure. There is no dead *qi* anywhere. To best practice *qi*-absorption, use the *zi*, *wu*, *mao*, and *you* hours. Exceptions: in the 3rd month of winter, the *zi* hour is no good, because it is too cold; in the 3rd month of summer, the *wu* hour is no good, because it is too hot. In all cases, adjust your intention to breathe slowly. If there is great cold in your belly, take in the morning and noon *qi*; if there is great heat, take in the midnight and dawn *qi*. [8b] To practice *qi*-absorption in the 3rd month of winter when it is very cold, use a small room with a charcoal brazier to warm it up before you start practicing. Then you will get a sense of balance and harmony in your belly. By the same token, when there is extreme heat in the summer, take in the *qi* of the moonlight for your practice; this will give you fresh coolness.

Every time you want to absorb your *qi*, always place your body in a state of calm and rest by inhaling and exhaling in gentle rhythm. Once you reach this state of calm and rest naturally, you can guide the *qi* immediately without paying too much attention to your breathing. If you find that you need to pay attention [to breathing], adding some healing exercises to enhance the breath will be most excellent.

When you first absorb your *qi*, take enough breath to feel satisfied and full. Once full, use healing exercises to help the process. This natural leads to cosmic peace within. Once in a state of cosmic peace, diseases or hardships will never again disturb you: you have reached Dao. [9a]

Someone who is good at using *qi,* when he breathes *xu* at water, it will flow backwards; at fire, it will go out; at a tiger or leopard, it will submit; at sores and ulcers, they will heal.

Formula for Curing the Myriad Diseases: To cure all kinds of ailments and diseases—if the disease is in the throat or chest area, use a pillow seven inches high; if it is beneath the heart area, use a pillow four inches high; if it is beneath the navel, remove the pillow. Exhale through the mouth, inhale through the nose—this is to disperse. Close the mouth to warm the *qi,* then swallow it—this is to enhance.

To relieve diseases associated with the head, lift the head.

To relieve diseases associated with the hip or legs, lift the toes.

To relieve diseases associated with the chest, bend the toes.

To relieve cold, heat, and other imbalances in the stomach area, hold the breath in the belly.

In all cases, use mainly the nose for breathing and you will find quick healing. [9b]

Healing Exercises [4]

1. Sit up straight with pelvis and legs engaged. Extend the arms and spread the fingers of both hands, pressing hard against the floor. Slowly exhale from the mouth and inhale through the nose. This will remove pain from chest and lungs. To swallow the *qi,* let it get warm, then close the eyes.

2. Kneel or sit upright with pelvis engaged, inhale through the nose and hold the breath. Rock the head back and forth thirty times. This will remove all emptiness, confusion, and dizziness from the head. Close the eyes while rocking the head.

3. Lie down on your left side. Exhale from the mouth and inhale through the nose. This removes all signs of unresolved blockages that have accumulated beneath the heart.

4. Kneel or sit upright with pelvis engaged. Slowly inhale through the nose while holding the nose with your right hand. This removes dizziness from the eyes. Should tears emerge, let go of the breath through the nose. It also helps with deafness and with headaches due to obstruction. In each case, the appearance of sweat is a good measure [10a]

5. Lie flat on your back. Slowly exhale through the mouth and inhale through the nose. This removes pressure from having eaten too fast. After-

---

[4] The same list also appears in the *Daoyin jing.* See ch. 5 below.

wards swallow the *qi* in small gulps. After ten swallows, let its warmth be your measure. If the *qi* is cold, it will make people retch and cause stomach pain. Inhale through the nose, counting to seven, ten, and up to a hundred, until you hear a big rumbling in your stomach. This will remove wayward *qi* and tonify proper *qi.*

6. Lie down on your right side. Inhale through the nose and exhale through the mouth in small puffs, counting to ten. Then rub both hands together to generate heat and massage the stomach with them. This will make the *qi* descend and leave. It also removes pain from the hips and the skin, and helps with depression.

7. Kneel or sit upright with abdomen engaged. Extend both arms straight up and raise both palms to the ceiling. Inhale through the nose and hold the breath for as long as possible. Repeat for seven breaths. This is called the King of Shu's Terrace. It removes ailments due to accumulations of *qi* beneath the waist. [10b]

8. Lie down on your belly. Remove the pillow and lift the feet [legs bent at knees]. Inhale through the nose for four, then exhale through the nose for four. At the end of each exhalation, let the *qi* come back to the nose very subtly, so softly in fact that the nose cannot feel it. This removes heat from the body and cures ailments associated with back pain.

9. Kneel or sit upright with pelvis engaged. Lift the left hand with the palm facing up, then do the same move with the right. Alternate the arms. This removes ailments associated with pain in the shoulders and the back as well as diseases caused by *qi*-accumulations.

10. Sit upright, interlace the fingers and warp them around the knees. Hold the breath and pulse the belly for two or three sets of seven. When the *qi* is full, exhale. Make the degree to which the *qi* penetrates the intestines your measure. Do this over ten years and you will look young even in old age.

11. Kneel or sit upright with pelvis engaged. Stretch to the right and left sides. Close the eyes and inhale through the nose. This removes head wind. Do this as deeply as you can. Repeat for seven breaths, then stop. [11a]

12. Kneel or sit upright with pelvis engaged. Inhale through the nose to the count of ten. This removes hunger and thirst from the belly and makes you feel full. Once satisfied, stop. If you are not yet satisfied, do it again. It is also good if there is cold in the belly.

13. Kneel or sit upright. Hold the hands as if shooting a bow, pulling them as far apart as you can. This can cure ailments in the four limbs, anxiety and depression, as well as back problems. It is best when done daily at a set hour.

14. Kneel or sit upright with pelvis engaged. Raise the right hand with palm up, then take the left hand and hold the left hip. Inhale through the nose. Work as deeply as you can and repeat for seven breaths. This removes cold from the stomach and helps with indigestion.

15. Kneel or sit upright with pelvis engaged. Raise the left hand with palm up, then take the right hand and hold the right hip. Inhale through the nose. Work as deeply as you can and repeat for seven breaths. This helps with blood contusions and the like. [11b]

16. [Kneeling and] With both hands pushing against the floor, raise the head. Inhale through the nose and swallow the *qi* ten times. This removes fever and helps with injured muscles and dead skin.

17. Lie down flat. Raise both legs and arms straight up. Inhale through the nose. Work as deeply as you can and repeat for seven breaths. Then shake and rock the legs thirty times. This removes cold from the chest and legs, helps with rheumatism in the body, and reverts coughs.

18. Lie down flat. Bend the knees and bring them in toward the head. With both hands hold the knees and engage the pelvis. Inhale through the nose. Work as deeply as you can and repeat for seven breaths. This removes fatigue, fevers, and pain in the thighs.

19. Sit up straight. With both hands hold the head, then turn and twist the torso, moving it up and down. This is called "opening the waist." It removes dullness and heaviness from the body and cures all diseases due to lack of pervasion.

20. Squat. Stretch out the right leg while holding the left knee with both hands. Engage the pelvis. Inhale through the nose. Work as deeply as you can and repeat for seven breaths. [12a] This removes difficulties in bending and stretching and helps with pain in the calves as well as with rheumatism.

21. Squat. Stretch out the left leg while holding the right knee with both hands. Engage the pelvis. Inhale through the nose. Work as deeply as you can and repeat for seven breaths. Now spread the left leg to rest wide on the outside. This removes difficulties in bending and stretching and helps with pain in the calves. According to one source, it also removes wind and helps with blurry vision and deafness.

22. Lie flat on your back. Extend both hands and let them intertwine and knead each other as if they were oiling cinnabar in a bag. This will lower moisture in the body and relieve difficulty in urination and heaviness in the lower abdomen. If there is heat in the belly, only exhale through the mouth and inhale through the nose. Repeat ten times, then stop. There is no need to

swallow in small gulps. If there is no heat in the belly, practice for seven breaths, then swallow the warm *qi* ten times and stop.

23. Lie on your belly with your face turned to one side. Press both heels against your hips. Inhale through the nose. Work as deeply as you can and repeat for seven breaths. This removes tension and pain in the legs muscle knots, and leg acidity. [12b]

24. Squat. With both hands embrace the knee caps. Inhale through the nose. Work as deeply as you can and repeat for seven breaths. This removes rheumatism from the hips and pain from the back.

25. Lie flat on your back. Stretch both calves and both hands, allowing the heels to face each other. Inhale through the nose. Work as deeply as you can and repeat for seven breaths. This removes dead skin, as well as cold and pain in the legs and calves.

26. Lie flat on your back. Twist both hands and both calves to the left, allowing the heels to meet. Inhale through the nose. Work as deeply as you can and repeat for seven breaths. This removes stomach ailments from undigested food.

27. Squat and engage the pelvis. With both hands pull at the heels. Inhale through the nose. Work as deeply as you can and repeat for seven breaths, always facing the knee caps. This removes rheumatism and retching/reflux.

28. Lie flat on your back. Stretch out the arms and legs, with palms and soles facing upward. Inhale through the nose. Work as deeply as you can and repeat for seven breaths. This removes tension and urgency from the belly. [13a]

29. Lie flat on your back. Hook the heel of your left foot over the first two toes of your right foot. Inhale through the nose. Work as deeply as you can and repeat for seven breaths. This removes cramps. If the heel is off and cannot reach the toes of the opposite foot, use a stick to complete the pose.

30. Lie flat on your back. Hook the heel of right left foot over the first two toes of your left foot. Inhale through the nose. Work as deeply as you can and repeat for seven breaths. This removes rheumatism.

31. If you have a disease on the left, kneel or sit upright with pelvis engaged and look to the right. Inhale through the nose, then exhale while counting to ten. Close your eyes while you do this.

32. If you have a disease beneath the heart, kneel or sit upright with pelvis engaged, lift the head and look up toward the sun. Inhale slowly through the nose, the swallow the saliva. Repeat thirty times. Keep your eyes open while you do this. [13b]

33. If you have a disease on the right, kneel or sit upright with pelvis engaged and look to the left. Inhale through the nose, then exhale while counting to ten.

The *Yuanyang jing* (Scripture of Primordial Yang) says: Always inhale through the nose, then hold the breath and rinse with it, swishing it [with the saliva] around the tongue, gums, lips, and teeth. Then swallow it. It is most excellent if in one day and night you reach to a thousand swallowings. Eat and drink little; if you eat and drink a lot, the *qi* will flow backwards. If the *qi* flows backwards, the hundred arteries will clog up. If the arteries clog up, the *qi* cannot be guided into a proper flow. If the *qi* does not flow properly, all kinds of ailments and diseases arise.

Xuanhe says: The will is the spirit of *qi*; *qi* is what fills the whole body. Manage it well and fulfill your life; manage it badly and destroy your body. Thus, by guiding *qi*, you eat little and are naturally balanced, your mind is stable and you are naturally calm, your will is firm and you are naturally connected [to the universe], your intention is focused and you naturally succeed—certain to reach immortality! To guide and absorb *qi*, carefully study this section and follow its instructions to the letter. This is how you reach Dao. [14a]

The Perfected says:[5] The way of Heaven can be overflowing and deficient; human affairs can be excessive and lacking. If you are in a position close to lack, unless you exert prudence, there is no way in the world you can overcome your difficulties and find salvation. Thus anyone who strives to nourish inner nature yet has no idea how to exercise prudence cannot by rights speak of the way of nourishing life and absorbing *qi*. Prudence is key! How can even sages not be aware of the dangers and taboos? So, always make awe and care your foundation. Without this foundation of awe and proper taboos, all sorts of affairs will be ruined and destroyed.

The *Scripture* says: Without awe for the majesty [of Dao], great majesty will arrive [to make you feel it]. Thus, in cultivating the self, if you do not show awe and care, your friends will desert you; in cultivating the family, if you do not show awe and care, the servants will despise you; in cultivating the state, if you do not show awe and care, inherent potency [virtue] will leave you. [14b]

Thus, awe and care are the gateway of life and death, the key to rites and good teaching. They are the cause of existence and perishing, the root of

---

[5] Here begins the section on "Prudence," identical with the first section of Sun Simiao's *Zhenzhong ji*. See ch. 7 below.

good and bad fortune. They are the prime source of all auspicious and inauspicious conditions.

> A gentleman without awe and care cannot reach rank and fame.
> A farmer without awe and care has fields that are not fertile.
> A craftsman without awe and care has his tools that do not work right.
> A merchant without awe and care cannot expand his business.
> A son without awe and care is insincere in his proper filial piety.
> A father without awe and care lacks the right love and concern.
> A minister without awe and care cannot develop valor.
> A ruler without awe and care has gods of soil and grain not at peace.[6]

To absorb *qi* and nourish inner nature, cultivate perfection and practice embryo respiration, study diligently and strive for Dao, work consistently to reach spirit immortality, note this: if you lose awe and care, your mind is confused and not ordered, your body is stressed and restless, your spirit is scattered, your *qi* is out of control, your will is excessive, and your intention deluded. Instead of living, you are dying; instead of resting, you rush around. Instead of succeeding, you fail; instead of good fortune, you meet with disaster. [15a]

Awe and care are like water and fire: you cannot forget them even for a minute. Without awe and care, even your children and brothers become your foes; even your wives and concubines turn into enemies. The highest state is being in awe of Dao, followed closely by being in awe of all beings, humans, and—finally—oneself. Thus:

> Who cares for himself will not be pushed around by others.
> Who is in awe of himself will not be controlled by others.
> Who is cautious about small things will not be afraid of big affairs.
> Who is controlled in dealing with near things will not be disappointed by far ones.

If you know this, you can travel on water without ever being attacked by monsters and dragons; you can travel on land without ever being harmed by tigers and robbers.

---

[6] A similar passage is ascribed to Sun Simiao in his official biography in the *Xin Tangshu* 新唐書 (New History of the Tang), 196:5ab (Sivin 1968, 117). See also ch. 7 below.

Now, the myriad diseases arise against the course of nature and people's lives are cut short against their destiny. This is for the most part due to the wrong use of food and drink. The havoc wreaked by food and drink exceeds even that of sounds and sights. Sounds and sights you can cut out, but over the years you cannot do away with eating and drinking. [15b] Moreover, rich foods and varied flavors come in hundreds of kinds. They all do battle with the *qi*, and if you put them under prohibition, they create an even stronger poison. The slow ones take several years before they lead to disease. The quick ones can create havoc fast and, bang, there's the end.

Thus, typically between summer solstice and fall equinox, do not eat any sort of fatty food or rich cake. They will create an obstruction, just like alcohol, broth, fruit, and melons, and at that time of the year you will not notice it before the disease arises. Then, after the fall equinox, you will notice a change in health and have much violent lowering of the *qi*. All because during summer you took too much cold food and drink and did not think about proper moderation. Then, when the disease arrives, people think it came about that very day. They do not realize that it grew very gradually. Thus taking precautions has to begin with the subtle and easy stages.

Now, those who wish to nourish inner nature, absorb *qi*, practice embryo respiration, and reach for Dao should: think little, reflect little, desire little, engage little, speak little, laugh little, mourn little, delight little, enjoy little, anger little, like little, dislike little. [16a] These Twelve Littles have to be accomplished by all who want to study Dao and nourish life.

> If you think much, the spirit disperses.
> If you reflect much, the will is defeated.
> If you desire much, the will is reduced.
> If you engage yourself much, the body is labored.
> If you speak much, the *qi* is struggling.
> If you laugh much, the organs are hurt.
> If you mourn much, the heart is constricted.
> If you delight much, the intention goes overboard.
> If you enjoy much, the will is confused and deluded.
> If you anger much, the hundred arteries are unsettled.
> If you like much, you are deluded and do not match principle.
> If you dislike much, you are anxious and have no pleasure.

Put a stop to these twelve excesses, lest they cause you to lose your life and ruin your *qi*. Only being free from excesses and free from doing too little will get you closer to Dao—they have difficulty in moderation. Thus hermits rarely get sick while travelers ail a lot. Farmers live to high old age while craftsmen die young—they experience too much. Ordinary people compete for benefits while Daoists are content with their lot. Ordinary people cannot be without desires and cannot be without affairs to deal with. They are always caught up in the ego-mind and in wild thoughts. If you purify yourself and reduce thinking, you will very gradually be able to rest from all that. [16b]

Fengjun Da [aka the Gray Ox Daoist] **says:**[7]

The body always move; your food always reduce.

In moving, never reach extremes. In reducing, never get to naught.

Eliminate fat and heavy things, control all salt and sour flavors.

Diminish thoughts and worries, lessen joy and anger.

Get out of being fast and rushing, watch out for sexual exhaustion.

In spring and summer drain [fields]; in fall and winter guard the larder.

Also: Avoid fish, game, fresh meat, raw substances, and cold items in large quantities and reduce them constantly. If people are too rushed, have them stop that. These things will bring forth great goodness.

If the mind always thinks of this goodness, it won't want to plot, cheat, or consider bad deeds, which all will cause great shame and reduce destiny. Be careful about them. Avoid them. Do not go against these rules.

Pengzu says: Heavy clothes and thick sleeves will prevent the body from feeling some hardship and invite disorders caused by wind and cold. Tasting meats, fatty foods, and sweets and getting intoxicated and very full will invite ruptures and congestion. Sexual infatuation, engagements with the opposite sex, and overindulgence in the bedroom will invite the misfortune of emptiness and wasting diseases. [17a] Luscious sounds and enticing music will move the heart and delight the ears but invite confusion and craziness. Racing, running about, and hunting in the fields invite the aberration of developing madness. Plotting military and business takeovers and taking advantage of others' disorder and weakness will lead into defeat through excess and nervousness. In all these, the sage guards against loss and understands that he should not even think about them.

Practicing long life and *qi*-absorption, do not do anything for a long time—walk, sit, listen, or look. Do not engage in heavy eating or drinking nor give in to worrying, sadness, or depression. Eat when hungry; drink

---

[7] A magical practitioner of the Former Han lived very long by eating only herbs and always rode around on a gray ox. See ch. 8 below for more details.

when thirsty. After each meal walk a few hundred steps. This is very good for you. At night, don't eat at all, or if you do, walk at least five *li* [1 mile] to avoid getting sick. Take care of your tasks during day or night, but avoid getting fatigued or you will sacrifice inner peace. Thus we say: Flowing water does not rot, a moving hinge does not rust. This is because they keep moving and do not rest.[8] [17b]

He also says: People who want to absorb their *qi* must know perfect balance and avoid getting lopsided. Thus we say: Long looking harms the blood, long sleeping harms the *qi*, long standing harms the bones, long walking harms the muscles, long sitting harms the flesh, far thinking and vigorous exercise harm the whole body, melancholy and sadness harm people, joy and pleasure harm people, going too far and not reaching far enough harm people, anger and unresolved conflict harm people, too much going after desires harms people, being upset by troubles harms people, irregular heat and cold harm people, imbalances in yin and yang harm people. All these can be remedied with various kinds of healing exercises.

If you can avoid the host of things that harm people and properly understand the arts of yin and yang, you have embarked on the way that leads to no death. Ordinary people only know how to crave the five flavors; they do not know that one can also drink primordial *qi*. The sage knows the poisonous nature of the five flavors; thus he does not crave them. He knows that one can properly absorb primordial *qi*; thus he shuts his mouth and does not speak, instead letting his essence and *qi* breathe within.

Anyone set on absorbing *qi* should carefully read this text from beginning to end and practice all its methods. This will complete the Great Dao!

---

[8] Here ends the section on "Prudence," also found in the *Zhenzhong ji*.

Chapter Five

Healing Exercises

Another area of specialization within longevity techniques is healing exercises as documented in the *Taiqing daoyin yangsheng jing* 太清導引養生經 (Great Clarity Scripture on Healing Exercises and Nourishing Life, DZ 818; see Despeux 1989). Like the *Jin'gui lu* ascribed to Master Jingli of the 4th century (see Loon 1984, 130), the text is recouped in two shorter versions in the Daoist Canon, one contained in the eleventh-century encyclopedia *Yunji qiqian* 雲笈七籤 (Seven Tablets in a Cloudy Satchel, DZ 1032; ch. 34), and another found in the compendium *Daoshu* 道樞 (Pivot of the Dao, DZ 1017; ch. 28) by the Daoist master and internal alchemist Zeng Zao 曾慥 (d. 1155) (trl. Huang and Wurmbrand 1987, 2:134-43).

Aside from previous medical practices and animal forms, the *Daoyin jing* stands out in that it presents exercise sequences associated with four major ancient immortals, all with first biographies in the Han-dynasty *Liexian zhuan* 列仙傳 (Immortals' Biographies). Important legendary figures of the Daoist tradition, they are Pengzu 彭祖, who allegedly ate only cinnamon and lived for 800 years through the Xia and Shang dynasties; Master Redpine (Chisongzi 赤松子), the Lord of Rain under the mythical Divine Farmer (Shennong 神農), best known for his magical powers of riding the wind; Master Ning (Ningfengzi 寧封子), the Lord of Fire under the Yellow Emperor, who was immune to heat and burning; and Wangzi Qiao 王子喬 who could travel through the universe at will. As different methods and sequences are ascribed to them, it is quite possible that these four ancient masters were representatives of different schools (Despeux 1989, 230).

The first mention of the *Daoyin jing* occurs in chapter 19 of the *Baopuzi*, but its materials mostly surface only from the 7th century onward. They

95

closely match a section of the *Zhubing yuanhou lun*, which repeats thirty of the fifty-five exercises associated with Master Ning (Despeux 1989, 229-30); the "Exercise" part of the *Yangxing yanming lu*, which probably dates from the mid-7th century (Stein 1999, 185; Maspero 1981, 542-52); the *Shesheng zuanlu* 攝生纂錄 (Comprehensive Record on Preserving Life, DZ 578; trl. Huang and Wurmbrand 1987, 2:75-90) by Wang Zhongqiu 王仲丘 of the mid-Tang, which lists six seated exercises ascribed to Master Redpine (Despeux in Schipper and Verellen 2004, 356); the *Huanzhen neiqi fa* 幻真內氣法 (Master Huanzhen's Method of Internal *Qi*, DZ 828, YJQQ 60.14a-25b), also from the mid-Tang, which has two methods of *qi*-control (Maspero 1981, 461n3); and various fragments of the *Yangsheng yaoji* as found in the *Ishinpō*.

Integrating various forms of exercises and modes of guiding the *qi*, the *Daoyin jing* brings the tradition to a new level of development, characterized by: the refinement and variation of medical exercises and animal forms; the organization of healing practices into integrated sequences and their ascription to legendary Daoist immortals; and the use of meditation techniques that integrate the guiding of *qi* with various body imaginings and Daoist visualizations. The text accordingly has three major kinds of instructions: methods for medical relief that constitute a development of those first found in the manuscripts; integrated sequences of practice that can be used to create healing but are more dominantly marked as methods of long life and immortality; and meditative ways of guiding the *qi* and visualizing the body which place the practitioner into a more divine and spiritual context. Within these three areas, the *Daoyin jing* first shows the systematic progress from healing through longevity to immortality, which becomes central in all later Daoyin forms and systems.

As regards medical relief, the *Daoyin jing* not only lists all six healing breaths (like the *Jin'gui lu*) but, following the standard correspondence system of Chinese medicine, associates them each with a particular organ and set of ailments, thus representing the system that has remained standard to the present day (Despeux 2006, 49). The text also lists a number of practices that are geared to what appear to be dominant ailments at the time: locomotive or gastro-intestinal, involving digestive troubles and sexual enhancement as well as joint aches (especially in the hips), arthritis, and swellings, often combined with fatigue. In a few cases, the exercises are geared specifically toward discomforts associated with too much food and drink, like the *Yangsheng yaoji*, addressed to an audience that is well off financially and concerned with the ills of civilization rather than with plain survival.

Also in line with the medical tradition, the *Daoyin jing* presents various practices associated with animals, in this case mostly water-based creatures, such as toad, turtle, and dragon. None match the famous Five Animals associated with the 3rd-century physician Hua Tuo 華佗, but some already appear in the medical manuscripts. Thus, the *Daoyin tu* mentions a Dragon Rise (#27) and a Turtle Move (#42), the latter depicted as a standing figure with both arms raised forward at shoulder height, while the *Yinshu* notes that Dragon Flourish is to "step one leg forward with bent knee while stretching the other leg back, then interlace the fingers, place them on the knee, and look up" (#19). Is also has a form called Leaping Toad (#37), which involves waving the arms up and down in rhythmical movement (Lo 2001a, 73). The latter features prominently in the medical work *Hama jing* 蝦蟆經 (Toad Classic), a text related to the *Huangdi neijing suwen* 黃帝內經素問(Yellow Emperor's Inner Classic: Basic Questions) that survived in Japan but probably goes back to the 7th century, if not before (Lo 2001a, 68-69). The toad, of course, is not only an aquatic creature but also the mythical animal in the moon and appears as the seventh of ten sexual positions in the Mawangdui manuscripts (Lo 2001a, 73). Its practice accordingly serves to improve breathing and open the pelvic area.

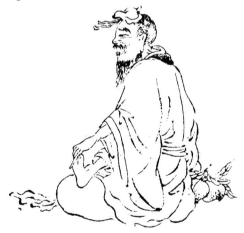

Fig. 9. Practicing a seated exercise

As regards integrated sequences of practice, the *Daoyin jing* outlines both, those undertaken from a single position and some that involve all different postures of the body. While some are geared toward medical healing, others serve overall health and the attainment of long life. Associated with various immortals, they are executed with controlled breathing and conscious *qi* awareness in all the different positions of the body, often combining standing, sitting, and lying-down postures in one set.[1]

In terms of more meditative energy work, the text recoups some Highest Clarity practices such as the absorption of lunar essence, also outlined in the *Shangqing wozhong jue* 上清握中訣 (Highest Clarity Instructions to Be Kept in Hand, DZ 140; 2.19a; Maspero 1981, 514) and in the *Dengzhen yinjue* (2.14a-16b; Maspero 1981, 514-15; Kohn 2008, 117). In addition, it presents several visualizations to ensure complete harmony of all aspects of the body. One of them is ascribed to Wangzi Qiao and called the "Eight Spirit Exercises." It involves a systematic vision of the body, seeing its different parts in different shapes and colors and becoming aware of the different psychological agents that reside in the organs. Although not entirely part of the Highest Clarity system of seeing body gods and palaces within, this it shows a creative and potent way of activating the key inner organs of the body. It can be considered a forerunner of the modern practice of the Inner Smile, which too has practitioners visualize the organs in their characteristic shape and color while releasing negative emotions and inviting advanced virtues into the self (Chia and Chia 1993, 85-102).

Along with integrating these various forms of Highest Clarity energy work, the *Daoyin jing* also presents exercises and methods of guiding the *qi* that have a more devotional component. According to one set, practitioners should focus on a divine radiance standing guard to their left and right and/or on the Ruler of Destiny as he takes up residence in the body with his two acolytes, resting there permanently and keeping the person alive. Another set instructs adepts to visualize how they fly about and divide their bodies. More than that, as adepts fly, they should always see people like themselves in front or behind. After many years of practice, they may even be able to talk to these divine entities to receive divine guidance and instruction as they traverse the otherworld.

To sum up, the *Daoyin jing* is a veritable treasure trove of healing exercises: from dominantly medical exercises that focus on physical movements and concentrated breathing through Highest Clarity energy work to the devotional practices of envisioning the body inhabited by gods and surrounded by divine entities. Healing exercises as seen here involve a wide-ranging collection of techniques that actively integrate the medical with the spiritual,

---

[1] For a detailed description and close examination of these sequences, see Kohn 2008, 98-127.

the functional with the devotional. The body is no longer merely an assembly of limbs and organs, nor even yet a combination of energy centers and pathways, but a multi-layered phenomenon, an intricate network that forms part of the cosmic patterns of the larger universe. Healing exercises and *qi*-practice cure the body but they also go beyond physical wellness and lead to the wholeness of Dao.

Translation

Healing Exercises [2]

[1a] **Master Redpine** was Rain Master under Shennong. He could follow the wind, freely rising up and sinking down. He was active well into the time of Gaoxin.

1.[3] When you first get up in the morning, loosen your hair and face east. [Standing up] begin by interlacing the fingers of both hands above your head [stretch up], then bend to the floor. Continue for five breaths. This expands the *qi*.

2. Lie down. Supporting your head with the right hand, touch the floor to your left with your left elbow [reaching over as far as you can].[4] Repeat on the other side, with your left hand supporting the head while the right elbow touches the floor. Continue for five breaths [on each side]. This releases muscles and bones.

3. With both hands hold your right knee and pull it toward your waist, raising your head at the same time to meet it. [Repeat with the left knee.] Continue for five breaths [on each side]. This releases the hips. [1b]

4. With your left hand push against your left knee as it is raised above the hip. Stretch your right arm up [and back] as far as you can. Repeat on the other side, with the right hand pushing against the right knee raised above the hip while stretching your left arm up. Do this for five breaths on each side. This releases the chest and belly.

---

[2] *Taiqing daoyin yangsheng jing* (DZ 818). Variants from YJQQ 34; *Daoshu* 28 (DZ 1017).

[3] The numbers of the exercises in the following presentation have been added by the translator.

[4] The comment in parentheses is based on the *Yunji qiqian* edition.

5. With your left hand press against your hip while stretching your right arm up [and back] as far as you can. Repeat on the other side, with the right hand pressing against the hip and the left arm stretching up [and back]. Continue for five breaths [on each side]. This releases the mid-belly.

6. [Sit up or kneel.] Interlace your fingers in front of the chest. Turn your head to the left and right. Hold your breath for as long as you can. This releases the face and ear muscles. It eliminates wayward *qi* and prevents it from reentering the body.

7. Interlace your fingers [behind your back and] below your hips. Turn your torso to the right and left as far as you can. This opens the blood arteries.

8. Interlace your fingers [in front of your body] and stretch your arms, while turning the torso to the right and left as far as you can. This releases the shoulders.

9. Interlace your fingers, reverse the palms, and stretch your arms above your head. Turn left and right in an easy rhythm. This releases the *qi* of the lungs and the liver. [2a]

10. Interlace your fingers in front of the chest. Stretch to the left and right as far as you can. This eliminates tense *qi* from the skin.

11. Interlace your fingers and bring the hands to the shoulders on the right and left. This releases skin-*qi*.

12. Stand up straight. Stretch your calves left and right. This releases leg-*qi*.

NOTE: These methods of Master Redpine serve to eliminate the hundred diseases, extend the years, and increase longevity. Always when you first rise in the morning spread a mat and face east. The exercises should be undertaken regularly every day. Over a longer period, you will feel a definite improvement.

Master Ning lived under the Yellow Emperor, whom he served as Pottery Master. He could stack up a fire, place himself in its center, and freely move up and down with the arising smoke. At the same time, his clothes would not even be singed.

Always practice between midnight and noon.

1. Loosen your hair and face east, make your hands into fists, and hold your breath for the count of one. Then raise your arms alternately left and right and stretch them until your hands cover the opposite ear. This will keep your hair black and prevent it from turning white.

2. Lie down and stretch, holding the breath for the count of two. Take the middle fingers of your hands and press them sharply into the meridians at the side of your neck. Repeat three times. This will brighten your eyesight.

3. Sit or kneel facing east and hold your breath for the count of three. Take the middle fingers of your hands and moisten their tips with saliva from your mouth. Rub them against each other for two sets of seven. Then gently massage your eyes with them. This will brighten your eyesight. [2b]

4. Sit or kneel facing east and hold your breath for the count of four. Then pinch your nostrils between your fingers. This relieves shortness of nasal breath due to too much flesh.

5. Sit or kneel facing east and hold your breath for the count of five. Click your teeth a number of times, then bend forward.

6. Lie on your side and hold your breath for the count of six. This relieves deafness in the ears and dizziness in the eyes.

7. Lie on your back and hold your breath for the count of seven. This relieves chest pains.

8. Squat. Wrap your hands around your knees and rise up on your toes. Hold your breath for the count of eight. This relieves all ailments between the chest and head, including those of ears, eyes, throat, and nose, as well as all wayward and hot *qi*.

9. [Lie down.] Remove the pillow. Curl your hands into fists and clasp them behind your head and briefly hold your breath. Rise up on your toes. Hold your breath for the count of nine, still facing east. This causes the *qi* to move up and down smoothly, opens and deepens its passage through the nostrils, and relieves emaciation and weakness.

Those who cannot follow the ways of yin and yang should not practice this.

The Frog Way of Guiding Qi

1. Kneel upright and move the shoulders to your right and left. Hold the breath for the count of twelve. This relieves fatigue. It is very effective. [3a]

2. Lie down on your side. Hold the breath for the count of twelve. This will alleviate phlegm and difficulty in swallowing. If the disease is located on the right side, lie on your right. If it is on the left, lie on your left.

3. To help with all kinds of undisclosed *qi*, practice three times a day, at sunrise, noon, and sunset. Always face the direction of the sun, stand up straight and hold the breath for the count of nine. Lift the head and inhale the essence and light of the sun. Swallow it nine times each. This will increase sexual essence a hundred fold.[5] This also helps to avoid harm from fire: when entering the fire, let the arms hang, and hold the breath.

---

[5] The fact that this is part of the Frog sequence is clear from the version in the *Yunji qiqian* (34.3a-4a). The *Daozang* version has a clear paragraph here, apparently

4. Face south. Crouch down and thread both arms under the bent knees to grasp the five toes of each foot with your palms. This intensifies the interior bends, benefits the hips, and opens the tail. It also relieves incontinence and excessive urination.

5. Sit with your legs spread, then cross the legs up and over to hold them with your hands. Interlace the hands within the crossed legs. Stretch as much as you can. This relieves irregularities in waking and sleeping and prevents *qi* and essence from leaking.

6. Interlace the fingers beneath the chin and pull the hands downward as far as you can. This benefits the lung-*qi* and relieves violent expectoration and coughs. [3b]

7. Raise both legs and press them toward the sides of the cheek bones while you press your hands down against the floor. This will help cure contractions and obstructions.

8. Raise the right hand and extend the left hand forward while kneeling on your right leg and holding the left leg [with the left hand]. This relieves all pains in the tail bone.

9. Raise both hands and interlace them behind the neck. Press them against each other strongly. This helps with pains below the waist.

10. Stretch out your left hand with the right hand underneath it. Press the thumb and fingers of the left hand as strongly as you can. Then stretch out the right hand with the left hand underneath. Press the thumb and fingers of the right hand as strongly as you can. This is good for arthritis in the bones and joints.

11. Hold both feet with your hands, your fingers placed right above the toes. This helps if you cannot reach the ground when bending from the hip. It is also good if you bruise easily.

12. Stretch the toes upward in this position. This helps with pain in the hip and back.

13. If you cannot turn your neck to look backward, raise your right arm above the head and bring it slowly forward and down. Then twist the torso, with the left arm placed on the floor. This will help you turn your neck to look backward.

14. Kneel on the floor and raise our left hand while the fingers of the right hand are placed near the left shoulder. Then twist to the right and left.

---

indicating a change in pattern. On the other hand, the *Yunji qiqian* does not have # 7 and ends with #14.

This stretches the sides and releases the knee and hip. It also helps with urinary blockages.

15. Face east and kneel in the direction of the sun. With your left hand salute the moon, raising the whole body. Then look toward the Northern Dipper and mentally ingest the *qi* of the moon. [4a] This helps prevent all sorts of evils from entering the head and thus prevents hardship and suffering.

16. With your right arm bent backward, stretch to the right and left as much as you can as if drawing a bow. This supplements insufficient *qi* in the five organs, allowing it to arrive properly.

17. Embrace your knees to bend the back. Stretch as much as you can. This helps the *qi* of the dantian to revert and nourish the brain.

18. Sit on the ground with legs extended, then knead the thighs and shinbones with your hands. Next, bring your head forward toward the ground. This balances the spine and with every strike benefits the roots of the hair, making it long and beautiful.

19. Sit on the ground and interlace your legs, then thread both arms underneath the bent knees and bring your head forward and down, so that the top of the head touches the knees. This relieves long-term cold, the inability to self-moisturize, and failure to hear unless people double their volume.

20. Sit quietly and hold your breath, while guiding the *qi* all through the body, from the head to the feet. This will relieve hurts and scars in the chest area, one-sided stiffness due to excessive wind, and all forms of rheumatism.

21. With all your might shake the shoulders while holding the breath for the count of nine. This relieves arm pains, fatigue, and improper flow of wind and *qi.*

The Turtle Way of Guiding Qi [6]

1. Cover the mouth and nose with your garment. Hold the breath for the count of nine. [4b] Lie down on your back and gently release the breath through the nose. This relieves nasal blockages.

2. Also, sit or kneel facing east, raise your head [like a turtle] and hold the breath for the count of five. Rub the tongue around the mouth until the

---

[6] Parts of the Turtle and Dragon Exercises are translated in Maspero 1981, 550.

mouth is filed with saliva, then swallow. Do two sets of seven repetitions. This relieves dryness and pain of the tongue.[7]

3. Reverse the palms and interlace the hands on the knees. Look up, stretching the neck like a turtle, then take the *qi* and envision it as a great yellow ball, thereby allowing the primordial *qi* to reach the cinnabar field. This frees the hips and spine from pain.

4. Pinch the nostrils between a finger and thumb, and hold the breath so that no air can come through. Guide the *qi* upward to the Niwan in the brain. This stabilizes the pattern of yin and yang and prevents fatigue [clears sinuses and brings oxygen to the brain].

5. Tightly holding the hair with the left hand, revolve the right arm over the top of the head. This is said to open the flow of blood and *qi* in the various channels, making each go to its root. It closes off overwhelming yang *qi* while preventing the yin *qi* from overflowing, making it clear and reliable instead. All this benefits the way of yin-yang.

6. Kneel upright and interlace your hands behind your back. This is called the sash tie. It relieves constipation and benefits the belly. It also relieves empty nakedness.

7. Kneel on the floor and interlace your hands underneath your shins. This relieves fullness of yin [eliminates all tension from the front of the body; brings the body forward into a contraction].

8. With both hands holding on to a rope, pull yourself up, then hang upside down, so that the legs are above the torso. This relieves dizziness in the head and craziness due to wind.

9. Pull up with both hands, reverse yourself, so your back is utmost, hanging from the rope. This relieves lack of concentrated essence and failure to digest properly.

10. With one hand pull yourself up on the rope while the other hand grabs hold of the legs. This relieves long-standing hemorrhoids and swellings in the tailbone area.

11. Sit on the floor with legs extended. Interlace the hands and pull the feet as strongly as you can. This relieves inactive bowels and acid reflux.

---

[7] The Turtle Pattern in the *Daozang* edition ends here. However, according to the *Yunji qiqian* (34.4b-5b), several exercises listed below in the *Daozang* (5b-6a) also belong here. I move them to accommodate the system of the *Yunji qiqian*.

The Wild Goose Way of Guiding Qi

Bow the head and bend the shoulders forward. Hold the breath for the count of twelve. Mentally push all remaining liquid and food in digestion from the lower body. This will aid natural healing.

The Dragon Way of Guiding Qi

1. Bow the head and look down. Hold the breath for the count of twelve. This relieves wind-induced itches and bad boils; it also prevents heat from entering the throat. To take best care of an ailment, do the exercises facing the sunlight.

2. Lie down. With both hands massage from the belly down toward the feet, then with your hands pull the feet under the arms. Hold the breath for the count of twelve. This relieves dampness and rheumatism in the legs and feet, as well as stiffness in the hips and back pain.

3. Interlace the fingers of both hands at the neck and stretch. This helps with all kinds of poison but will not relieve too much *qi* in the belly, which needs a proper form of exhalation.

Ways of Inhaling Lunar Essence :[8] To inhale the essence of the moon, always practice at new moon and full moon, when the moon rises and sets, stand upright facing the moon. Hold the breath for the count of eight. [5a] Turn the head upward and inhale the essence of the moonlight. Swallow it eight times. This will expand your yin-*qi*. Especially if practiced by a woman, her yin-essence will increase to overflowing and she can conceive.

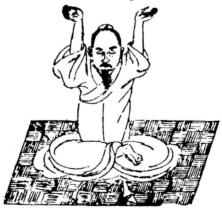

Fig. 10. Raising both arms.

---

[8] This heading and the beginning of the following sequence are based on the *Yunji qiqian* edition (34.6a).

1. If you fall into a river, raise both hands and arms and hold the breath. this prevents drowning

2. Face north. Sit with your legs spread wide and hold the toes of both feet with your hands. This relieves "bent-rabbit" paralysis and tension in the muscles of the tail bone.

3. Sit with legs spread, thread your arms through the bent knees and place the hands on the floor. Then put pressure legs as they are bent over the arms and lift the tailbone off the floor. Guide the *qi* to this area to help you. This relieves incontinence and pain in the breasts.

4. Lift the legs and cross them as high as you can, then with both hands placed on the floor, lift the tailbone. Going along with the breath as much as you can, lift the legs further, interlacing them above the head. This relieves sadness and fullness in the belly and eliminates the Three Deathbringers. It benefits the five organs and quickens both spirit and *qi*.

5. Sit cross-legged. With both hands lift the feet as high as you can, bringing the shins to horizontal. This relieves *qi* blockages and hip pain. It also prevents cold disorders from moving up or down and affecting the kidney *qi*.

6. Sit cross-legged. With both hands lift the toes of the feet, then bend down to bring the head forward as much as you can. This opens the *qi* of the five organs. [5b] It helps with ears that don't hear, eyes that are not clear. If you do it over a long period of time, it will even make your hair grow back to black.

7. Lie down flat on your back. Curl your hands and make them both into fists. Hold the breath out and move them down along your legs, the heels sticking firmly to the bed. This cures knotted muscles, cramps, and paralysis.

8. Bring both hands back, lift yourself into a squat, and place the hands beneath your armpits. This cures fullness in the chest, dizziness, and stiff hands.

9. Remove the hands and place them on the knees, then lift the head and look up like a turtle. Take in the *qi* and send it to the great yellow [spleen], while guiding primordial *qi* into the elixir field. This makes the hips and spine to cease hurting.

10. With your thumb and forefinger tightly close the nostrils and hold the breath out, making it move up to the Niwan Palace inside the brain. This causes your yin and yang to go on and on without tiring.

11. With your left hand tightly grasp your hair; stretch the right hand back to the middle of the nape of the neck. This makes the *qi* in the blood

vessels flow back to their root points and contains the *qi* of great yang, preventing yin from becoming excessive and staying clear. It greatly benefits the way of yin and yang.

12. Sit up straight and interlace your hands behind the back. This is called "tighten the girdle." It helps with constipation, benefits the stomach, and relieves empty nakedness.

13. Sit on the ground and interlace the hands, then drop them to the ground while still joined. [6a] This helps with an excess of yin.

14. With both hands grasp a hanging rope and turn like a winch; come to hang by the rope upside-down, with the feet above. This helps with dizziness in the head and with vertigo.

15. Reverse the grasp of both hands and pull up, so the back is above; hang on to the rope and sway naturally. This helps with inability to concentrate and food not going down well.

16. With one hand above grasp the rope, and with the other below grasp the feet. This helps with long-term hemorrhoids in your behind.

17. Sit on the ground while stretching both legs straight out, then with both hands joined pull at your feet as hard as you can. This helps with inability to retain food and vomiting.

Master Ning says: If you wish to practice healing exercises and guide *qi* in order to eliminate the hundred diseases, prolong life, and prevent old age, always keep your mind concentrated on the One and revert your elixir in the elixir field. What brings people to life is the elixir; what saves them is the practice of reverting it. If [the elixir is] complete, you will extend your years. If it lost, however, you will wither and decay.

Thus the practice of healing exercises eliminates all wayward *qi* from the limbs, skeleton, bones, and joints. Only proper *qi* remains in residence, becoming ever purer and more essential. [6b] Practice the exercises diligently and with care whenever you have time. If you do them both in the morning and at night, gradually your bones and joints will become firm and strong, causing the hundred diseases to be healed.

Even if you contract a wind-induced disorder that settles in firmly, a major wind-ailment that causes paralysis, so that your ears go deaf and no longer hear, your head is delirious and crazed, adverse *qi* rises up into your hips and spine, so they are wrecked with pain—you can use the chart and look at the illustrations to locate the core of the disease, then guide the *qi* there, practice the exercises, and with focused intention eliminate the disease completely.

Guiding *qi*, you can enhance your energy deep within; doing the exercises, you can cure your four limbs without. The Dao of nature is such that, as soon as you diligently activate it, Heaven and Earth come to protect you.

Pengzu's Supine Practice for Nourishing Immortality: Pengzu was a high official under the Shang dynasty. He lived through both the Xia and Shang dynasties—altogether for over 700 years. He lived primarily on cinnamon and thereby attained Dao.

1. In your residence, loosen your clothes and lie down on your back. Stretch your hips and lengthen the sacrum. Breathe five times. This stretches the kidneys, relieves diabetes, and helps with yin and yang. [7a]

2. Stretch out the left leg while holding the right knee and pressing it into the torso. [Repeat on the other side.] Breathe five times [on each side]. This stretches the spleen and eliminates all cold and heat from the heart and belly as well as all wayward and obstructed *qi* from the chest.

3. [With legs straight up in the air] pull the toes of both feet with your hands. Breathe five times. This eliminates all potential hernias and digestive trouble from the belly. It also benefits the nine orifices.

4. Raise your torso toward the toes. Breathe five times. This stretches the hip and the spine. This relieves localized pain and stiffness. It also improves hearing.

5. Turn your feet so the toes face each other. Breathe five times. This stretches the heart and lungs. It eliminates coughs as well as ailments due to rising or reverse *qi*.

6. Turn your feet so the heels face each other. Breathe five times. This tenses the thighs, thereby cleansing the *qi* of the five networks. It benefits the intestines and stomach, and eliminates wayward *qi*.

7. Bend your left shin and press it against the right knee [with right leg straight up]. [Repeat on the other side]. Breathe five times [on each side]. This stretches the lungs and eliminates *qi*-depletions caused by wind. It also sharpens the eyesight.

8. Extend the shins all the way to the toes. Breathe five times. This prevents muscle cramps.

9. Grasp the knees with both hands and bend them in so they are directly above your heart. Breathe five times. This relieves hip pain.

10. Turn both feet to the outside. Repeat ten times. Then turn both feet to the inside. Repeat ten times. This restores you from fatigue.

NOTE: This method of Pengzu to do healing exercises for nurturing immortality while lying down serves to eliminate the hundred diseases, extend the years, and increase longevity. The practice works in ten sections of five breaths each, i.e., fifty breaths in all. Repeating the exercises five times, moreover, one reaches a total of 250 breaths. It should always be undertaken between midnight and cock crow or dawn, but never after a meal or a bath.

Wangzi Qiao's Eight Spirit Healing Exercises: This, too, will extend the years and increase longevity by eliminating the hundred diseases. It goes as follows:

Lie on your back with your head on a pillow four inches high, your feet five inches apart, and your hands three inches from the body. Untie your clothes and loosen your hair. Let go of all thoughts and calm your intention.

Slowly inhale through the nose and exhale through the mouth. Allow each breath to reach its fullness before you start again. If you want to rest, first exhale completely. Do not strain to do the long breath. As you practice over time, it will become naturally long.

Make the breath come and go so softly and so concentrated that your ears do not hear it and your nostrils are hardly aware of it. If it gets too long, pull it back a little. Whether you're aware of it or not, continue for about a hundred times, moving the belly and swallowing the *qi*. [8a] Eventually there will be a sound on the outside, which signals the completion of practice. Once you have completed the practice, how will you ever get sick again?

The throat/windpipe is like a succession of white silver rings, stacked twelve levels deep. Going downwards, one reaches the lungs, white and glossy. They have two leaves reaching tall in front, and two leaves hanging low in the back. The heart is connected to them underneath. It is large up top and pointed below. All over it is shining red like an unopened lotus bud hanging down from the lungs.

The liver is connected to it underneath. Its color is a clear green like a male mallard's head. It has six leaves that envelop the stomach. The two leaves in front reach up tall, while the four leaves in the back hang down low. The gall bladder connects to it underneath, like a green silk bag. The spleen is in the very center of the belly, enwrapped from all sides. It is bright yellow like gold, lustrous and radiant. The kidneys look like two sleeping rats lying back to back, curled up with elbow to navel and as if they wanted to stretch out. Their color is a thick, glossy black. Fat streaks run through them, so that the white and black glow jointly.

The stomach is like a plain sack. If you think of it bending and folding, its rightward bend will remain free from all afflictions through dirt and filth. The liver houses the spirit souls; the lungs house the material souls; the heart houses the spirit; the spleen houses the intention; the kidneys house the essence. [8b]

Because of this, they are called the "containers of spirit." If you cultivate these containers of spirit, the hundred channels will be in harmony and any waywardness and sickness will have no place to go. The small intestine is nine feet long. It resembles the nine provinces.

NOTE: "One text says: the nine regions. The large intestine is twenty-four feet long."

If in your practice of healing exercises you want to remedy an empty condition, keep your eyes closed. If you want to alleviate a full condition, keep them open. The reason for this is that, if the practice is hard, the *qi* is exercised properly. In all cases, practice for seven breaths, then stop. Very slowly walk back and forth, taking a total of 200 steps, then sit down and swallow the *qi* in small gulps five or six times. It makes no difference if you repeat it again the same way. The gymnastic stretches will efficiently relieve your various symptoms and ailments.

Lie down on your back, loosen your hair as prescribed, then softly take in the breath through the mouth, allowing the belly to expand as much as possible. Interrupt the flow of breath briefly, before letting it out again through the nose. Do this for several sets of ten, and whatever in the body is empty will be strengthened; whatever is full, will be dispersed. Close your mouth, gather the warm *qi* and swallow it. After doing this thirty times, there will be rumbling in the stomach. Stop at this point. Very slowly walk back and forth for 200 steps. If you ailment is not better after this, repeat the exercise. [9a]

If the ailment is located in the throat or chest, work with a pillow with a height of seven inches. If it is below the heart, use a pillow that is four inches high. If it is below the navel, do away with the pillow altogether. In this position, if you breathe through the mouth and not through the nose, we speak of expansion. If you keep your mouth closed and swallow the warm *qi*, we speak of dispersal.

To Cure All Sorts of Diseases by Holding the Breath: To relieve headache, look up and pull the head back. To relieve hip and leg pain, stretch the toes of the feet. To relieve chest pain, curl the toes of the feet. To relieve shoulder pain, pull up the shoulders. To relieve cold and heat or other discomforts in the stomach, whether a centered cold or an overall heat, always hold the breath and extend the belly. When you want to breathe, slowly breathe in through the nose. Repeat until you achieve a cure, then stop.[9]

---

[9] Here follows the same list of 33 exercises as in *Jingui jing* 9b-13b. They are translated above in ch. 4.

From Wangzi Qiao's Exercise Chart: [13b] For seven days, stretch out the left leg while bending the right knee, pressing it toward the inside for five breaths. This relieves spleen-*qi* and eliminates heat and cold from the heart and belly. It also cures pathogenic tension in the chest.

From Pengzu's Exercise Chart: For this practice, begin by loosening the hair, then sit or kneel facing east, curl the hands into fists and hold the breath for one cycle. Raise the arms right and left in gymnastic rhythm, then with the hands cover the ears and with your fingers tap the meridians on the sides of the ears five times. This helps people's vision to be clear and lets their hair stay black. It also eliminates all wind from the head.

Formula for Cleansing *Qi*: The Formula says: People's five inner organs each have their proper *qi*. At night, when they sleep, the breath is closed in, so that after waking up in the morning when getting ready to absorb *qi*, you first need to revolve the *qi*. This is to allow complete digestion of the evening meal and elimination of old, stale *qi*. Only after doing this can you absorb your *qi* in proper harmony.

To revolve *qi*, first close your eyes and curl your hands into fists. Lie down flat while looking up, then bend the arms so that the two fists are placed between the nipples. Place the feet on the mat to raise the knees, then lift the back and buttocks. [14a] Hold the breath in, then drum the Ocean of *Qi*, causing the *qi* to revolve from the inside to the outside. Exhale with *he*. Do one or two sets of nine repetitions. This is called cleansing the *qi*. Finish this and go on to practice balancing *qi*. Sit facing east and hold the breath for the count of four. Click the teeth for two sets of seven. This will also help with various forms of toothache.

Formula for Swallowing *Qi*: People come to life in this physical body because they are equipped with the primordial *qi* of Heaven and Earth. Every time they swallow and breathe in or out, the interior *qi* mingles with the external *qi*, and the *qi* from the Ocean of *Qi* naturally follows the exhalation and rises all the way into the throat. What you have to do is to wait until the very end of the exhalation, then abruptly close the mouth, drum [pulse] the abdomen, and swallow the *qi* back down. This causes a gurgling sound like water dripping. In men, the *qi* descends on the left side of the body, in women on the right. It passes the twenty-four articulations [of the esophagus], going drip-drip like water. [14b] If you can hear this clearly, the internal and external *qi* look after each other perfectly and will separate as appropriate. Use your intention to send the *qi* along and with your hand massage its passageways, making it go quickly into the Ocean of *Qi*. The Ocean of *Qi* is located three inches beneath the navel; it is also called the lower cinnabar field.

When you first begin your practice of *qi*-absorption, the Upper Heater may not yet be open. In that case, use your hands to massage its area and thereby make the *qi* descend all the faster. Once it flows through nicely, there is no more need for the massage. Instead, you may get to a point where you just close your eyes and swallow the *qi* three times consecutively. One rinsing of the mouth and swallowing of *qi* as it is mixed with the saliva in the mouth is called "rain activity." When you first begin to absorb *qi*, and the *qi* is not flowing quite through yet, practice every swallow separately and do not try to swallow three times consecutively. Wait until the *qi* is open and clear, and only then very gradually add to it until you get to a small level of attainment. After about one year it will be open and clear, and in three years you will reach complete attainment. [10]

1. To practice healing exercises and *qi*-absorption: Stand up straight against a wall and hold the breath. Guide the *qi* from head to feet, then stop. This cures ulcers and scabs, great wind, one-sided paralysis, and other kinds of ailments. Some also say that you can guide the *qi* from feet to head for this practice. [15a]

2. Lie on your back, close your mouth, pulse the jaw and the belly, and make the *qi* fill the mouth so you can swallow it. At the time, create an intention that moves the *qi* toward the back. It is most wondrous to do this every morning and evening.

3. Squat on the ground leaning against a wall. Hug your knees with both arms, bend the head forward, and hold the breath out for the count of nine. This cures neck pain and problems in the hips and legs. Some say it also helps with fatigue.

4. Stretch both arms to the right and left. Hold the breath out for the count of nine. This cures fatigue in the arms and prevents mental *qi* from getting out through the nodes.

5. Sit or kneel upright, look up to the sky, and exhale deeply to expel all *qi* from being drunk on wine and satiated with food so that you can again be hungry and sober. This is best done in the summer months. It causes people's body temperature to be moderated evenly.

6. Sit or kneel upright, expand your nostrils, take in *qi*, and guide it internally to below the navel. Since the opening is small, regulate it very

---

[10] Each of the following items is introduced with *daoyin*, "healing exercise."

slowly. [15b] Hold the breath to eliminate all knots and tensions. It is best done when you are joyful and during the hot summer months.

7. Slightly incline the head, breathe softly, then interlace the hands and move the arms to the right and left. Hold the breath for the count of twelve. This will help digestion, make people feel light, and increase essence. Spirit should match the *qi* and not be entered. Another version of the same practice says: To properly guide the *qi,* slightly incline the head and squat down to hug your knees. With a rope tie yourself up to keep the head down. Hold the breath for the count of ten. This aids digestion and makes the body feel light.

8. Raise both hands as if lifting a thousand-pound rock, right and left moving well together. Doing this regularly, the entire body will be free from disease.

9. Place both hands on the ground, contract the body, and bend the spine, then lift up. Repeat this move three times. Doing this exercise every day will tonify and increase *qi* and extend your years. The best time to do it is when there is no one around. It also involves holding the breath in, then ingesting it once and exhaling so softly that the ears cannot hear it. If you are exhausted or fatigued, use *si* to exhale. [16a] If you have cold-based troubles in the organs, use *chui.* If you have a heat-based condition, use *hu.*

10. To practice the snake form, hold the breath in while lying down flat on your back. Then rise up, squat, and face the dominant direction. In this pose, hold the breath out. If you eat little, this will create pervasion and openness and help you use *qi* for your main nourishment. Then saliva will flow as a sweet juice, emerging like a spring and safely stored for the winter. The Jade Liquor in the Flowery Pond is sweet like candy. Diligently practice this and never have a single doubt. This will allow you to be active in spring, lubricated in summer, and harmonious in winter. For your inner organs, close your eyes and see a light in front of them that then revolves within.

11. *He* is the breath associated with the heart, and the heart governs the tongue. If the mouth is dry, even well assembled *qi* cannot pervade the body, thus allowing various forms of wayward *qi* to enter. Heaven will take are of that. If there is great heat, open the mouth wide. If there is little heat, keep the mouth lightly closed. Also, use your intention to measure it suitably. If you do it beyond being cured, however, the practice will caused renewed diminishing.

12. *Hu* is the breath associated with the spleen, and the spleen governs the central pulse and belongs to the phase earth. [16b] If the *qi* is a little bit hot in the belly, the intestines are very full, or there is melancholy in your mind, use *hu* to cure it.

13. *Xu* is the breath associated with the liver, and the liver governs the eyes. If the eyes are runny and red, use *xu* to cure them.

14. *Chui* is the breath associated with the kidneys, and the kidneys govern the ears. If the hips and knees are cold or weak, use *chui* to cure it.

15. *Si* is the breath associated with the lungs, and the lungs govern the nose. If cold and heat are not in harmony, use *si* to cure it.

He, hu, xu, chui, and *si* are each used for one of the five inner organs. Use them to the best of your ability.

16. Your sleep platform should be high to prevent earth *qi* from rising up and attacking you as well as to keep demon *qi* from invading your body.

17. [17a] Never be hasty or aggressive. Haste and aggression are robbers of the entire body.

18. Never face north or turn your back on the gods. If there is a violation in any affair, do not speak of it. On a *haizi* day, never face north to swallow the *qi*. This will reduce your destiny.

19. Visualize the Ruler of Destiny with two acolytes to his right and left. Practice until you can see him always.

20. Visualize a divine radiance both wide and bright on your sides. Make sure you can see it always, day or night.

21. Visualize your five inner organs with their characteristic shape and color, thus allowing the *qi* to flow evenly through the body.

22. Visualize the gods of the five organs with their appropriate colors, each in his specific place. From here on down, the human body is completely based on the five organs.

23. Visualize the gods of the five organs transform into dragons or fish.

24. Visualize the kidney *qi* below the navel in bright red and white and see it move along the spine, up to the head, and back down again to pervade the entire body. [17b]. This is called "reverting essence."

25. Visualize the heart as a fire like the Dipper. Let the will block out all bad *qi*.

26. Visualize yourself flying about and dividing your body. As you fly, always see people like yourself in front or behind you. After practicing this for a long time, you may even be able to talk to them, but make sure you face north or south as you start the conversation.

NOTE: The above was collected on the basis of notes from Master Ning's *Daoyin tu*. It has some similarities with Daolin's *Daoyin yaozhi*.

1. Lower the head and with both hands hold on to your feet. Hold the breath for a count of twelve. This helps with the digestion of grains, makes people's bodies feel light, and increases essence and *qi.* All wayward *qi* and nasty diseases cannot enter.

2. Squat with both hands joined, then stretch the feet up and down. Hold the breath for a count of five. This helps with inflammation and ulcers in the nose and mouth as well as with the five different kinds of piles. [18a]

3. Sit with your knees tied together, then place both hands on top of the knees and stretch the hip as far as you can while raising the head. Hold your breath for the count of three. This helps with the skin.

4. Sit cross-legged, interlace the fingers, reach up above your head, then stretch the head and bring it forward so as to touch the ground. Hold the breath for the count of five. This makes your *qi* strong and increases it.

5. Kneel upright and bend the arms back so that the hands embrace the nipples. Rock right and left, then hold the breath. This helps to extend destiny and allows you to stay young forever.

6. Sit upright and with both hands embrace the knees, placing them right in front of your chest. Hold the breath for the count of three. This will help with hip pain, kidney problems, and any discomforts in the back and spine.

7. Sit like a winnowing basket [with legs spread wide] and with your hands hold the five toes of the feet. Come forward as far as you can and reach the head toward the ground. Hold the breath for the count of twelve. This cures pain in the head, neck, hip, and back. It also makes people's hearing keen and their vision bright.

8. Sit cross-legged, interlace the fingers of both hands, place them underneath the head, and stretch them as far away as possible. Hold the breath for the count of six. [18b] This alleviates hip pain and difficulty in turning or raising the head.

9. With both hands rub the belly, then hold the feet while squatting on the ground. Hold the breath for the count of twelve. This helps with rheumatism in the knees, difficulty in walking smoothly, and with hip and back pain.

10. Stretch out both legs and with both hands hold the toes of the feet. This helps with hip pain due to stagnation and eases other forms of blood stagnation and bruises.

11. Bend both legs and, while sitting, lying down, or standing, and take hold of the toes. This helps with hip and back pain.

12. Lie down flat on your back. With both hands massage the belly toward the feet, then pull the *qi* up again, still using both hands. Hold the breath for the count of twelve. This helps with rheumatism and dampness in the legs as well as with hip and back pain.

13. With your left hand quickly pull your hair while your right hand pulls against the neck. This aids the activity of yin and yang.

14. Sit up straight and interlace your hands behind your back, stretching them away. This helps with digestive problems.

15. With one hand raised up and holding to a hanging rope, take the other hand to touch your feet. This help with piles and swellings.

16. Squat crouching forward and wrap both arms around the knees. In this position, bend your head forward. Hold the breath for the count of nine. [19a] This helps with neck pain, fatigue, hip pain, and various other joint discomforts.

17. Sit upright, look up at the sky, and exhale all stale *qi* from overeating and too much wine into immediate digestion. Done in the summer, this also helps people to stay naturally cool.

18. With the thumbs of both hands pinch your two nostrils. Hold the breath. This keeps people's yin-yang from getting tired. From here, turn the feet out ten times, then turn them in ten times. This helps with all empty or diminished conditions and augments *qi*.

Master Redpine's seated exercises, if done regularly, will help your hearing to be keen, your vision to be bright, and your years to be extended to great longevity, with none of the hundred diseases arising. The exercises are as follows:

1. First, [sit or] kneel upright and stretch out both arms before you, palms open and fingers turned out.

2. Interlace the fingers, stretch the arms away and roll the body to the right and left.

3. With the right hand on the hip, reach the left hand up and above the head. Repeat on the other side. [19b]

4. With the right hand stretched out backwards, use the left hand to grasp the hip from the front. Repeat on the other side.

5. Alternate the right and left arms stretching forward, then bend them back to grasp the hips from the back.

6. Raise both hands up with vigor.

Chapter Six

Eating for Long Life

Food and drink being the second major area of *qi*-intake next to breathing, dietetics play an important part in the longevity tradition. There are three levels of practice. The first is eating normally, using the same food stuffs as society at large but paying more attention to the various energetic constellations affecting health: seasonal change, local produce, and personal needs. The second level involves a more specialized diet to cure specific conditions or maintain a subtler level of health, such as those involving food cures or the Daoist monastic diet. The third deals with different forms of fasting and is generally known as "avoiding grain" (*bigu* 辟穀); it involves herbal supplements, breathing practices, and different ways of guiding *qi* to allow long-term fasting and the transformation of the body's energy system. In all cases, diet is just the pinnacle of an overall life-style adaptation.

Thus, for the first, eating normally but with close attention to *qi*, practitioners should breathe deeply, eat moderately in accordance with the seasons, move smoothly, exercise without exertion, and match their activities to the body's needs. They should partake of both yin and yang substances. Yin foods tend to grow in the earth and in dark, shady locations; they are sweet in flavor, fatty in consistence, and rich in potassium. Yang foods grow in air and sunshine; they are salty in flavor, lean in consistence, and rich in sodium. Yin foods include raw food, leafy vegetables, fish, and mellow tasting substances; with their cooling, moisturizing, and decongesting effect, they promote fluid production while mitigating heat accumulation. Yang foods include anything fried, boiled, fatty, or spicy, as well as meats; they are warming, drying, and stimulating in nature. Managing the cooking fire, they generate heat in the body and stimulate circulation (see Anderson 1988, 188-89; Farquhar 2002, 65).

Within this general system, food has three major properties:

1. stimulating (yang/heating/qi-enhancing)—e.g., apricots, barley, cherries, pineapple, plums, celery, coconut;

2. calming (yin/cooling/qi-calming)—e.g., bananas, tofu, cucumbers, eggplant, lettuce, mushrooms, pumpkins, tomatoes, watermelon;

3. neutral (neither yin nor yang/qi-maintaining)—e.g., apples, cabbage, carrots, papaya, grain, beans, eggs (Lu 1996).

These properties are associated with the four seasons, with geographical locations, with people's ages, and with particular mental states. Thus, foods eaten in spring should be stimulating and neutral; in summer, they should have a calming and cooling effect; in the fall, they should serve to retain fluid (more meats); and in winter they should stimulate and warm the body. In other words, food is used to balance the pattern of the seasons, and people should favor yin foods in yang times and yang foods in yin times. By the same token, foods also balance the geographic situation of a person, so that people in hotter climates should take more yin foods, while people living in colder, more northern, places should eat more yang. However, at all times one should avoid raw and cold substances, since their extreme yin properties deplete the system, weaken the spleen, and harm the small intestine.

Another modification of the food intake is according to age. Young people tend to be warmer, more energetic, and more yang in quality, while older folks have increased yin. Small children, being the most yang, often crave sweets to mellow their yang-*qi*. Older people, on the contrary, tend to like meats, stews, and warming foods to counteract their yin-nature. Beyond this, food also has an effect on the mental attitude. If we lack in confidence and depend much on others, more yang food may be indicated; if we tend to be aggressive, assertive, and stubborn, a mellowing yin-rich diet would be beneficial. Overall, yang foods increase valor and strength, while yin foods will have a calming and slowing effect (Craze and Jay 2001, 19, 23).

On a subtler level, practitioners rely on the system of the five phases, matching the flavor and quality of their food to the demands of the seasons and their inner organs—the yin organs that store *qi* (organ1) and the yang organs that move and transform it (organ2). The overall pattern is as follows:

phase	organ1	organ2	season	flavor
wood	liver	gall bladder	spring	sour
fire	heart	small intestine	summer	bitter
earth	spleen	stomach	Indian summer	sweet
metal	lungs	large intestine	fall	spicy
water	kidney	bladder	winter	salty

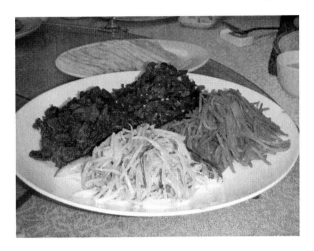

Fig. 11. Vegetables matching the five phases

A classical document that contains detailed prescription on a month-to-month basis is the *Sun zhenren sheyang lun* 孫真人慑養論(Preserving and Nourishing [Life] According to Perfected Sun, DZ 841) by the Tang physician and alchemist Sun Simiao (see ch. 7 below), translated here. It spells out specific guidelines for each month, presenting the overall pattern, specifying foods that match the changes of the five phases in the course of the year, and listing behavioral taboos along the lines of a Farmer's Almanac, such as when to get a haircut, take a bath, or go on a journey.[1]

In addition, and on a second level of eating for long life, food is also used as medicine by itself, in a practice known as dietary therapy, described variously as food cures (*shiliao* 食燎), nutritional therapy (*shizhi* 食治), and medicated foods (*yao'er* 樂餌) (Engelhardt and Hempen 1997, 1; Lo 2005, 163). It means selecting food stuffs and forms of preparation in the conscious attempt to balance *qi* and alleviate or cure medical conditions. Paying attention to food qualities as expressed in color and inherent temperature, making sure of the proper saturation with flavor, and seeing to the addition of *qi*-modifying ingredients (such as herbs and minerals) in accordance with the organs and *qi*-flow of the body are all factors which distinguish the medical from the culinary (Lo 2005, 176).

---

[1] Similar guidelines also appear in the 6th-century *Qimin yaoshu* 齊民要術 (Essential Arts for the People's Welfare), which contains 260 recipes. See Sabban 1996; Huang 2000, 123-24; Lo 2005, 166. For more classical works on seasonal adjustment, see Huang 2007, 70-73. For a modern perspective, see Engelhardt and Hempen 1997, 617-20.

To determine which dietary measure should be taken for what condition is the task of traditional Chinese diagnostics. Physicians analyze the state of the patient's *qi*-flow, using—besides obvious immediate impressions and questions about symptoms and case history—tongue inspection, pulse analysis, and abdominal palpation (see Kohn 2005, 63-74; 2010a, 61-65). They then recommend certain foods and herbal supplements while prohibiting others. People also increasingly self-medicate with food so that, in recent years a new trend in culinary culture has evolved: medicinal restaurants serving medicated dishes (*yaoshan* 藥膳) that bolster and tonify *qi* as part of nutritional therapy or personal self-care (Farquhar 2002, 51).

Another form of a more specialized longevity diet is religiously based: monastics of both Buddhism and Daoism eat vegetarian and avoid the five strong vegetables—onions, scallions, leeks, shallots, and garlic—thus ensuring a steadier flow of calmer energy in the body (Kohn 2010a, 83-87). They also tend to avoid alcohol, sugar, and caffeine; anything cold, canned, frozen, and irradiated; as well as all artificially colored, preserved, sprayed, or chemically treated foods (such as sodas). On the other hand, they use mostly local food, adapt their food choices to the seasons, and are careful about the energy that goes into the food during the cooking process.

Kitchens should be light and airy, comfortable rooms that create a happy work environment. The design should match the rules of traditional Feng Shui and apportion light, water, and fire in the proper manner (Miles 1998, 35). All base materials and utensils, moreover, should match the requirements of naturalness and clarity. Kitchen staff should cultivate a calm, meditative, and cosmically aware attitude and put good wishes and positive energy into anything they handle (Kohn 2010a, 73-77). Monastic kitchens are highly successful, both in terms of quality and efficacy of food, thus leading to the increased popularity of Buddhist, and more recently also Daoist, restaurants in Taiwan as well as on the mainland.

On a third level, the most efficient way to use food for long life is by avoiding it altogether. Known as *bigu*, the procedures for doing so involve a multiplicity of practices, most importantly dietary changes, herbal formulas, breath control, and the conscious guiding of *qi*, such as outlined earlier. Medieval sources divide into two major camps, those that favor the application of herbal formulas and those that rely entirely on working with *qi*.

The earliest source on herbal formulas is the *Lingbao wufuxu* 靈寶五符序 (Explanation of the Five Numinous Treasure Talismans, DZ 388), a complex text in three scrolls edited over several centuries, part of which go back to the Han (see Arthur 2006a; 2009). The second scroll is entirely dedicated to immortality recipes, the essence of which is further summarized in the

Taiqing jing duangu fa 太清經斷穀法 (Ways to Give Up Grain Based on the Scriptures of Great Clarity, DZ 846), translated here. The text contains materials that go back to the Han dynasty and refers to various recipes in the *Baopuzi* and *Wufuxu*. It was probably compiled in the late Six Dynasties (Lévi in Schipper and Verellen 2004, 99; Kohn 2010a, 145-49).

Key ingredients include: asparagus root (*tianmen dong* 天門冬), grown in Shandong and Sichuan, which is tonic, stomachic, and expectorant, inducing sweat; atractylis (*shu* 术), grown mainly in Zhejiang which is warming and stomachic, a stimulant, tonic, and diuretic that staves off old age; China root fungus (*fuling* 茯苓), also called "excrescences," the mushroom-like growth on tree roots considered a transformed resin, which is peptic, nutrient, diuretic, and quieting; Chinese lycium (*gouji* 枸杞), a shrub native to the northern plains which has tonic, cooling, and life-prolonging properties; jade bamboo (*weirui* 萎蕤), a northern plant with cooling, sedating, and tonifying properties; mallows or malva (*kui* 葵), a strong diuretic used to clean the stomach and lubricate internal passages; pine tree (*song* 松) in various forms, such as sap, seeds, or roots, considered nutritious, life-enhancing, and strengthening; sesame (*huma* 胡麻; *jusheng* 巨勝), introduced from the West, with cooling, expectorant, and laxative properties; yellow essence (*huangjing* 黃精), also know as Solomon's Seal, a mountain plant that looks like bamboo and is also called "hare bamboo" or "deer bamboo" with strong medicinal properties that make it useful as a tonic and prophylactic (see Stuart 1976; see also Arthur 2006b; Eskildsen 1998, 60-66; Huang 2007, 55-58; 2008, 100-29).

Traditionally preparation included cleaning, chopping, pounding, and cooking of these various substances which were then mixed in various combinations and formed into pills or decoctions with binding ingredients such as alcohol, yeast, honey, and soy paste as well as various animal fats (see Arthur 2006a). The resulting drugs were then taken on a regular basis while gradually eliminating ordinary food stuff to eventually be given up also for a complete fast during which only *qi* was ingested.

The alternative way was to focus largely on breathing and the internal guiding of *qi* and saliva using only a minimum of dietary supplements. This method is known as "eating *qi*" (*shiqi* 食氣) which involves the dedicated, disciplined practice of breathing exercises, which in turn become the bridge to the ultimate level of living on *qi* through the technique of "absorbing *qi*" (*fuqi* 服氣). The difference between the two is that eating *qi* replaces ordinary foodstuffs with refined foods, potent formulas, and breathing without essentially changing the body's respiratory and digestive systems. Absorbing *qi*, on the other hand, does away with food and herbs, shuts down the lungs and spleen, activates the kidneys and heart to a new level of yin-yang interchange, and thereby transforms the body's system to a primordial level that functions on a purely internal energy exchange (Jackowicz 2006, 78-79; see also Huang 2007, 59; 2008, 130-46)

In either practice, adepts inhale *qi* through the nose, then hold it in the mouth to form a mixture of breath and saliva. They rinse the mouth with it to gain a feeling of fullness, allowing the *qi* to envelope the tongue and teeth. Next, they consciously swallow it, visualizing the mixture as it moves through the torso into the inner organs. Once the *qi* is safely stored in its intended receptacle, they exhale. The more frequently they perform the practice, the more efficient it is; soon they can give up all solid foods.

Many medieval texts present these methods. The work partially translated here is the *Taiqing tiaoqi jing* 太清調氣經 (Great Clarity Scripture on Balancing *Qi*, DZ 820), probably of Tang origin, whose descriptions closely match those in other medieval sources, such as the *Jin'gui lu*, *Daoyin jing*, and *Yangxing yanming lu* included in this volume.[2]

Translation

Monthly Guidelines[3]

[1a] In the **first** month, kidney *qi* is susceptible to sickness, while lung *qi* wanes. It is best to reduce salty and sour flavors and increase spicy food. This will help the kidneys and supplement the lungs. To calm and nourish stom-

---

[2] On the text, see Lévi in Schipper and Verellen 2004, 369. Earlier translations appear in Huang and Wurmbrand 1987, 80-86, 96-98; Kohn 2010a, 150-58. Other texts that contain similar instructions include *Huanzhen xiansheng fu neiqi juefa* 幻真先生服內氣訣法 (Master Huanzhen's Essential Method of Absorbing Internal *Qi*, DZ 828, YJQQ 60.14a-25b); *Taiwu xiansheng fuqi fa* 太無先生服氣法 (Master Great Nonbeing's Method of *Qi*-Absorption, DZ 824; YJQQ 59.8b-10a); *Yanling jun lianqi fa* 延陵君煉氣法 (Lord Yanling's Method of *Qi*-Refinement, YJQQ 61.25a-26b); *Yanling xiansheng ji xinjiu fuqi jing* 延陵先生集新舊服氣經 (Master Yanling's Scripture Collecting Old and New [Methods of] Absorbing *Qi*, DZ 825). See Maspero 1981, 460-61; Kohn 2008, 118-21.

[3] *Sun zhenren sheyang lun* (DZ 841).

ach *qi*, moreover, do not expose yourself to cold and frost nor get extremely warm and heated. Rise and retire early to relax body and spirit.

In terms of diet, avoid raw leeks, since they diminish people's fluids and blood. Do not eat raw pepper, which may lead to chronic conditions and can cause the face to attract wind. Do not partake of hibernating animals: this reduces destiny. Nor should you eat the meat of wild beasts like tigers, panthers, and foxes. This causes agitation in people's spirit and souls.

The 4th day of this month is good for plucking out white hairs. The 7th day is good for quieting thoughts and contemplating perfection, and doing retreats to increase good fortune. On the 8th day, take baths but avoid long journeys.

In the **second** month, kidney *qi* fades, while liver *qi* becomes dominant. It is best to reduce sour flavors and increase salty food. This will help the kidneys and supplement the liver. It is also good to rest the diaphragm and eliminate potentially infectious liquids through frequent urination and perspiration. This serves to disperse the clustering *qi* of dark winter. [1b]

In terms of diet, avoid vegetables with yellow blossoms and those pickled in vinegar, since they cause chronic conditions. Do not take garlic, large or small, which may lead to *qi* obstructions and thus prevents openness in the joints and passes. Do not partake of mallows or chicken eggs, which may block people's blood and *qi*, dissipating essence. Nor should you eat the meat of wild beasts like rabbits, foxes, and badgers. This causes agitation in people's spirit and spirit souls.

The 8th day of this month is good for plucking out white hairs. On the 9th day avoid eating all kinds of fish—this is a great danger that all students of immortality avoid. The 14th day is not good for long journeys. Generally, moreover, to maintain proper *qi* in the season of spring, be moderate in your consumption of alcohol and keep your inner nature safe and secure.

In the **third** month, kidney *qi* is already at rest, while heart *qi* gradually approaches. Wood [liver] *qi* is in position of dominance. It is best to reduce sweet flavors and increase spicy food. This will support essence and increase *qi*-flow. Be careful to avoid westerly winds, since they tend to disperse the structure and make the body mellow. Rather, keep inner nature calm and at peace. Also, to go along with the Dao of Heaven, do not engage in killing or capital punishments.

In terms of diet, avoid vegetables with yellow blossoms. Do not eat raw mallows, since it tends to overextend people's *qi* and increases the chance of water pox. [2a] Do not eat pig's liver, since at this time the liver spirit is dominant. Do not partake of chicken eggs: they cause confusion which may last all your life.

The 3rd day of this month has a strong taboo against eating the five kinds of intestines and the hearts of the hundred vegetables. Eating them causes Heaven and Earth to be lost. The 6th day is good for taking baths. The 12th day is ideal for plucking out white hairs. On the 27th day avoid long journeys. However, it is a good day to do retreats and meditate on perfection.

In the **fourth** month, liver [*qi*] is still susceptible to sickness, while heart *qi* gradually grows stronger. It is best increase sour flavors and reduce bitter food. This will supplement the kidneys, help the liver, and balance stomach *qi*. Do not curse or expose yourself to the stars and lunar stations; avoid wind from the north and west, and do not eat garlic. Any of these will harm your spirit and spirit souls as well as diminish gall bladder *qi*.

In terms of diet, avoid raw scallions, since they cause people's tears and saliva to increase and phlegm to develop. Do not eat chicken in any form, since it may give rise to ulcers and tends to reverse primordial *qi*. Also, do not eat eel, which is generally bad for people.

The 4th day of this month is good for taking baths and plucking out white hairs. The 7th day is good for quieting thoughts, calming the mind in contemplation, and doing retreats. They will by necessity lead to good fortune and blessings. But make sure to avoid long journeys on this day. [2b]

In the **fifth** month, liver *qi* is at rest, while heart *qi* is dominant. It is best to reduce sour flavors and increase bitter food. This will enhance the liver and supplement the kidneys. It also stabilizes essence and softens *qi*. Get up and go to sleep early. When you pass water, make sure not to expose yourself to stars and lunar stations. Do not stay in humid places, since they attract disease-inducing *qi*.

In terms of diet, avoid leeks and scallions, since they cause chronic conditions by harming the spirit and diminishing *qi*. Do not eat raw garlic, which may lead to xxx and can cause the face to attract wind. Do not eat the meat of horses or any kind of game, since it causes agitation in people's spirit and *qi*.

The 5th day of this month is good for doing retreats and purifying meditation, but make sure to avoid looking at the blood of any living being and maintain a fast. The 16th day has a strong taboo against all kinds of desire and sexual activity. Violation will lead to an early death and cause major harm to the spirit. Also on this day, do not undertake long journeys. The 27th is good for taking baths and plucking out white hairs.

In the **sixth** month, liver *qi* wanes, while spleen *qi* dominates alone. It is best to reduce bitter flavors and increase salty food. Also, make sure to moderate the intake of rich and fatty foods. This supplements the liver and helps the kidneys as well as enhances muscles and bones. [3a]

Beyond this, be careful of east wind: its attack may cause paralysis in hands and feet. Do not wash your hands or feet in icy water and do not eat any mallows: either may cause water pox. In terms of diet, avoid dogwood, since it causes *qi* blockages.

The 6th day of this month is good for doing retreats and taking baths. It is also a good day for moving earth and undertaking construction. The 24th day is good for plucking out white hairs, but bad for long journeys. The 27th is good for taking baths, quieting thoughts, and the contemplation of perfection, as well as for undertaking all kinds of quiet and withdrawn activities.

In the **seventh** month, liver and heart *qi* are lessened, while lung [*qi*] is dominant. It is a good time for cultivating peace in emotions and inner nature. It is best to increase salty flavors and reduce spicy food. This helps the *qi* and supplements the muscles. It also nourishes the stomach and spleen. Do not expose yourself to extreme heat or indulge in ice and cold, yet try to avoid breaking into a great sweat.

In terms of diet, avoid dogwood, since it causes *qi* blockages. Do not eat any pork, as it may diminish spirit and *qi.* Also, in this month, do not think about evil affairs—this is a great taboo of the immortals.

The 5th day of this month is good for taking baths. The 7th day is good for cutting off all thoughts and doing retreats. The 9th day is good for repenting past deeds and offering prayers for new blessings. [3b] The 28th day is good for plucking out white hairs. On the 29th day avoid long journeys.

In the **eighth** month, heart *qi* wanes, while lung *qi* and metal become active. It is best to reduce bitter flavors and increase spicy food. This will help the muscles and supplements the blood. It also nourishes both heart and liver. Do not expose yourself to disease-inducing winds, lest your bones and flesh develop boils that may turn into persistent sores.

In terms of diet, avoid small garlic, since it harms people's spirit and *qi* and agitates spirit and spirit souls. Do not eat pigs' stomach, which may lead to bronchitis in the winter, potentially lasting the better part of the year without letting up. Also, do not eat chicken, since it diminishes spirit and *qi.*

The 4th day of this month is bad for trading animals that have hoofs or need to be shod. This is a great taboo of the immortals. The 18th day is good for doing retreats and sitting in meditation as well as other auspicious activities. It is a time when the celestials widely bestow success and good fortune. The 21st day is good for plucking out white hairs, but very bad for long journeys. If you go away on this day, you will not return. On the other hand, it is a good day for taking baths.

In the **ninth** month, yang *qi* has declined and yin *qi* is greatly empowered. Violent storms come frequently, so take care to avoid all invasive and disease-inducing winds. [4a] It is best to reduce bitter flavors and increase salty food. This will supplement the kidneys and enhance the liver. It also helps the spleen and assists the stomach. Do not expose yourself to wind and frost, and make sure not to indulge in intoxication and satiation.

In terms of diet, avoid leafy vegetables, since they may harbor worms you cannot see. Do not eat ginger and garlic, which diminish people's spirit and *qi*. Make sure not to have any vegetables grown in frost or any type of gourd, as they cause harm to people's hearts. And avoid all mallows, since they tend to promote water pox. Do not eat dog meat: it lessens the years and causes an early death.

The 9th day of this month is good doing retreats. The 16th day is good for taking baths and for plucking out white hairs. On the 27th day, avoid long journeys. It is called the day of enclosure.

In the **tenth** month, heart and lung *qi* are weak, while kidney *qi* gets stronger and abundant. It is best to reduce spicy and bitter flavors to nourish the kidneys and prevent harm to the muscles and bones. Do not puncture the skin and avoid vainly undergoing acupuncture and moxibustion, lest the blood stagnates and the fluids do not move.

In terms of diet, avoid raw peppers, since they diminish people's blood and arteries. Do not eat raw scallions, which may increase phlegm. Also, do not partake of bear meat or pork and stay away from leafy vegetables: all these may weaken your complexion. [4b]

The 1st day of this month is good for taking baths. On the 4th and 5th days, do not execute punishments. This is a great avoidance of the immortals. The 10th day is bad for long journeys. The 13th day is good for plucking out white hairs. The 15th day is good for doing retreats, sitting in meditation, and contemplating perfection. One will by necessity receive good fortune and blessings. On the 20th, by all means avoid long journeys.

In the **eleventh** month, kidney *qi* becomes dominant, while heart and lung *qi* wane. It is best to increase bitter flavors and cut out salty food. This will supplement and support lungs and stomach. At this time, do not apply moxa to belly or back, and make sure not to expose yourself to scorching heat in any form. Also, be very careful to avoid thieving and disease-inducing wind. Its attacks cause swellings in people's faces as well as potentially severe pain in hips and lower back.

In terms of diet, avoid the meat of badgers, since it harms people's spirit and spirit souls. Do not eat any snails, mussels, crabs, or turtles, which diminish primordial *qi* and increase intestinal worms. Do not partake of pickled vegetables grown over the summer, since they cause head wind and may enhance water pox. Stay away, moreover, from raw vegetables, since they may cause chest pains.

The 3rd day of this month is good for doing retreats and sitting in meditation. The 10th day is good for plucking out white hairs, but not good for long journeys. It is ideal to use the time to contemplate the good and the heavenly, thereby to attract good fortune and dispel disasters. The 16th day is good for taking baths. [5a]

In the **twelfth** month, earth [*qi*] is dominant, while water *qi* returns to being inactive. It is best to reduce sweet flavors and increase bitter food. This will supplement the heart and balance the kidneys. Do not expose yourself to frost and dew and avoid any strong leakage of body fluids or sweat.

In terms of diet, avoid mallows, since they may cause water pox. Do not eat raw scallions, which may lead to chronic conditions. Also stay away from turtles.

Herbal Supplements [4]

Pine Root: Take eastward growing pine root, peel it to remove the white skin, chop fine, fry, then pound it into a paste. Eat your fill and you can eliminate all grains. Should you be thirsty, just drink water.

China Root Fungus: Take China root fungus, scrape it to take off the black skin, then pound the branches and place them into an earthenware jar to soak in good-quality wine. Tightly seal the lid with dirt and keep the mixture buried for fifteen days. When you open it, the mixture should be firm like a cake. Cut it into lumps the size of chess pieces and take a day. You can also crumble it and take it in an inch-sized spoon. You will no longer feel hunger and thirst, be free from all diseases, and extend your years.

Take five pints of fungus branches, seven pounds of oily pine sap, five pounds of white wax, three pounds of white honey, two pints of Sichuan thyme, and steam them all together as if you were steaming a picul of grain. [5] When it is well cooked, take it out and form it into pills the size of cypress seeds. Take ten of them, gradually decreasing their number until you feel no more hunger. After ten days, you can limit yourself to one pill. Do not over-eat! But you can drink a little wine.

Atractylis: Take one picul properly cured atractylis, rinse and wash it, then pound it. Soak it overnight in two piculs of water, then boil it until the

---

[4] From *Taiqing jing duangu fa* (DZ 846).
[5] Measurements include: pints (*sheng* 升 = ab. 0.7 liters), pecks (*dou* 斗 = ab. 7 liters), pounds (*jin* 斤 = 597 grams), and piculs (*dan* 石 = 72 kilos).

liquid is reduced by half. Add five pints of clear wine and boil again. When
the mass is down to one picul, wring it out and remove the dregs. Next, simmer it over a low flame, adding two pints of soy branches and one pint of
asparagus root. Mix it all into pills the size of crossbow pellets. Take three in
the morning, once a day. Living in the mountains or on a long journey, you
can take them with you replace food. You will be able to withstand wind and
cold, extend your years, and be free from all diseases. This method was used
by Cui Yezi 崔野子.[6] Oh, and make sure to take the skin off the asparagus
root before adding it.

Yellow Essence: Take one picul of minced yellow essence and steam it
in two-and-a-half—or, alternatively, six—pints of water, simmering it all day.
When dusk arrives, it will be done. Once well-cooked, take it out and cool it.
With your hands, press it and make it into small pieces. Put them into a
wineskin to ferment, then extract the juice. Take the sediment and let it dry,
then put it into a pot and form it into pills the size of chicken eggs. Take one
pill three times a day. This will help you to eliminate grains, expel the hundred diseases, become light in body, stay vigorous, and avoid aging. Your
dosage should be regular, do not take more or stop in the middle of the
course. Should you be thirsty, just drink water. This method is of highest
excellence. It comes from the *Wufuxu* [2.21ab].

Jade Bamboo: Always pick the leaves in the 2nd or 9th months. Chop
them, then let them dry before curing and taking them. Use an inch-sized
spoon three times a day. You can also prepare the herb into cakes like you
would Yellow Essence. When you take it, guide its *qi* through the channels.
It strengthens muscles and bones, cures interior wind, heals tendons, knits
flesh, and will also smooth out wrinkles and create a good complexion.

Asparagus Root: Take three piculs of asparagus root, peel it and discard
the skin, then thoroughly soak it, pound and wring it until you extract one
picul of juice. On a small fire, simmer it down to about five pints of boiled
extract. Add one pint of white honey and two pints of steamed sesame
[*Wufuxu*: that has been boiled so it is fragrant and has a golden hue]. Stir the
mixture without resting, then make it into pills the size of soybeans or into
round crumb-cakes about three inches in diameter and a half inch thick.

---

[6] An immortal of the Six Dynasties, Cui has a biography in *Lishi zhenxian tidao
tongjian* 歷世真仙體道通鑒 (Comprehensive Mirror through the Ages of Perfected
Immortals and Those Who Embody the Dao, DZ 296), by Zhao Daoyi 趙道一 of
around the year 1300 (7.13b; see Lévi in Schipper and Verellen 2004, 99).

Take one piece a day. After one hundred days, you will no longer feel hungry, your skin and flesh will be moist and glossy, [*Wufuxu*: your white hair will return to black, lost teeth will re-grow, and you can extend your years]. You can also add three pints of Yellow Essence juice and cook it all together. This recipe is most excellent. It comes from the *Wufuxu* [2.30b-31a].

Sesame: Take any amount of fat black sesame, sift, clean, and steam it. Let the steam rise so it envelopes you completely. After a while take it out and dry it. Repeat this process nine times. It is best to do it three times per day and continue the procedure for three days to make a total of nine rounds. Dry the mixture, then place it in a mortar bowl, moistening it with a little hot water, and pound it until it becomes white. Again dry it and sift it to remove excess skins. Steam it once more until it becomes fragrant, then mash it under your hands to sift out coarse parts. Use two or three pints daily, as you see fit. You can also mix it with honey and form it into egg-sized pills. Take five of these daily. You can also mix it with sugar or dissolve the mixture in wine.

Gradually reduce the dose. After one hundred days, you will be free from disease. After one year, you will have a glossy complexion. After five years, you will be invulnerable to fire and water, and when you walk you will be as swift as a horse. The *Baopuzi* says: "This is not contained in the Jiangdong edition. The recipe was used by refuges at the disorder in the first year of the Yong'an reign period [in 264, at the end of the Three Kingdoms period]. I obtained and recorded it on 8/1 in Yongxing 2 [305 CE].[7]

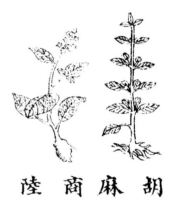

Fig. 12. Poke root and sesame

Assorted Grains: Mix one pound each of the following ingredients: non-glutinous rice, paniceled millet, buckwheat, sesame, and steamed soybeans; add one pound of white honey, fry it and soak it in cold water. Then make the mixture into pills the size of plum pits that you can swallow in one gulp. You will not be hungry to the end of your days. This comes from the *Wufuxu* [2.36a].

---

[7] This citation is not contained in the *Baopuzi* as transmitted today. See also Lévi in Schipper and Verellen 2004, 99.

Take one pint common millet and three pounds red stone fat [cinnabar], mix and soak them in water, then leave the compound in a warm place for two or three days until a coat forms on top. Next, pound it into pills the size of plum pits and take three per day. You will no longer feel hungry. Should you be thirsty, just drink water. You will also be able to walk as far as a thousand *li* without getting tired. This comes from the *Wufuxu* [2.35a].

Direct Internal Preservation: Take three pints of very fresh bean sprouts, place them in your hands, then visualize a radiance spreading through your body, warm and beautiful. Eat the sprouts, swallowing them quickly so they can be ingested. After fifty to a hundred days, you will not feel hungry any longer. Should you be thirsty, just drink water. Make sure not to overeat; rather, keep reducing the amounts.

To take two pints of steamed bean porridge, use the following method: eat time first face the sun and bow repeatedly, then swallow one pint at a time. Revolve each mouthful around the mouth, then swallow it. Repeat this process three times on the first day. On the next day, split one pint into three portions. Children should use half the amount.

To Return to Eating Grains and Stop Taking Herbal Formulas: While taking herbal formulas for internal preservation or after eliminating grains, do not take any extraneous items. Should you be thirsty, just drink little sips of cold water. If you wish to give up the diet and return to eating grains, first take a decoction from mallow seeds and lesser formulas, then you can start eating again. Begin by taking one serving of thin rice porridge three times a day. After two more days, take two servings, increasing the amount to five servings after three more days, then seven servings after yet another three days, and finally to one pint after three more days. Continue like this for one month and you will be ready to eat ordinary food.

Mallow Seed Decoction: Take one pint mallow seeds and one pound pork fat. Boil in five pecks of water until the liquid is reduced to two pints. Remove the sediments and take it very, very slowly. Feel it sink down to fill [the belly], then stop. You can also mix it with rice to make thin porridge. It is also excellent if drunk with Sichuan thyme.

Giving Up Ordinary Food [8]

[9b] To live on *qi*, it is best to work after you wake up from sleep, right from around midnight to the fifth watch [3-5 a.m.]. Balance the breath, inhaling and exhaling in proper measure and with due attention to the breathing rhythm.

Rinse your mouth with the numinous fluid [saliva], then lie down on your back, make your hands into fists, and block [the *qi* opening at] the soles of the feet. [10a] Support your head with a pillow and breathe, keeping your mind stable and following the movement of the breath without interruption as it comes in and goes out, passing through gate [nose] and doorway [mouth]. Then close the mouth firmly and become aware of the internal *qi*, pulling it up carefully into the mouth. Softly drum [the belly] and swallow it down, using your intention to guide it or using your hands to rub it from above the heart to the lower belly. Then again balance the breath six or seven times before you proceed to swallow it once more, as before using your hands to guide it by rubbing [along the front of the torso]. Stop when you have completed twenty rounds of *qi*-work in this manner.

During daylight hours, again find suitable times to sit or lie down and rest in perfect calm and serenity. Practice the swallowing for at least ten rounds. Make sure to balance the breath in between each swallowing, breathing steadily forty to fifty times, then swallowing slowly and carefully. Even if you are not busy at all, do not do all the swallowings at the same time. Also, make sure each time to use your hands to rub the front of the torso, guiding the *qi* downward while also using your intention to send it on its way. Then examine yourself. If the Upper Heater is open, the *qi* will move easily below the navel. If not, the *qi* will stay in the chest and heart area.

Pay particular attention to meal times and see whether the upper torso feels empty and if there is a feeling of flow below. If this is the case, the *qi* is flowing freely. [10b] Then you can go ahead and eat. However, do not eat if you are not in fact hungry, and when you do eat, do not fill up completely, since fullness hinders *qi*-absorption. After the meal, wait until the area between heart and belly feel slightly empty, then again absorb your *qi* by practicing a set of twenty swallowings. Do the same at the evening meal. Every day repeat this process around the same time, regardless of whether you are

---

[8] *Taiqing tiaoqi jing* (DZ 820), 9b-14b and 22b-22b. Subheadings added by the translator.

walking, standing, sitting, or lying down. Complete a hundred days like this. Always remember: Every time you swallow *qi*, use your hands to disperse it and practice at least ten balanced breaths in between. This will maximize the effect.

Levels and Precautions: In the beginning it is common that the Triple Heater is not quite clear and the various passes are not open. As long as that is the case, obstructions are common and you won't be able to take in much *qi*. Increase your practice by three times five swallowings every ten days until the first hundred days have passed. After 150 days, again increase by four times five swallowings, until you reach 200 swallowings in a day. Once you have done the practice for a whole year, the *qi* will easily flow, passes and joints will be open, your skin and flesh will be moist and glossy, and your hair pores will be free and clear.

Having reached this level, you just need to wait until your stomach feels empty, then do three times five swallowings as appropriate. You may do them successively, without balancing the breath in between, and there is no more need for adhering to a rigorous daily schedule. [11a] Just do not overdo it: no more than 300 swallowings a day.

After three years of practice, the *qi* will flow freely all around, completely pervading the entire body. Your five organs will be well nurtured, your bones solid, your marrow full, and your skin glossy and rich. At this point, there is no more limit to the number of swallowings, and you should be able to eliminate grains with ease.

Should you go into fasting before the three years are up, you will suffer from the five exertions and seven injuries,[9] reducing the potency of your inner organs and causing the hundred joints to dry up and wither. The process will not work unless you cultivate the *qi* very gradually and never give in to the temptation of cutting out grains abruptly to quickly attain long life. It also won't work unless you eliminate all thoughts of involvement in worldly schemes, of satisfying the six senses, and of going after wealth and sensual pleasures.

Also, if you give in to a hungry stomach, letting go of grains only reluctantly and without sufficient supplementary formulas, you will cause new ailments to arise and the myriad diseases to assemble. If your thoughts and desires do not die, how can you ever reach attainment?

Another point is that, after practicing *qi*-absorption, you need to make sure you know how to eat properly. Every day at breakfast, eat a little unflavored watery porridge to balance the spleen-*qi* and provide sufficient fluids

---

[9] These are listed in the *Yangxing yanming lu* (2.3a). See below, ch. 8.

to last you through the day. At noon, eat one or two unflavored slices of bread and maybe some broth that contains onions or scallions. [11b] Do not eat them hot, though. If you are hungry in the evening, take a few unflavored dumplings that you have boiled for twenty or thirty minutes. Again, make sure not to eat to fullness but three to five mouthfuls less. It is best always to leave the table with a feeling of slight emptiness in the stomach.

If you fill up in one batch, the passage of *qi* is blocked and it cannot flow, wasting a whole day's work. To prevent this, also avoid all greasy, fatty, and sticky foods as well as raw vegetables, root plants, and anything old, stale, smelly, or suchlike. Also, never take anything that has turbid *qi* [slaughtered and killed].

In the first thirty to fifty days, it is unavoidable to have occasional twinges of hunger. If you catch yourself thinking of food, immediately balance the breath and practice the *qi* method, then gradually your belly will feel rich and moist and you won't be tempted to think of the hundred flavors.

When we speak of taking porridge, bread, or dumplings, in all cases eat them in accordance with your schedule and convenience. There is no need to rely on a specific daily regimen of eating, but for the most part your order of food intake should follow the above outline. Establish your own schedule and rhythm and take mostly unflavored watery porridge with little bits of boiled rice here and there. This will be most excellent. [12a]

Once you have begun to successfully ingest *qi*, your Triple Heater will be clear, the stomach apertures will be open, and the five organs will be in perfect harmony. Then sweet saliva arises and the Jade Pond will be luscious. At this point any food you take will taste delicious, just like to a person just recovering from illness. The tendency at this point is to get greedy and no longer know when it is enough: it all just tastes so *good*! Curb this urge. If you give in to it, great harm will come. So, initially you must pay great attention to the times and amounts you eat.

Now, every time you eat, you are bound to ingest some toxins as well as excess heat from the five flavors. For this reason, after every meal open your mouth wide and exhale with the *he* breath. This will lessen the hot *qi* in the mouth and prevent future afflictions. Also make sure to limit your intake of salty, spicy, sour, and other strong flavors. In fact, it is best to avoid them altogether. This may be hard in the beginning, but not for long. Within even ten to twenty days, you will notice a numinous spring of sweet fluid gushing forth, which would not happen if you ate salty or spicy foods. Practicing *qi*-absorption, you will further find that your five organs are juicy and full and that your proper *qi* sinks down to chase out any bad energies, which duly leave through the lower orifices.

To avoid harm to the already purified stomach area, you should also not eat anything sticky or greasy nor anything raw or hard. [12b] Should you inadvertently take a mouthful of such a substance, you will feel a slight pain wherever the morsel comes to rest in your system. With continued effort and a deeper awareness of your inner workings, you will realize this naturally.

To sum up: Eat only soft and well-cooked food. That is most excellent. And after every meal always exhale with *he*.

Supplements: Each time you eat rice, first swallow twenty or thirty raw peppercorns with some water. Only then eat the rice. Should you feel pain or fullness after a meal, you can take ten additional peppercorns. The pepper will move the Triple Heater activity downward and chase out all sorts of bad *qi*. It will also dissolve any food remnants left behind in the intestines.

Similarly, you should take two or three peppercorns if you feel a sense of dense and cloying [depressed] *qi* in the heart and chest area during your guiding of proper *qi*. They will in due course dissolve this feeling. The benefits of simple peppercorns are truly beyond words.

Another way to deal with bouts of fullness, a cloying feeling, or a sense of *qi* stagnation is to practice quiet-sitting and balancing the breath. The feeling will disperse quickly and the *qi* will leave through the lower orifices.

Some old texts say that one should stabilize the *qi* and not allow it to leave. In the old days when people first practiced, they accordingly stabilized the *qi*, holding on to it as much as possible. [13a] However, after a short period of time, they would feel a tension in their bellies, be beset by worries, and imagine themselves dying. The two lower orifices directly connect to the nose and mouth above. Thus, when there is stale or bad *qi* in the five organs, it must sink down to leave. Why should one stabilize and hold on to it?

Stabilizing the *qi* prevents it from flowing freely and leaving the body. If it does not flow freely and is prevented from leaving, pain results. This is so because, when the stale *qi* has not yet left and fresh *qi* suddenly enters, the two *qi* clash with each other and create discomfort. If is thus not necessary [or advisable] to stabilize the *qi*. Much better to have it flow freely and leave properly.

Also, every day try to drink one or two cups of liquor on an empty stomach, as your disposition allows. This is really good. But make sure that you do not get to the point of getting intoxicated or maudlin. It is even better if you can slowly sip three to five cups of liquor every day, greatly aiding your *qi*-work. In all cases, the liquor should be clear and of good quality.

When you first start taking it, don't drink more than one mouthful. Be prepared for the *qi* to be unsettled for a few days.[10]

On another note, if something delightful happens to you and you wish to celebrate by drinking, you can also do so, using the method described below. The reason why ordinary people get intoxicated or maudlin when they drink liquor is that it is usually made toxic by fermenting yeast and when that toxic *qi* enters the four limbs, there is intoxication. [13b]

To drink properly, do the following: When you sit with five or ten people and the cup gets passed around, reaching you every so often, drink when your turn comes and every time afterward open your mouth and exhale with *he* seven or eight times. This way the liquor's toxin will be expelled and dispersed. Should more than one cup arrive at your place at the same time, open your mouth very wide and exhale with *he*, but if there is only one cup at a time, be subtle about it.

Generally, whenever you exhale, accompany the leaving breath with a subtle *he*. Like this you can make it through a whole banquet without stopping your practice of balancing the breath. Even better: If you can usually drink three pints, that day you can stomach ten, yet without getting inebriated and without losing the good taste of the liquor throughout the evening. Even if you drank for a whole day, the taste would not diminish. Eventually you will go to sleep, and after you wake up you swallow the *qi* and balance the breath again as described above.

Social Situations: On another note, there may be a sudden burst of *qi* leaving the body through the lower orifices at an unexpected time, such as during a meal, when with an invited guest, while riding on horseback, or when with honored relatives. So, if the *qi* comes then, what to do? You must find a suitable way to let it escape. If you keep it tight and fail to let it leave, [14a] it will reverse its course and move back into the intestines where it will cause stomach pain and irritate the heart and chest area. If not dispersed over a long period, even one colonful of contained *qi* can cause confusion, depression, and pain.

Should you, due to public or private affairs, have no time to undertake longevity practice, make sure to at least avoid meat and the five strong vegetables. Then, even if *qi* leaves through the lower orifices, it will not be very smelly. Once you have started the practice of avoiding grain, on the other hand, whether there is one instance of flatulence or more, the escaping *qi* will be entirely without odor.

---

[10] Huang and Wurmbrand interpret this to mean nausea, followed by a purging of the system through vomiting (1987, 84).

Also, make sure to avoid any contact with birth, dirt, pollution, and various forms of serious illness. They all massively reduce proper *qi*. Should you walk along a public street and unexpectedly encounter any form of such bad *qi*, immediately enclose the *qi* [by holding your breath] and pass by quickly. Should this be impossible, drink a bit of clear liquor or have a small bite of meat or a strong vegetable. This will create a block. Should you have actually taken in some bad *qi* and begin to feel restless and ill at ease, practice balancing the breath to expel it.

Another precaution: Do not shout out loud, sing, cry, or wail. If in your social life you cannot avoid a situation of mourning, make some small appropriate noises but do not cry excessively. [14b] Should you feel the *qi* move upward and create a lump in your throat, do not repress it but let it rise up to a certain point, then swallow it back down. Once it has reached the belly, again take in fresh *qi* and swallow it. Repeat this three or five times. This will help you settle down. You can also help it disperse by rubbing the front of your torso down with your hands.

Taking a bit of pepper and some liquor will completely relieve the situation. However, if you are it by a sudden sob that you cannot move down, then do not force yourself to swallow. This would only cause an obstruction in the Upper Heater. Rather, breathe slowly and with conscious intention, then examine yourself. If the *qi* has not yet dispersed, do not eat, since any eating or sense of fullness will prevent you from doing a proper swallowing. Eat only after you have swallowed a few times. Otherwise, you are inviting disease.

Also, at each swallowing hold the breath and block the nose. When inhalation and exhalation are regular, use the intention to send the *qi* outward. Then watch it on the inside. It moves down the left side of the torso, along twenty-four notches. As it descends one notch at a time, you can hear it like water dripping, clear and rhythmical. If there is no sound it is because you ate something oily or heavy or did not follow the proper procedure. If it does not dissolve soon and you work more with your *qi*, it will create internal pressure and lead to disease. [15a] Be very careful! . . .

Giving up Ordinary Food: [21b] If you want to fast for a period, just use the [breathing and swallowing] method spelled out earlier. After three years, your five organs will be well nurtured, your bones will be solid and your flesh full. The hundred spirits return and maintain residence, your blood arteries are open to free flow, your *qi* passageways are loose and wide, and your various body energies circulate smoothly without obstruction. You will feel light and completely renewed every day.

Once you reach this point, you naturally find yourself having less and less desire to smell the aroma of the five flavors and hardly ever think about food. It will be not difficult at all to stop eating altogether. [22a]

Worldly people tend to be greedy for pleasure and love profit. They cannot stop their thoughts and widely search through recipe books for formulas to take for grain abstention. When such herbal concoctions first enter the stomach, they do in fact create a feeling of fullness for a period of time. However, once their effect is exhausted, hunger will come back with a vengeance. This creates a vicious circle without end.

In addition, this tendency constantly keeps the mind involved with thoughts of formulas and the quest for apparent harmony in daily affairs. Moving to and fro, forever restless, such people do not have even a moment's rest. Their strength feeble, their thoughts drained, they continuously increase troubles and vexations and don't even need to invite misfortune to arrive. Also, even though they take various concoctions and things, how can they suddenly eliminate eating? So, some will suck on fruit pits to increase vigor while others ingest more complex concoctions to simulate fullness.

In fact, all you need to do is increase your breath-balancing practice, keep yourself well, and nurture peaceful thoughts. The exhausting toil of chasing after the right formulas, the demeaning effort of refining various concoctions—they all strain people for months and years and uselessly labor essence and spirit. How can they ever attain the reversal of aging and a return to youth? If you just don't eat rice, how can you call it "giving up food"?

Indeed, there are lower-level practitioners who can't even live without grains and still work in the world by taking herbal formulas to supplement their system. Yes, they will gain some minor benefits. But higher-level practitioners do not do anything like this. [22b] They just take in *qi* over long periods and as they perfect their practice, they come to fast naturally. Sensing that their stomachs are empty, they just swallow *qi*. Never worried whether early or late, they have no obstructions or hindrances. Swallowing whenever they feel the need, they have no limits or boundaries. They become naturally aware of their proper rhythm and timing and won't even need lots of practice sessions anymore. As they absorb their *qi* like this for a long time, they naturally reach the stage of eliminating eating. They thereby attain complete self-liberation and freedom from vexations in all they do.

To sum up: In the beginning stages of practice, if you want to take some herbal formulas to supplement your *qi*-absorption, by all means do so. However, the tendency is that those who get into taking the supplements often do not practice *qi*-absorption and make the quest for, and ingestion of, herbs their main objective.

Chapter Seven

The Gods over Your Shoulder

The Tang dynasty (618-907) has often been called the heyday of Chinese civilization. It established the first stable rule after many centuries of division and violent unification under the Sui, and much of its culture was dedicated to unification and integration. This was obvious not only in the political realm but also in the world of thought and religion, leading to integrated organizational structures and worldview systems, such as the Three Caverns that organized the Daoist priestly hierarchy and the various encyclopedias that described Daoist thought.[1]

The longevity tradition was no exception. Its greatest organizer was Sun Simiao 孫思邈.[2] Born near Chang'an in 581, he was a precocious child and easily acquired an extensive knowledge of the classics and philosophers as well as of Buddhist and Daoist scriptures. Since he suffered from various ailments he also developed a strong interest in medical matters. As an adult, he trained in classical Chinese medicine, then traveled widely to collect ancient books and recipes all over the country. He was also ordained as a Daoist of the Celestial Masters, the lowest level of the Three Caverns. Between 605 and 615, he engaged in various alchemical experiments to find the elixir of immorality. His main activities as a healer date from 616 to 626, and it seems that he turned to writing in the following decades. In 659, having become quite famous as a physician and master of long life, he joined the retinue of

---

[1] On Daoist organization under the Tang, see Barrett 1996; Kohn and Kirkland 2000. The main encyclopedias are the *Sandong zhunang* 三洞珠囊 (A Bag of Pearls from the Three Caverns, DZ 1139; see Reiter 1990) and the *Daojiao yishu* 道教義樞 (The Pivotal Meaning of the Daoist Teaching, DZ 1129; see Wang 2001).

[2] Details of Sun's life are outlined in Sivin 1968, 82-96; Engelhardt 1989, 266; Sakade 1992, 2; Kohn 2008, 129-33.

Emperor Gaozong in an informal capacity. After about fifteen years, he requested permission to retire from the court on account of illness and presumably died in 682. Today he is widely venerated as the King of Medicines (Yaowang 樂土). His most important writings are in the medical field, especially his *Qianjin fang* 千金方 (Prescriptions Worth a Thousand [Ounces of] Gold) series: extensive collections of detailed medical information that date from the 650s and are still actively used by physicians in China today.[3]

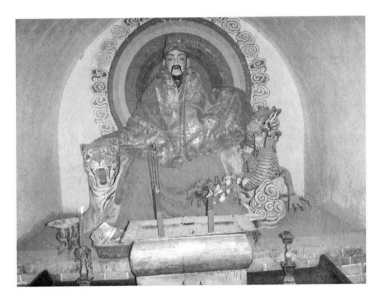

Fig. 13. Sun Simiao as God of Medicines

Several other extant works deal specifically with long life. Besides the *Sheyang lun* on monthly dietary recommendations translated above (ch. 6), Sun is credited with two brief general outlines on how to best live one's life: the *Fushou lun* 福壽論 (On Happiness and Long Life, DZ 1426), a presentation of the workings of destiny and various ways to enhance it; and the *Baosheng ming* 保生銘 (On Preserving Life, DZ 835), a concise treatise extolling moderation, a regular life-style, and virtuous attitudes. He is also the author of a concise overview of longevity methods, the *Sheyang zhenzhong*

---

[3] For more on these texts, see Despeux 1987. The *Qianjin yaofang* is contained in the Daoist canon (DZ 1162, 1163). See Despeux in Schipper and Verellen 2004, 339-40.

fang 孫真人枕中方 (Pillowbook of Methods for Nourishing Life, YJQQ 33, DZ 837).[4]

While the texts recoup much found in earlier sources, they present several themes that are new in longevity literature: destiny as defined as one's proper lot; personal ethics and appropriate conduct in daily life; and behavior as monitored by officials in the otherworldly hierarchy.

According to this understanding, long life is a direct function of the genetic make-up and talents one brings into this world, described as inner nature (*xing* 性), in combination with the physical strength, social circumstances, and overall situation in life one receives from Heaven, defined as destiny (*ming* 命). While inner nature manifests in one's principle (*li* 理), the "inner beacon" that guides one's direction, destiny appears concretely in one's lot (*fen* 分), the chances and opportunities one has in life. This terminology picks up concepts first outlined in the *Zhuangzi* and specified in detail by its commentator Guo Xiang 郭象 (d. 312). He defines lot as the share one has in Dao which manifests in inner nature, while principle is the overall structuring factor of life, described in terms of destiny.[5]

Inner nature, says Guo Xiang, "is what people rely on spontaneously without ever being conscious of it" (DZ 745, 2.35b). It is the way people are naturally, their inherent psychological makeup, which is entirely independent of knowledge or consciousness. It has nothing to do with people's subjective wishes or concrete hopes, but is there and cannot be changed. Obtained at birth, any enforced change of inner nature must result in suffering, as much as any development along its lines will be to the good. In a sense, inner nature is therefore very restricting, very limiting; this should be so because it represents the individual's participation in Dao. Everyone has a natural intuitive sense of what is good and bad in a particular situation. But people have for generations distorted their inner natures, their feeling and idea of themselves. Therefore they continue to strive for things that are not appropriate for them.

Destiny, on the other hand, is parallel to principle; it is the life that one is ordered or destined to have by heaven. "That which one is given is one's destiny," Guo Xiang says (4.11a). Destiny is there to be accepted, not to be

---

[4] The *Fushou lun* is probably the same as the *Fulu lun* 福錄論 (On Happiness and Prosperity), ascribed to Sun in the early bibliographies. Its full title is *Tang Taigu Miaoying Sun zhenren Fushou lun* 唐太古妙應孫真人福壽論 (Treatise on Happiness and Long Life by the Perfected Sun Miaoying of Great Antiquity of the Tang. See Despeux in Schipper and Verellen 2004, 743; Sivin 1968, 132.

[5] On Guo Xiang and his understanding of share and destiny, see Robinet 1983; Knaul 1985a; 1985b; Kohn 1992, 70-80.

changed. It orders human existence in exactly the same way that principle structures the universe. It determines every individual's birth, age, opportunities, chances—all the outer circumstances of his or her life. Destiny means the concrete conditions of life; inner nature means the basic psychological character of the individual. Respectively representing nurture and nature, destiny and inner nature are together responsible for the development of the individual's life. Both should be fulfilled, not counteracted. The more one works along with one's destiny and stays within one's lot, the better one realizes oneself, and the more contentment, happiness, and perfection one experiences. The more one tries to avoid it, the harsher the realities of life appear (Kohn 1992, 72).

Sun Simiao strongly agrees with this outlook, but defines the parameters slightly differently. Where Guo Xiang sees lot and principle as the dominant cosmic factors and looks upon inner nature and destiny as their manifestation in human life, Sun reverses this pattern and places inner nature and destiny on the more cosmic level while lot and principle are what people face in concrete reality. He also reverses the connections: instead of linking inner nature with lot and destiny with principle, he connects inner nature with principle—the beacon that shines within and guides the person from the inside-out—and destiny with lot—the specific role one comes to play in one's social and economic setting, one's determination of goals and success from the outside-in. Sun's system has remained standard: the concepts of inner nature and destiny, expanded to indicate the psychological and physical determinants of the individual, became dominant in internal alchemy and have remained so until today.

According to Sun Simiao it is impossible to attain long life unless one stays within the boundaries of one's lot and avoids violating it. Health is one among various functions of happiness and good fortune—*fu* 福, the same word in Chinese—which in turn are directly related to karma and depend on the good and bad deeds one performs in life. Violations of one's lot, moreover, mean moral transgressions and acts that hurt others, which leads to his other main point, the observation of major precepts (such as against killing, stealing, cheating, and sexual misconduct) as well as of various taboos that bring life into cohesion with the flow of cosmic energy. Any acts committed on this earth, moreover, are closely monitored by the gods of the otherworldly administration who keep detailed records and adjust one's health, fortune, and life expectancy—destiny—accordingly.

Ever since the Shang dynasty, the Chinese have conceived of their supernatural world in bureaucratic terms. First there was just an "elaborate hierarchy of ancestors, each with his specific jurisdiction" (Shahar and

Weller 1996, 4), later various celestial administrators, such as the Ruler of Destiny, already mentioned in the *Shujing* 書經 (Book of History), kept "a record of the moral behavior of men and bestowed upon them either a long or a short life" (Eberhard 1971, 179; Yü 1987, 383). Although assumed originally to have been patterned on bureaucratic structures in the real world, the otherworldly administration is now understood as the foremost expression of a basic religious model which helped to create "an ordering control over the world" (Shahar and Weller 1996, 8). Administrators and their offices are predictable and reliable; bound by intricate rules, they can yet be circumvented, bribed, or tricked if only one understands their nature and that of the rules they follow (Campany 2005). As a result, both cosmic and personal crises can be dealt with efficiently, giving people a large measure of control over their lives and nature (Keightley 1978, 224).

By the early middle ages, the celestial administration had extended its reach to include agents deep within the individual person, notably the Three Deathbringers who regularly report people's deeds to the Department of Destiny. Human beings had also figured out the exact amounts that would be added to or detracted from their life expectancy. As the *Baopuzi* says, "For more important misdeeds, 300 days are deducted from our lives. For lesser sins, three days are taken off" (Ware 1966, 115-16). The *Chisongzi zhongjie jing* 赤松子中戒經 (Essential Precepts of Master Redpine, DZ 185) of the 4th century describes human life energy as contained in a "perfected talisman of Great Unity" (*taiyi zhenfu* 太一真符), a smidgen of pure starry essence the Ruler of Destiny places on people's foreheads. The essence then changes in accordance with the subtractions made by the gods:

> If they subtract one year, the star [essence] on the person's head becomes lackluster and he or she runs into lots of difficulties. If they take off ten years, the star begins to fade and the person encounters disasters and disease. If they subtract twenty years, the star is extinguished and the person runs into legal trouble and is imprisoned. If they make a deduction of thirty years, the star dissolves and the person dies. (2ab; Kohn 1998, 841)

The text then lists specific numbers of good and bad deeds as registered in the otherworldly ledgers and the consequences one can expect on earth. For example, bad deeds have the following results:[6]

---

[6] *Chisongzi zhongjie jing* 5ab. Similar lists appear also in Tang literature, notably in the *Yaoxiu keyi* 要修科儀 (Essential Rules and Observances, DZ 463), 12.11b-12a, 12.10a-11a; and Du Guangting's 杜光庭 (850-933) *Yongcheng jixian lu* 墉城集仙錄 (Record of the Assembled Immortals in the Heavenly Walled City, DZ 783), 1.4a-6a. More specific lists for Daoist monastics are found in the *Fengdao kejie* 奉道科戒

1	intention not calm and at peace
10	energy and strength hollow and declining
20	body afflicted by much sickness and disease
30	nothing planned comes to pass
40	constant difficulties, facing decay and destruction
50	never finding equal partner
60	line of descendants dies out
70	harmed by yin demons
80	disasters of water and fire, being burnt and drowned
90	poor and cold, in distress and weak, hungry and going mad
100	harmed by energy of heaven, affairs bad, prison, execution
200	harmed by energy of earth, robbed and stripped by brigands
300	descendants humble and common
400	descendants poor and lowly, destitute and begging
500	descendants cut off family line
600	descendants blind and deaf, mute and mad
700	descendants rebels, unfilial and criminal
800	family has ministers and unfilial sons, cause destruction and beheadings to entire clan
900	family has demonic and evil people, cause destruction to their own and other clans
1000	descendants malformed and crooked, looking like maimed animals or wild birds

This thinking strongly informed Sun's understanding of the celestial administration and its impact on human life and health, making the celestial connection and the proper observance of one's lot a key point in his presentation. In addition, he also emphasizes that it is best to live in moderation, stay away from dangers, avoid all stressful speech and thought, balance the five flavors, and observe the taboos of sun, moon, and the four seasons. By living calmly and in harmony, *qi* and spirit remain within the body and one can live in health and happiness for extended years. He spells out further details on how best to align oneself with the rhythm of Dao in physical and breathing practices and by matching one's food to the seasons—all themes that recoup earlier longevity sources.

(Rules and Precepts for Worshiping the Dao, DZ 1125; trl Kohn 2004c). For a study of this quantification of fate, see Kohn 1998.

Translation

Happiness and Long Life [7]

[1a] Sages embody Dao and never act intentionally.
The wise know what causes misfortune and never cheat.
Achievers divine destiny and never pursue anything.
Believers protect their faith and maintain themselves in stillness.
Carers maintain benevolence and are modest and respectful.
Literati are diligent about their scholarship and rest at ease in reverence.
Ordinary folk obscure cosmic principle and act illicitly and wrongly.
Dummies hold on to their stupidity and never dread anything.
Petty people go against Dao and forever keep acting intentionally.

Happiness [good fortune] comes from the accumulation of bringing forth goodness. Unhappiness [misfortune] comes from the accumulation of bringing forth no good. Demons and spirits cannot cause misfortune for people; nor can they deliver happiness and good fortune. It is only when people accumulate a lot of no good that they ruin their destiny.

In wealth and honor, high-handed grabbing leads to violating your lot. In poverty and low status, sneaky stealing leads to violating your lot. The gods keep a close record—people just don't realize it! [1b] The divine ledgers, moreover, create consequences in the otherworldly ledgers, [leading to early death]. On the other hand, if people's principles and internal beacon are upright and they die, it is because their allotted destiny is used up.

The poor often live longer; the rich often die young. The poor living longer is because in their state of poverty, destitution, and continuous hardship they never have enough and thus give the celestial administrators no reason to punish them. The rich dying young is because they go after things aggressively and indulge in luxury and excess, thus getting their destiny cut short. In other words, Heaven tends to diminish excess and supplement insufficiency. [2a]

There are also those poor and destitute, hungry and cold, exposed and naked, their corpses without proper burial. They are people whose heart is not auspicious. They lack in virtue, thus they are poor; they lack in heart, thus they die. Heaven didn't do anything to kill them—they themselves brought about their violent death. They cannot live in harmony with others,

---

[7] *Tang Taigu Miaoying Sun zhenren Fushou lun* (DZ 1426).

appreciate the protection and support of Heaven and Earth, or honor the light and presence of the sun and the moon. [1b] Just as the *Huangting nei-jing jing* says: "Human beings have over 10,000 gods that reside in their bodies." The Three Deathbringers, Nine Worms, Lads of Good and Evil all keep records and file reports, continuously feeding information into the underworld ledgers.

In dummies and crazy people, the body gods are insufficient; in sages and enlightened ones, they are in excess. They cannot use one or two faults and take time off people's destiny, but if their inherent dignity is vilified or slandered, if they see violence, censure, and degradation, they can delete people's names from the ledgers [of life]. Thus, if people are afflicted with a serious disease, it is largely because their principles and internal beacon are out of synch with the divine law. If their principles and internal beacon are not upright, yet they don't die, this is because there is still some destined longevity left and has not yet been exhausted. Still, they are not worthy of being called human.

They violate their lot when it comes to rank and office, carriages and horses, wives and concubines, property and real estate, [farming] grain and silk, trade and business—the gods recording each and every instance. They continue this behavior for three, five, ten, even twenty years, never stopping their excesses. In due course, the gods pursue them and they die. [2b]

Violating one's lot in rank and office means that one sits in state like on a high peak, always taking gifts and bribes. Feeble in virtue and clinging to their position, people like these aggressively pursue [gain] and abscond with the funds. As they continue to pursue their aggressive acquisition, they inevitably become hard. Once they are hard, they violate their lot. Soon they are beleaguered by disasters, diseases, and death. The gods keep a close record—people just don't realize it!

Violating one's lot with regard to carriages and horses means buying horses at bargain prices, then wanting then to excel. People like these feed and water their horses at irregular intervals, whip and beat them without constraint, make them run and gallop without pause, never acknowledging that they might be exhausted from all that urging and racing nor understanding that they are weary after having run near and far. The gods keep a close record—people just don't realize it!

Violating one's lot in terms of wives and concubines means that one engages in many love relationships with extensive expenditure and involvement. The path to lasciviousness and debauchery inevitably leads to pride and dissipation. Excessively decked out in gold and kingfisher blue, abundantly covered in fragrant ointments, they nastily belittle the patterns and colors [of other's clothes] and continuously overindulge in jewels and delicacies. When others do it, it's wrong; when I myself do it, it's fine. When others do it, it's tough; when I myself do it, it's fun. The gods keep a close record—people just don't realize it! [3a]

Violating one's lot with regard to maids and servants means treating what is good as worthless and what is right as wrong. People like these have no sympathy when their servants suffer and never allow them to enjoy themselves. They whip and flog them, never asking how submissive and downtrodden they already are; they insult and shame them, never asking whether they are close or distant. Of all these instances of violating one's lot the gods keep a close record—people just don't realize it!

Violating one's lot in terms of property and real estate means that one continuously builds spacious mansions, always trying to push the price down and punishing the workmen. People like these use illegally acquired wealth to forever repair and remodel their homes. The work has to be outstanding; the decorations have to be splendid. At the same time, chisels and hammers drain their strength; wood and stone labor their spirit. They do not realize the inherent poverty of their walled compounds, the inherent baseness of their luscious dwellings. Of all these instances of violating one's lot the gods keep a close record—people just don't realize it!

Violating one's lot when engaged in [farming] grain and silk means that one rushes planting and delays harvesting. People like these exhaust their workers and burden their supporters, just to pile up their hoardings in gigantic granaries. Toiling excessively year after year, they fill up their thieves' dens like birds feathering their nests and rats filling their burrows, until their warehouses and estates are overburdened with debt and they sink into deep oppression. Of all these instances of violating one's lot the gods keep a close record—people just don't realize it! [3b]

Violating one's lot when it comes to clothes and adornments[8] means that one owns tons of clothes in all kinds of colors and designs yet, despite this overflow, continues to have new ones made. People like these have trunks and wardrobes without limits so that poverty and cold never reach them. They never consider the shame of being naked and exposed, the possibility that one may not have enough cloth and silk. Quite like worms, fish, and rats, their mouths feed on blue-black decay and rot. Of all these instances of violating one's lot the gods keep a close record—people just don't realize it!

---

[8] Reading *shi* 飾 (adornments) for *shi* 食 (food).

Violating one's lot with regard to food and drink means that one gets to eat and is ready to go anywhere on land and water, gets to drink and is ready to break into music and song. People like these try to reduce their food expenses while buying large quantities.[9] Bran and coarse food are not good enough for them, and they keep wasting good meals, having their servants and maids toss them into mud. Of all these instances of violating one's lot the gods keep a close record—people just don't realize it!

Making a good profit in trade and business is not in violation of one's lot, but harming people in going beyond a reasonable profit is. Making exceptional profits is a sign of good fortune, but petty people cannot receive them with ease. Those who violate their lot in this respect scorn what is cheap (4a) and only value what is expensive. Another person's stupidity becomes their illicit gain. If they use illicit gain to make a living, they are courting misfortune; if they use lucky deals to make a living, they are courting disaster. On the other hand, if they do what is right for their lot to make a living, they are blessed; and if they yield to others to make a living, they are truly fortunate.

People's death is never caused by external circumstances, pain or disease. It only comes from the accumulation of lots of unkindness and vast amounts of ill, causing the gods to pursue [and punish] the individual.

If people make amends for their transgressions and repent their faults, do many good deeds of benevolence and kindness and engage in sympathy and caring, virtue will come to fill them and they can survive even in the dark realm of the otherworld, even if they may not be able to entirely escape the disasters caused by their past burdens.

If they do not do this, their misfortune [unhappiness] increases daily, just as their longevity is curtailed sharply. They may still have an overabundance of gold, but their good fortune has already run out. Also, any illicit, unrighteous wealth being bought in blood, it causes nothing but trouble above and leads to an early burial below. Behaving like this to me is like being a tramp [floating cloud]: nothing is ever enough for them to think of themselves as wealthy.

Yet again, if people venerate hidden virtues and do not cheat, the sages will know them, the wise will protect them, [4b] Heaven will love them, people will delight in them, and demons and spirits will respect them. They can rest in their wealth and never lose it; relax in their high positions and never lose them. Misfortune cannot reach them, and their longevity will not be curtailed. Aggression and thievery, disasters of fire and water will be

---

[9] Reading *shi* 賒 (buy on credit) for *shi* 世 (world).

completely eliminated from their lives. They are bound to preserve their life
and live out their heaven-ordained years in peace and plenty.

Preserving Life [10]

If people exercise their bodies, the hundred ills cannot arise.
If they never drink to intoxication, the host of ailments stays away.
After a meal, walk a hundred steps and massage the belly a few times.
For sleep avoid high pillows, and spit or cry without looking back.

Cut your nails on *yinchou* days and give your hair a hundred strokes.
When satiated, urinate standing up; when hungry, pass water squatting down.
In walking and sitting avoid the wind; in your residence avoid small nestings.
Never face north to urinate, and throughout life remain obscure and hidden.
Observe taboos on sun and moon, stay away from dangerous fire and water.
At night wash the feet before retiring; after dinner don't eat another snack.

Consideration and forbearance are of highest value;
Cheating and gossip kill family relations.
Thinking and worrying most harm the spirit;
Joy and anger all upset the breath.

Regularly remove all nasal hairs; always avoid spitting on the ground.
Rise as soon as day breaks; when getting up, put the left foot first.
Through the day avoid disasters, get rid of wayward *qi*, stay away from evil.
Focus on performing the Seven-Stars Step: live a long and happy life.
Sour flavors harm the muscles; pungent flavors reduce good *qi*.
Bitter flavors diminish the heart; sweet tastes injure the will.
Salty flavors hinder long life—don't give in to cravings for one or the other.
In spring and summer, go with ease; in fall and winter, stabilize your yang.

Sleep alone to guard perfection; remain cautious and tranquil at all times.
Wealth and brocades all have their proper lot: know enough for best profit.
Aggressive acquisition is a great affliction: few desires keep you safe.
Qi and spirit remain naturally present and you can learn the Dao completely.

Write this on your wall or door and teach it well to other worthy fellows.

---

[10] *Baosheng ming* (DZ 835).

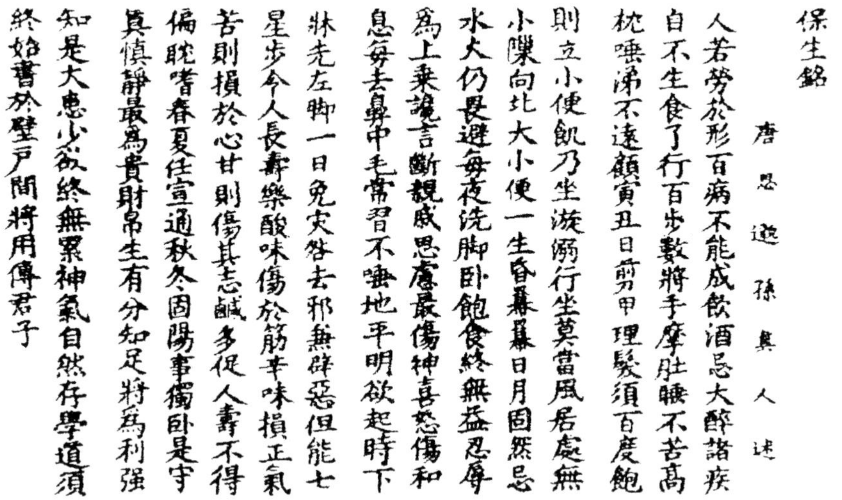

保生銘

唐思邈孫真人述

人若勞於形百病不能成飲酒忌大醉諸疾
自不生食了行百步數將手摩肚皖不苦高
枕唾涕不遠顏寅丑日剪甲理髮須百度飽
則立小便飢乃坐游溺行坐莫當風居處無
小隙向北大小便一生昏暮暮日月固然忌
水火仍畏避每夜洗脚卧飽食終無益忍辱
為上乘魂言斷視慮最傷神喜怒慈傷和
息每去鼻中毛常習不蜘地平明欲起時下
牀先左脚一日免災咎去邪無辟惡但能七
星步令人長壽酸味傷於筋辛味損正氣
苦則損於心甘則傷其志鹹多促人壽不得
偏眈嗜春夏住宣通秋冬固陽事獨卧是守
真慎靜最為貴財帛生有分知足將為利強
知是大患少欲終無累神氣自然存學道須
終始書於壁戶間將用傳君子

Fig. 14: Sun Simiao's "On Preserving Life"

The Life-Preservation Pillowbook [11]

Preface

[1a] Methods for nourishing life and restoring inner nature as found in the scrolls of texts are exceedingly numerous. Some of them are obscure and subtle, esoteric and secret, raising suspicions in the unenlightened mind, notably things like spirit soaring, inner observation, mystery excursions, and perfection plucking. Complex, they cannot be reached with lesser wisdom. One has to constantly think of how best to pursue and organize them, and only then can one reach them. If you cannot hold them steadily in your will, if you don't dedicate your heart fully to work on them, you will never be able to experience any of these arts. Previous errors compound and make them even harder to pursue—the ways of nourishing [life] and protecting [inner nature] gets farther and farther away, eluding you completely. [1b]

For this reason, practitioners learn to enter a state of submersion [in chaos] where all boundaries are merged. They cut off mentation and rest in a state free from all thinking. Xi Kang awakened to this great attainment and wrote about it [in his *Yangsheng lun*]. Others, unprepared for the depth, approach this in order to experiment, but they take one good look and get scared.

---

[11] *Sheyang zhenzhong fang* (YJQQ 33). DZ 837 variants noted in brackets.

Taking all this into consideration, I have selected certain methods in this brief work to represent key techniques found in the literature. Although they are hidden from ordinary discourse and to a certain degree esoteric, they are all easy to understand and easy to practice, supplementing any previous gaps. Studying them, there is no need to avoid the emotions or desires in your inner nature—just follow what you can and go with the times; there is no need to give up the joys of eyes and ears—just practice looking around and inquiring carefully.

The instructions are terse, but the applications are vast.

The effort is small, but the gains are huge. [3a]

All the methods and descriptions I have laid out here have been around for a long time. Trying to find and go after more esoteric ways is not likely to provide any additional benefits. Also, unless a technique is based in utmost wonder and utmost spirit, I have not included it in this work.

With sincere faith and sincere effort, I have compiled the materials for the first time in the following sections to make their vast benefits accessible to future generations. Avoid offending the Dao: be careful not to transmit the work vainly and do not pass it on to undeserving people, lest they be lost within three generations. I have compiled them in five sections to make one scroll. If you are of like mind as myself, treasure and practice them!

1. Prudence

[This section is identical with *Jin'gui lu* 14a-17a, translated in ch. 4 above.]

2. Prohibitions

From the Immortals' Scriptures
In general, *jiayin* days are when ghosts and demons move about and when essence and spirit are easily compromised. [5b] On those days, do not cohabitate with or speak directly to your spouse. Rather, use the time to take cleansing baths and stay awake and alert.

While taking herbal supplements, do not eat garlic, pomegranates, pig's liver, dog meat, or pork.[12] While taking herbal supplements, do not observe the common taboos of the north.

Whenever you enter the mountains, before you have gone a hundred paces, walk backwards for a few steps. When you have completed a hundred paces, turn around and start climbing. This way, the mountain sprites will not dare to harm you.

---

[12] "Pork" appears only in the DZ edition.

If you are serious about pursuing immortality, at all costs avoid looking at corpses or cadavers. [DZ: This is greatly inauspicious.]

Be particularly careful on the 1st day of the 3rd month, [13] and definitely do not share the same space with a woman.

[DZ: Do not sleep during the *jiazi* night in the mid-winter season.]

Preventing the Ten Self-defeating Actions [6a]
1. Do not delight in debauchery.
2. Do not steal or bring about misfortune and evil.
3. Do not intoxicate yourself with wine.
4. Do not fall into foulness and torpor without containment.
5. Do not eat the flesh of animals associated with the day of your parents' birth.
6. Do not eat the flesh of animals associated with the day of your own birth.
7. Do not eat the flesh of the six domestic animals.
8. Do not eat any raw meat or five the strong vegetables.
9. Do not kill any living beings, even insects and worms
10. Do not relieve yourself facing north.

There are the ten basic precepts of immortality. [14]

Immortals' Taboos [15] [DZ 5a]
11. Do not take off your clothes while facing north.
12. Do not curse or abuse anyone while facing north.
13. Do not execute stern punishments on the festivals of the Eight Nodes.[16]
14. Do not get angry on new or full moon.
15. Do not eat crab or shellfish on the six *jia* [crab] days.
16. Do not eat chicken on *bingshen* days.
17. Do not eat pheasant on *bingwu* days.
18. Do not get drunk on *yimao* days.
19. Do not eat fish on the 9th of the 2nd month. [5b]
20. Do not eat the animal intestines or plant cores on the 3rd of the 3rd month.
21. Do not cut down trees or decimate shrubs on the 8th of the 4th month.
22. Do not watch anything bloody on the 5th of the 5th month.
23. Do not move earth on the 6th of the 6th month.

---

[13] The DZ here has "during the 3rd and 1st months."

[14] This list is also translated in Engelhardt 1989, 284.

[15] The following section seems corrupt in the YJQQ, where it is about half as long as that in the DZ. I follow the latter.

[16] These are the solstices, equinoxes, and points in between—the beginnings of the seasons in the Chinese calendar.

24. Do not think evil on the 7th of the 7th month.

25. Do not sell or trade in hoofed animals on the 8th of the 8th month.

26. Do not move beds or mats on the 9th of the 9th month.

27. Do not punish debtors on the 5th of the 10th month.

28. Do not take baths on the 11th of the 11th month.

29. Do not fail to burn incense and remember the Dao on the last three days of the 12th month. [17]

All of these taboos and regulations are important prohibitions imposed by the celestials and enforced under the close supervision of the Three Bureaus [of Heaven, Earth, and Water]. Committing any of these acts on the days specified is a grave offense indeed. They cause people's three spirit souls to hate each other, their seven material souls to compete against each other, and in general are things that the womb gods detest. On days when the Three Bureaus learn about you commitment of bad deeds, they will send nightmares to disturb your cinnabar heart and roaming sprites to seize your vermilion towers. Your essence and fluids will be offended and upset; your body gods and perfected will be disturbed and confounded. [6a]

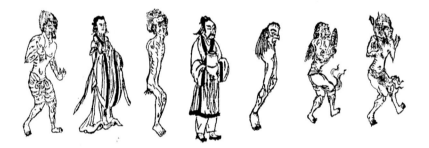

Fig. 15. The seven material souls.

[So it is better to] go along with the numerous prohibitions and genuinely acknowledge [the importance of] following the taboos. If you can honor and cultivate them, you will soon develop immortal aptitude. If you fail to observe them, on the other hand, you will be harmed and suffer defeat.

---

[17] This set of 29 rules goes back to Highest Clarity and first appears in the *Lingshu ziwen xianji* 靈書紫文仙忌 (Immortals' Taboos According to the Purple Texts Inscribed by the Spirits, DZ 179), 1b-3a. The original version, revealed by the Azure Lad, has detailed explanations in terms of what the actions will do to the body gods for the first ten items. For complete translations, see Bokenkamp 2007, 362-65; Kohn 2004b, 73-74.

The celestial officials and great divinities prohibit consuming raw meat and bloody flesh, cooking the six domestic animals, tanning skins and feathers, and eating garlic and strong vegetables. All these harm and disturb the primordial [*qi* of the] womb; their stench offends the infant gods. Be very careful!

As long as you seriously study the Dao, do not exchange clothes, including shoes, socks, caps, and skirts. This is highly inauspicious. Also, do not condole with others who have suffered bereavement, get close to a corpse, or come into contact with polluting situations or substances.

If there are people around who worship the Six Heavens or pay homage to the demon spirits of the mountains and rivers, do not stay at their house or partake of their food. Do not wear their clothes and do not put on their kerchiefs. In general, avoid the inferior *qi* of corpses and pollution, stay far away from the movement of evil winds.

On the festivals of the Eight Nodes do not stay in mixed company but use the time to focus your essence and pursue the wondrous. Do not step into polluted areas, [6b] always burn fragrance and incense and take frequent baths. Go against this and suffer exhaustion and defeat; be careful about it and fly off in ascension.

Now, as regards the arts of the female elixir, control of the inner quarters, and the bedchamber; the practices of the intermingling of yellow Dao and red *qi*; the essentials of the intake and expulsion of [the rhythm of] seven and nine; the methods of male and female reverting the elixir in [the pattern of] six and one—although they come under the name of "immortality," the perfected of Highest Clarity do not accord them nearly the same power. Although they equally lead to transformation, the Highest Lord does not value them particularly. They have a tendency to pollute the immortals and spoil the perfected, and should not be seen in the jade towers of Heaven. [They are like] high mountain tops and icy roads that see lots of tumbling carriages. Pursuing these arts, you will likely turn into a confused earth immortal.

If you wish to set your will, focus on your study, nourish your spirit, and practice immortality, you should take frequent baths and enhance your numinous *qi*. While studying the Dao, you are under close supervision: every time you develop a desire or hold a secret, each word, each deed is reckoned with—and each reckoning may cost you three days of life. [7a]

Do not participate in the morning services unless you have clean clothes. Do not enter or leave the oratory improperly: rinse your mouth and burn incense upon entering and do not look back after leaving. While rinsing and swallowing saliva, always close your eyes and focus inward. While writing petitions and talismans always face north; do not employ ordinary brush or ink and always first burn incense.

If you hear chirps or bleats, howls, or cries in your ears or if, while rising with water, you notice claps of thunder or sounds of drumming; also, if you smell the stench of decay or the odor of blood in your nose: these are unlucky signs.

Should that happen, quickly burn incense, take a bath, and fast for three days. Visualize the Imperial Lords of the Three Primes, asking them for protection. It is also good to perform some secret good deeds for others. Unless you do things for others, you won't be able to do anything—feel compassion for the orphaned, have pity for the impoverished, support those in danger, or assist the fallen. [But if you do,] all evils will naturally dissolve.

[7b] When you sell herbal supplements, do not bargain with others over the price, but rather follow the local leader. As a seller, also, do not be chatty or exhibit jealousy. People will take notice.

Now, joy and anger reduce the will; distress and grief lessen inner nature; luxury and floweriness compromise inherent potency; yin and yang [sexual activity] exhaust essence. All these are greatly tabooed in Dao studies and massively avoided among immortality methods. Rather, properly maintain your robes and capes and in general pursue constancy. Know that if you always burn incense you will find steadiness without confusion.

Practicing perfection, you need to be completely free from the impulses of emotions and desires, of fantasies regarding male and female. As long as ideas of "red and white" [intercourse] occupy your breast, the perfected will not respond and the numinous ladies and highest worthies will not descend. If you give free rein to passions, you will never get beyond the first level. As long as you are entrapped by yin energies, you will be unable to cultivate the ultimate Dao.

I myself used to be given to strong feelings. Relying on these methods, I found that things changed swiftly. Thus I know that the Dao of perfection should not be pursued in partnerships; essential words should not be heard by fools. Be very careful! Be very careful!

3. Healing Exercises

[YJQQ 8a] Always with both hands massage and rub the entire face. This causes people to have radiance and glossiness, and prevents the arising of wrinkles and discolorations. If you do this for five years, your complexion will be like that of a young girl. Massage the face for twice seven times, then stop.

When you get up in the morning, balance the *qi*. To do so, sit up straight and interlace the fingers behind the neck. Face south and raise the head, resisting this movement with your interlaced hands. Repeat this three or four times. This will make your essence harmonious and open your blood arteries. By doing this you will prevent all sorts of diseases.

Next, [stand up and] bend the body forward, stretching all four extremities and extending the sides by rotating to the right and left. Shake the hundred joints. Repeat three times.

Again, when you first wake up, rub the neck, the four sections of the face, and the ears with the soft inside of your hand, then cover the entire area with a hot, moist towel. Next, comb your hair and massage the top of your head for a good long time, then move both hands over the face and the eyes, covering them for a good while. This will make your eyes naturally bright and clear and prevent all wayward *qi* from accosting you. [8b]

When you are done with all this, swallow the saliva thirty times, guiding it deep inside the body. To count the number of repetitions as you swallow, maybe press your ears to the right and left. This way you won't lose count and at the same time prevent deafness in the ears and stuffiness in the nose.

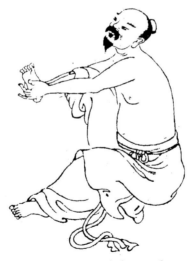

Fig. 16. Practicing daily stretches.

Always, during the time of rising, living *qi* swallow the saliva twenty-seven times while pressing on any area of the body that is sore or painful. To do so, sit down, close your eyes, and inwardly envision the five organs and six viscera. With prolonged practice you will naturally become clear, discerning, and adept.

Place your middle fingers on the inner corner of the eyes against the bridge of the nose. [NOTE: The inner corners of the eyes connect to the brightness of the pupils.] Then hold the breath and allow the *qi* to come through. Once you feel the *qi* [as a pulse], look around to exercise your eyes, and repeat once more. If you do this regularly, you will be able to see as far as ten thousand miles.

With your hand massage the small hollow behind the eyebrows. [NOTE: This place is where the *qi* flows to the eyes.] Repeat this for three sets of nine. Also, using both palms and fingers, rub the eyes all the way to the forehead, [9a] reaching as far as the ears. Do thirty repetitions without losing track of count or time.

After this, stroke the hands upward against the forehead for three sets of nine. Begin by moving upward from the center of the eyebrows and into the hairline. Prolonged practice will help you attain immortality. Also, when you cultivate this, make sure not to interfere with the Flowery Canopy. [NOTE: The Flowery Canopy indicates the eyebrows.]

4. Guiding *Qi* [18]

In pursuing immortality, there are three great methods: preserving essence,, guiding *qi*, and taking herbal supplements. Each of these comes in several levels, from the shallow to the profound. Without encountering a perfected or passing through periods of effort and hardship, one cannot know them sufficiently.

Also, the arts of preserving essence come in several hundred forms; the recipes for herbal supplements each have a thousand variants. In all cases, use persistent effort and labor but do not make the practice a forced duty.

By guiding *qi* you can cure the hundred ills, root out infections, stop serpents and wild beasts, prevent sores, [9b] rest under water, eliminate hunger and thirst, and in general extend life. Its most important form is embryo respiration, which means that one no longer breathes through mouth and nose but lives like an embryo in the womb. Reaching this, the Dao is complete.[19]

Once you are competent in the application of *qi*, you can exhale with *xu* at water, and it will flow backwards; at fire, and will go out; at tigers and wolves, and they will crouch down without moving;[20] at sores and ulcers,

---

[18] This section has some passages identical with the *Jin'gui lu* sections, "Formulas on Guiding *Qi*" and "The Way of Guiding *Qi*" (7a-9a).

[19] This echoes *Baopuzi* 6; Ware 1966, 114. See also Kohn 2008, 89.

[20] This is also found in *Baopuzi* 8; Ware 1966, 139.

and they will heal. Also, if you hear that someone has been bitten by a poisonous insect, even if you are nowhere near the person, you can exhale with *xu* at him from a distance, chanting: "I point at you with my hands: male left, female right! You may be over a hundred *li* away, but all is cured!"

Also, if someone has been bitten and is already sick from the poison, you can just swallow [saliva] for three or nine sets of nine times on his behalf, matching the nine cosmic *qi*, and the person will soon be fine.

[Everyone has this innate ability.] It is just that people for the most part are rushed and hectic, and only rarely can be calm and tranquil. Thus they find it hard to cultivate Dao.

The basic techniques of guiding *qi* should be practiced in a secluded chamber with the doors closed. Lie on a raised bed or comfortable mat, [10a] with a pillow about 2.5 inches high. Stretch out on one side, close your eyes, and hold your breath in, so that it naturally comes to stay in the chest area. If someone were to place a goose feather at you nostrils, the feather should not move. Do this for a count of 300, and your ears will stop hearing, your eyes will stop seeing, and your mind will stop thinking. Then slowly release the breath.

As long as you still partake of fresh and cold food, the five strong vegetables, fish and meat, or are still given to emotions, such as joy and anger, anxiety and rage, you may guide the *qi* all you want but it will not stay in and won't do you any good. On the contrary, it will increase *qi*-based ailments and cause superior energy to leak or flow the wrong way.

If you cannot hold the breath, start slowly and gradually increase the time. Begin with a count of three, then go on to five, seven, nine, and up to a dozen. Continue to increase the time further until you get to twenty: this is a lesser cycle. 120 make a greater cycle. As you do this, you will find an overall increase in healing and well-being.

Always practice after midnight and before noon, at the time of living, rising *qi*. As you hold the breath, keep count mentally and silently, without your ears hearing anything. If you are worried about losing track or getting confused, use your fingers to keep count.

[10b] In breathing practice, always exhale much and inhale little; always inhale through the nose and exhale through the mouth. If there is severe weather—heavy fog, strong winds, or extreme cold—do not practice *qi*-guiding. Just enclose the *qi* and keep calm; that will give best results. As Pengzu says:[21] "Reaching for Dao means being free from vexations. Just don't think or reflect, and your mind will always remain unlabored."

---

[21] A similar citation also appears in the *Yangxing yanming lu*. See ch. 9 below.

If you faithfully practice healing exercises, *qi*-guiding, embryo respiration, and visualization of body gods, you can reach a thousand years. If in addition you take the great medicine of the golden elixir, you won't wither even if Heaven itself comes to an end.

Always practice pure fasting and abstention from ordinary food, replacing it increasingly with visualizing the sun and the moon in your mouth. Work with the sun during the day and with the moon at night.[22] See either one as a large disk: the sun red and with nine rays of purple radiance; the moon yellow with ten white rays. Imagine yourself swallowing the essential sap of those rays, always practicing in complete silence and without voiced counting.

Also, whenever you undertake this visualization, let the sun and the moon move around your face and settle in the Hall of Light [between the eyebrows]. The sun should be on the left, the moon should be on the right. See the two luminants merging *qi* with the two pupils in your eyes, creating a state of open pervasion. Thereby you will effect a wide circulation of vital essence and greatly benefit your spirit and spirit souls. As a result, the Six Ding gods will come to serve you while celestial troops provide you with all-round protection. This is the Dao of perfection.

If you feel nervous during nightly practice or when going to sleep, [11a] visualize the sun and the moon circulating around your head and settling in the Hall of Light. After a short time, the hundred specters will vanish. Also, if you live in the mountains, at midnight of the 5th day of each month visualize the sun in your heart. Having entered through your mouth, it vibrantly illuminates your entire body. Radiate jointly with the sun and become aware of your heart and belly shining brightly with a celestial hue.

To conclude this exercise, rinse and swallow the saliva nine times. Do the same also on each 15th and 25th day. You will find your joints opening up and your face glowing with a jade-like complexion. Also, men should work more with the sun; women, with the moon. Doing this regularly without fail makes your senses keen and you inner organs bloom.

---

[22] The DZ version is quite corrupt here, not even completing the sentence but moving into a detailed discussion of various foods and herbal and mineral recipes, which seems to be taken from another text. It does not speak of *qi*-guiding again or contain a section on "Guarding the One."

5. Guarding the One

To practice guarding the One, understand first that in your head, there is the Hall of Light one inch in from between the eyebrows, followed by the Cavern Chamber at two inches and the upper elixir field at three inches.[23] The latter matches the middle elixir field in the heart and the lower elixir field in the abdomen, located 1.2 inches below the navel. In each of these centers resides a divine being, clad in formal garb of a specific color and called by a unique name.[24] In men, the divinity measures nine tenths of an inch; in women, six tenths.

In the old days, the Yellow Emperor traveled to Mt. Emei and was received by a divine lord in a jade palace. The Emperor asked him about the Dao of the Perfect One. The Lord said: "Long life and ascension to the immortals all come from working with the golden elixir. Guard the body and repel old age, and you will come to rest with the Perfect One. Thus the immortals value it highly."

Now, all meditation and visualization should be done thousands of times, always carefully keeping the multitude of vexations and the variety of troubles at bay. Anyone who properly understands guarding the One will remain free of them with no problem.

The immortal master said: "If you take the great medicine of the golden elixir, even before you transcend this world, the hundred forms of wayward *qi* won't dare to come near you. If you take lesser medicines made from herbs and shrubs or ingest the eight minerals, you will get rid of all diseases and extend your years, but you won't be able to eliminate other nasty situations, such as being oppressed by demons, summoned to [the realm of the dead at] Mt. Tai, disregarded by the mountain gods, or attacked by local sprites. Only by working with the Perfect One can you avoid fearing any of these."

---

[23] These are the first three of the nine palaces in the head. For details, see Kohn 1991; Kalinowski 1985.

[24] The text has a note here, saying that this information is based on the *Huangting jing.* See Homann 1971.

Chapter Eight

Nourishing Inner Nature

While Sun Simiao was undoubtedly the first and foremost of Tang organizers of longevity ideas and practices, the most important text to present the integrated tradition is the *Yangxing yanming lu* 養性延命錄 (On Nourishing Inner Nature and Extending Life, DZ 838; abridged in *Yunji qiqian* 32.1a-24b), translated in this and the following chapters. The text presents a summary of nourishing life practices in six sections: General Concepts, Diet, Taboos, *Qi*-Absorption, Healing Exercises, and Sexual Control. Some Song bibliographies attribute it to the first Highest Clarity patriarch Tao Hongjing, others—as well as the text's preface—link it with Sun Simiao. While the style is somewhat reminiscent of the former, its integrative tendency, certain key concepts, and several passages also found in Sun's other works relate it to the latter. The multitude of documents cited and its close relation to Sun suggest that it is a mid-to-late Tang reconstitution drawing closely on Sun's works. [1]

The first and longest section of the text presents a comprehensive overview of previous works and interpretations of the longevity tradition. It begins with the ancient classics, *Zhuangzi, Daode jing*—also cited as "Laozi says" and by Laozi's more formal (mid-Tang) name *Hunyuan daojing* 混元道經 (Chaos Prime's Scripture on the Dao)—and *Liezi*. In all cases, it uses their commentaries: Xiang Xiu 向秀 and Guo Xiang 郭象 on the *Zhuangzi*,[2]

---

[1] See Despeux in Schipper and Verellen 2004, 345-46. Previous translations include: the entire text in Japanese, with ample annotation translation (Mugitani 1987); in English, sects. 2 (Switkin 1987), 4 (Jackowicz 2003), and 6 (Wile 1992, 119-22).

[2] On Xiang Xiu's take on the *Zhuangzi*, see Kohn 1992, 107-08. For detailed discussions of Guo Xiang, see Knaul 1985a; 1985b; Robinet 1983.

Heshang gong 河上公, Yan Junping 嚴君平, and Yin Xi 尹喜 on the *Daode jing*, and Zhang Zhan 張湛 on the Liezi.[3]

A text closely related to this group is also the *Hunyuan miaozhen jing* 混元妙真經 (Chaos Prime's Scripture of Wondrous Perfection), variously cited in medieval sources as a work in the philosophical tradition. Topics of fragments include: the proper morality in government and self-cultivation; right accordance with the rhythm of the times; the way to lead an orderly family and community life; how to be careful in speech and avoid over-stimulating the five senses; how to understand the spontaneity of nature and be equally soft and yielding; how to cultivate oneself, maintain good health, and keep the spirit(s) at peace in the body. However, the text is also denounced in anti-Daoist polemics as an adaptation of the *Lotus Sutra*, and quite possibly was edited later to be more philosophical, only to be lost completely in the late Tang (see Kohn 1995b, 204-05).

From these Daoist philosophical sources, the *Yangxing yanming lu* next moves on to more generic literati texts that deal with longevity, notably the works by Xi Kang, but also Sima Tan's 司馬談 preface to the *Shiji* 史記 (Records of the Historian), the *Kongzi jiayu* 孔子家語 (Kong Family Annals), and the *Bowu zhi* 博物志 (Record of Wide Ranging Matters).[4] In addition, it takes recourse to the medical classics, such as the *Huangdi neijing suwen*, the *Shennong jing* 神農經 (Scripture of the Divine Farmer), and the *Mingyi xubing lun* 名醫敘病論 (Famous Physicians Explain Disease). All these it cites

---

[3] Passages from Heshang gong's commentary are found in ch. 1 above. Yan Junping, aka Yan Zun 嚴遵, is the author of a Han-dynasty commentary of the *Daode jing*, known as the *Laozi zhigui* 老子指歸 (Pointers to the *Laozi*, DZ 693); see Robinet 1998. Yin Xi is the legendary Guardian of the Pass, who requested that Laozi write down his philosophy before emigrating to the west. He is associated with a text cited here as *Laojun Yin Shi neijie* 老君尹氏內解 (Yin's Esoteric Explanation of Lord Lao), which is probably identical with the *Laozi jiejie* 老子節解 (Sectioned Interpretation of the *Daode jing*), a 3rd-century commentary that survives in fragments (Robinet 1977, 49-55). The passage cited here is also found in the *Yangsheng yaoji* 養生要集 (Stein 1999, 174), the longevity work of the *Liezi* commentator Zhang Zhan (see ch. 2 above). Cited passages from the *Liezi* are from chs. 1 and 3 (Graham 1960, 25, 62).

[4] For a discussion and translation of Xi Kang's works, see Holzman 1957; Henricks 1983. For a brief outline of the *Shiji*, see Nienhauser 1986, 689-92; a full translation appears in Watson 1968b. *Kongzi jiayu* is a collection of Confucian sayings compiled by Wang Su 王肅 (195-256). For a discussion and selected translations, see http://www.chinaknowledge.de/Literature/Classics/kongzijiayu.html. The *Bowu zhi* is a collection of odd records and myth compiled by the scholar-official Zhang Hua (232-300). A complete translation appears in Greatrex 1987.

with passages that show how people's shortened destiny has primarily to do with life-style, moderation, and lack of emotional constraint.[5]

Beyond this, the *Yangxing yanming lu* also cites two apocrypha, probably dating from the Later Han, that connect to the mysterious "River Chart" and "Luo Writ," magic squares revealed by a dragon and turtle surfacing in the Yellow and Luo Rivers respectively. Understood as keys to cosmic secrets and empowerment, they are at the root of Daoist talismans and actively connect people to the greater flow of celestial *qi* (Robinet in Pregadio 2008, 483-85; Saso 1978). The texts, which are not otherwise documented, are the *Hetu dishi meng* 河圖帝視萌 (Emperor's River Chart Exegesis) and the *Luoshu baozi ming* 洛書寶子命 (Precious Orders of the Luo Writ). The passages from the texts deal with good fortune in relation to Heaven; they also appear in other longevity sources, notably *Ishinpō* 27 and *Yunji qiqian* 35.

Following the same tradition, three titles cited in the text are listed in Ge Hong's library as described in *Baopuzi* 19, but have not survived as independent text. They are the *Huanglao jing xuanshi* 黃老經玄示 (Mysterious Pointers of the Scripture of the Yellow Elder), the *Daoji* 道機 (Central Pivor of Dao); and the *Xianjing* 仙經 (Immortals' Scripture). The passages cited from these texts relate people's health and sickness to destiny, on the one hand, emphasizing that each one is born with a particular destiny and innate constitution, on the other hand, insisting that we do have control. Especially the *Xianjing* is cited with a statement found in section 26 of the *Xisheng jing* 西升經 (Scripture of Western Ascension, DZ 726) that insists that "my life is my own; it does not depend on Heaven" (Kohn 2007, 56, 249).

Last, but not least, the text cites four works that can be connected to the Highest Clarity tradition. First is the *Zhongjing* 中經 (Central Scripture), which might be an abbreviation for *Laozi zhongjing* 老子中經 (Central Scripture of Laozi, DZ 1168, YJQQ 18-19), a technical treatise that, like the equally quoted *Huangting jing*, describes the gods in the human body (see Schipper 1979; Lagerwey 2004). Another work is the *Dayou jing* 大有經 (Scripture of Great Existence, DZ 1314), a 4th-century text that deals with the cosmology of heavens and the body (Kohn 1995, 101). The third is the

---

[5] The *Huangdi neijing* is the prime classic of Chinese medicine. It is translated, among others, in Veith 1972; Ki 1985; Ni 1995. The passage cited here appears in Veith 1972, 97-98. The *Shennong jing*—cited with a passage on food and personality that closely resembles the citation from the *Kongzi jiayu* and echoes distinctions made also in the *Laozi shuo fashi jinjie jing* 老子說法食禁戒經 (Prohibitions and Precepts on Ceremonial Food, Revealed by Laozi, DH 80), an early Tang text on Daoist food prohibitions found at Dunhuang; Kohn 2004b, 93) and the *Mingyi xubing lun* are not otherwise known.

Xiaoyou jing 小有經 (Scripture of Lesser Existence; otherwise unknown), with a passage also found in *Ishinpō* 29.

Taking these various sources together, the *Yangxing yanming lu* documents the integrative and overarching nature of the longevity tradition, showing just how seamlessly it combines the ancient Daoist philosophical tradition and its medieval expansion with literati aspirations found among historians, poets, and Confucians, plus esoteric apocryphal interpretations of the classics, technical works on immortality, and Highest Clarity revelations.

The same variety is also evident in the personages cited. Besides the various commentators to the Daoist classics, the *Yangxing yanming lu* makes reference to various figures—legendary and historical—that again shows the broad scope of the tradition:

Pengzu 彭祖, a famous ancient immortal with biographies in the Han-dynasty *Liexian zhuan* (Kaltenmark 1953, 82-84) and in Ge Hong's *Shenxian zhuan* (Campany 2002, 177), whose statements are equally found in the *Yangsheng yaoji* (Stein 1999, 172);

Huangshan 黃山, the Lord of Yellow Mountain, who appears in the *Shenxian zhuan* as a follower of the long-lived Pengzu (Campany 2002, 181);

Feng Heng 封衡, aka Junda 君達, often also called Qingniu daoshi 青牛道士 (Gray Ox Daoist), a magical practitioner of the Former Han mentioned in the *Han Wudi neizhuan* 漢武帝內傳 (Inner Biography of the Han Emperor Wu, DZ 292) as a personage who lived very long by eating only herbs and always rode around on a gray ox—an animal of high age with a particularly shiny black-gray-bluish coat (Schipper 1965; Smith 1992) and also described in the *Shenxian zhuan* (Campany 2002, 149, 399; see also Stein 1999, 114) as well as cited in the *Jin'gui lu* (ch. 4 above);

Chen Ji 陳紀, aka Yuanfang 元方, a long life practitioner of the Later Han who is mentioned in ch. 29 of the *Hou Hanshu* 後漢書 (History of the Later Han) and also cited in the *Yangsheng yaoji* (Stein 1999, 187);

Han Rong 韓融, zi Yuanchang 元長, also of the Later Han mentioned in *Hou Hanshu* 62 (Stein 1999, 115) and cited in the *Yangsheng yaoji* (Stein 1999, 195);

Zhong Changtong 仲長統, another master of Later Han origins with biographies in *Hou Hanshu* 49 and in ch. 21 of the *Sanguo zhi* 三國志 (Record of the Three Kingdoms) (see Ngo 1976; DeWoskin 1983);

Hu Zhao 胡昭, *zi* Kongming 孔明, a master of long life under the Wei state of the Three Kingdoms (Stein 1999, 114), cited with a passage also found in the *Yangsheng yaoji* (Stein 1999, 171);

Zhi Dun 支遁 (Shi Daolin 釋道林), a Buddhist monk and active proponent of longevity practices in the early 4th century, credited with a major text on healing exercises, the *Daolin lun* 道林論 (Despeux 1989, 231; Kohn 2008, 137);

Zhaiping 翟平, mentioned in the bibliographic section of the *Suishu* as the author of a *Yangsheng shu* 養生術 (Methods of Nourishing Life).

These many various sources and personages by and large agree on certain fundamental principles of nourishing vitality. Human life is the coming together of spirit and body, provided by Heaven and Earth through the venue of the parents. It comes with certain set parameters, such as a predestined destiny and certain inborn characteristics, but its absorption is entirely up to the individual. If people stay within their parameters and use their Heaven-given energy and qualities prudently, they can easily live to high old age and even make it to the biological limit of 120. If they enhance their natural predisposition with deep breathing, healing exercises, medicinal supplements, and meditations—"floating their mind in emptiness and stillness"—they may well double or even quadruple this lifespan.

However, most people become victims of the senses, get involved in social strife and competition, engage in excessive food and sex, give rise to the six destructive emotions—anger, hatred, worry, fear, sadness, and euphoria—and thus in various ways diminish their energy and squander their essence. This leads to intense stress, psychological tensions, physical fatigue, and eventually results in sickness, disease, and early death, defined as the separation of spirit and body, followed by their ongoing transformation in different realms of nature and the otherworld. It also tends to come with moral shortcomings and bad deeds, which are duly recorded by the celestial administration, adding yet another level to the person's burdens. The first step and prime way out is to let go and relax, stay away from sensory engagement and social strife. As the text has it most pertinently: "Hermits never get sick; salesmen are full of afflictions."

Translation

Nourishing Inner Nature and Extending Life[6]

Preface

[1a] Human beings are noblest among creatures because they are equipped with *qi* and contain numen. What human beings value most is life. Life is the foundation of spirit; the body is its tool. If you use spirit a lot, it gets exhausted; if you exert the body a lot, it perishes.

Now, mentally float in emptiness and stillness, let go of worries, rest in nonaction, ingest primordial *qi* after midnight, practice healing exercises in a calm setting, support and nourish life without fail, take healthy food and efficacious herbs—if you do all this, then a hundred years of vigorous longevity are your proper due. On the other hand, foolishly waste your intention to indulge in sights and sounds, apply your wisdom to scheme for rank and wealth, suffer a loss and harbor it permanently in your chest, rush about so you cannot even keep up with yourself, never heed the rules of rites and deportment, eat and drink without moderation—if you stumble along like this, how can you possibly avoid the afflictions of harm and early death?

Understanding this, I have practiced cessation and observation and entered subtle states of mind. I have also carefully studied various essential collections on nourishing life, [1b] such as those formerly created by dedicated disciples such as Zhang Zhan and Shi Daolin, as well as those by the likes of Zhaiping and Huangshan. All these works relish the heroic and the marvelous and encourage people to focus their will on treasuring personal training. In addition, I have examined the rules of long life followed by perfected beings as presented in various tales and immortal scriptures.

I have also obtained the various arts of life enhancement associated with Pengzu and Lord Lao, arts that reach back as far as the Divine Farmer and the Yellow Emperor and have been transmitted to us from the Wei and Jin dynasties. They focus on increasing the benefits of nourishing life and how to lessen the impact of later afflictions. I first made a detailed record of the various books, so that I could create an abstract and extract their most essential methods while eliminating all extraneous and irrelevant matters. I then classified everything according to heading and topic, divided it into two scrolls,

---

[6] *Yangxing yanming lu* (DZ 838), preface and section 1.

and placed three sections in each of them. I am calling this compendium the *Yangxing yanming lu*.[7] In all of this, I received support and help from those with the right karmic connections. If there were some who differed from or denigrated my work, I endeavored to "make all things equal."

1. General Concepts

[1a] The *Shennong jing* (Scripture of the Divine Farmer) says: Those eating grain are wise and bright; those eating refined minerals are stout and long-lived; those eating fungi extend their years and do not die; those eating primordial *qi* Earth cannot bury and Heaven cannot kill; Thus if you take medicinal supplements, you will end with Heaven and rank with the sun and the moon. . . . [8]

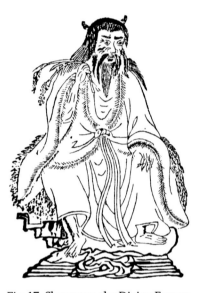

The *Zhuangzi*, in his chapter on "Nourishing Life" [ch. 3] has:

Your life has a limit.

Xiang Xiu comments: All that life is endowed with has a limit, but wisdom has none.

Fig. 17. Shennong, the Divine Farmer

Xi Kang says [in the *Da Nan Yangsheng lun*]: Desiring without thinking stimulates inner nature; bringing forth impulses with conscious awareness activates wisdom. When inner nature is stimulated, it goes along with beings as it encounters them; if there is just the right amount of this, there won't be any excess. When wisdom follows along with its activation, there is no pursuit; it gets tired, but does not reach its end. Thus the afflictions of the world tend to be from wisdom being activated rather than from inner nature being stimulated.

If you use what is limited to pursue what has no limit, you will be in danger.

---

[7] The part on "dividing into two scrolls and placing three sections" is not found in the *Yunji qiqian* edition. On the other hand, it calls the final text *Yangxing yan-nian lu*, replacing *ming* 命 (life) with *nian* 年 (years).

[8] The next page (1b-2b) contains chapters 6 and 50 from Dao*de jing* with Heshang gong's commentary. For their translation see ch. 1 above.

Guo Xiang comments: Using limited inner nature to pursue unlimited wisdom, [3a] how can one attain it and not run into trouble? If you understand this and still strive for wisdom, you will be in danger for certain.

Xiang Xiu notes: You will be in trouble with wisdom. It is like understanding the danger and yet going for an attack. One will be in danger.

Who has attained the essence of life does not bother with what life cannot do. [ch. 19]

Xiang Xiu says: What life cannot do means what lies beyond the scope of a person's inner nature.

Zhang Zhan says: Life has its principle and is naturally complete. Doing anything that exceeds one's lot is using the limited to pursue the limitless.

Who has attained the essence of destiny does not bother with what wisdom cannot reach.

Xiang Xiu says: When destiny is exhausted, there is death. This is the right way.

Zhang Zhan notes: As one strides along with the principle of life one can fully exhaust all one is originally endowed with. How could wisdom know this?

The *Liezi* (Book of Master Lie) [ch. 1] says: When young, not worrying about proper conduct; when grown, not competing with others; throughout life at peace in poverty; in old age continuing to reduce desires; throughout relaxing the mind and working the body: this is the way of nourishing life.

It also [ch. 3] notes: [3b] The whole body filling and emptying, ebbing and flowing along at all times: thus you can pervade Heaven and Earth and go along with the myriad creatures.

Zhang Zhan says: This refers to people being completely open to the energetic flows of yin and yang. In harmony in the beginning, in harmony in the end, calm the spirit and let go of wild imaginings: this is the way of life. From beginning to end in harmony, spirit and the will never scatter.

The *Huanyuan miaozhen jing* (Chaos Prime's Scripture of Wondrous Perfection) says: Human beings always lose Dao; Dao never loses them. Human beings constantly reject life; life never rejects them. Thus nourishing life means to be careful not to lose Dao. Practicing Dao means to watch out not to lose life. This way one causes life and Dao to preserve and to guard each other.

The *Huanglao jing xuanshi* (Mysterious Pointers of the Scripture of the Yellow Elder) has: As Heaven's way moves and transforms, it goes along with the myriad beings and never ends. As people's way moves and transforms, their bodies and spirit diminish and die. As they turn spirit on and activate essence, they soon exhaust it and go into decline. The body originally brings forth essence; essence is also created by spirit. If one avoids activating it in life, one can match one's inherent potency [virtue] with Heaven; if one does not let it change along with the spirit, one can join Dao.

The *Xuanshi* further says: Transforming by means of the body is attaining deliverance from the corpse.[9] [4a] The spirit separates from the body and the two are no longer together. They may follow the beasts or fly up like the birds, enter the ocean and turn into crabs, going along with the yin-yang energies of the seasons. Changing along with the *qi* one can hope for life; changing along with the body one will face great danger.

Yan Junping, in his *Laozi zhigui* (Pointers to the *Laozi*) says: Float the mind in emptiness and stillness, tie the will to the subtle and wondrous, rest your thinking in a state of no desires, give up all plans in favor of nonaction: doing this you can master life, extend destiny and live as long as Dao.

The *Dayou jing* (Scripture of Great Existence) says: Someone asks, "To begin we all commonly arise beyond nonbeing, to end we all receive *qi* from yin and yang. We receive bodies and material souls from Heaven and Earth, we are born and grow through food and breath. Still, there are the ignorant, the wise, the strong, the weak, the long-lived and the die-young. Who is doing is that? Heaven? People?"

I explain: The nature of our bodies and lives, whether we are ignorant or wise—that is due to Heaven. Whether we are strong or weak, live long or die early—that is the making of man. The way of Heaven is spontaneous, self-so; the way of people is ego-focused. When we are first conceived in the womb, our *qi* is full and complete. After birth, we receive breast milk and have ample. Growing up, we crave fancy flavors and they are never enough. Once adults, we are constantly subject to the enticements of sights and sounds. [4b] If we exercise moderation, we can be strong and live long.

On the other hand, when the *qi* at conception is empty and scarce, when there is insufficient breast milk after birth, when we still crave fancy flavors and can never get enough and are given lasciviously to the enticements of sights and sounds, then we will end up weak and die young. Yet again, if our life is strong and full, and we add some exercises and nourishing practices into the mix, then our years will go beyond all expectations.

---

[9] This involves leaving an object behind as one transforms into an immortal. For details, see Robinet 1979; Cedzich 2001

The *Daoji* (Central Pivot of Dao) has: People take birth with life expectancies that can be long or short. This is not just a spontaneous occurrence but is directly related to whether we are careful with our bodies. If in food and drink we go beyond the limits, know no bounds in lasciviousness and entertainment, go against the rhythms of yin and yang, let our spirit soul and spirit run wild, then our essence will be depleted and our destiny declines as the hundred diseases grow wild. Then we will not be able to live out our full longevity.

The *Hetu dishimeng* (Emperor's River Chart Exegesis) says: Insulting Heaven's timing brings bad luck; following Heaven's rhythm means good fortune. In spring and summer enjoy mountains and high places; in fall and winter rest in low regions and deep hide-outs. Good fortune is beneficial and brings great happiness, a long life without limits.

The *Luoshu baozi ming* (Precious Orders of the Luo Writ) notes: The ways people of antiquity cured diseases was to create internal harmony with sweet spring [saliva], moisten themselves with primordial *qi*. Their herbal supplements were neither astringent nor bitter; they tasted sweet and were full of flavor. They would take their fluids and flow them through their five inner organs, [5a] tie them into their hearts and lungs. Thus their entire bodies would be free from afflictions.

The *Kongzi jiayu* (Kong Family Annals) says: Those who eat meat are valiant, daring, and cruel—like tigers and wolves. Those who eat *qi* are spiritual, bright, and long-lived—like immortals and holy tortoises. Those who eat grain are wise and celestial. Those who do not eat at all are spirits who never die—they just swallow their breath and remain free from all thoughts.

The *Zhuan* (Commentary) says: Those who eat miscellaneous things suffer from the hundred diseases and die young. The less we eat the more open our minds are and the easier it is to increase our years. The more we eat, the more obstructed are our minds and the more we lose in years.

The Grand Historian Sima Tan notes [in the preface to the *Shiji*]: Life is the foundation of spirit; the body is its tool. If you use spirit a lot, it will be exhausted; if you exert the body a lot, it will perish. I have never heard of one whose spirit and body were declining early and who yet managed to live as long as Heaven and Earth. Thus, what gives people live is the spirit; what the spirit relies on is the body. When spirit and body separate, the person dies. Once dead, he cannot come back to life. [5b] Once separated, they cannot come back together. For this reason, the sages of old valued them highly.

Now, the way of nourishing life has many rules regarding the great return. If you cannot meet all of them, just thinking about them helps. Every time you go against ordinary patterns you further withdraw from common paths. Just make sure to overcome precedents and catch yourself in all possible transgressions: that is already half the effort. As a disciples who dedicates his minds to this fully, how can you not pursue this?

The *Xiaoyou jing* (Scripture of Lesser Existence) says: [10] Think little, reflect little, desire little, work little, speak little, laugh little, mourn little, delight little, enjoy little, anger little, like little, dislike little. Practicing these twelve signifies a small level of nourishing life.

If you think much, the spirit is endangered. If you reflect much, the will is dispersed. If you desire much, you your volition is diminished. If you work much, the body gets tired. If you speak much, the *qi* is contrary. If you laugh much, your organs are harmed. If you mourn much, the heart is exerted. If you delight much, the intention overflows. If you enjoy much, you forget you sometimes make mistakes and get deluded. If you anger much, the hundred channels are unstable. If you like much, you fall into error and disorder. If you dislike much, you are sad, distressed, and desolate. Unless you eliminate these twelve "much" attitudes, you lose the foundation of life. [6a] Once free from them, you are close to being perfected.

In general, those who are generous and laid-back live long; those who are stingy and uptight die young. It is the difference of being relaxed and at ease versus labored and tightfisted. A farmer, long-lived and rich, versus a burglar pestered by endless cravings—that in essence is the experience of "little" versus "much." Hermits never get sick; salesmen are full of afflictions—that in essence is the difference between duty and ease. For this reason, while ordinary people compete for profit, Daoists rest in their homes.

Hu Zhao, *zi* Kongming, says:[11] Let the eyes not see any improper sights; let the ears not hear any ugly words; let the nose not smell any disgusting stench; let the mouth not taste any harsh or toxic flavors; let the mind not plan affairs of deceit: all these shame the spirit and reduce long life. Also, if you constantly breathe deeply when at home, humming and whistling morning and night, you will certainly attract a thousand proper energies.

Now, it is quite common that people are not able to fully attain freedom from desires and usually do not manage to be free from affairs. Just try to be harmonious in mind, reduce your thoughts, keep your body at rest, and let go of worries. This will first eliminate all disturbances to the spirit and harm to your inner nature. It is the key art of maintaining your spirit endowment. [6b]

---

[10] The following is a variant version of the Twelve Littles. See ch. 2 above.

[11] This and the following also appear in *Ishinpō* 23 as from the *Yangsheng yaoji.* See Stein 1999, 171, 174, 195.

The *Huangting jing* (Yellow Court Scripture) [Wai 1] has: "The clear water from the Jade Pond drips to the Numinous Root. All who cultivate this will live long." [The commentator] Ming adds: Take food and drink in natural rhythm. The more natural it is, the more it becomes the Flowery Pond. The Flowery Pond is the saliva in the mouth. Inhale and exhale as prescribed, then swallow it down and you won't be hungry any more.

The *Laojun Yin Shi neijie* (Yin's Esoteric Explanation of Lord Lao) says: As the saliva drips down, it becomes a sweet spring. If you collect it consciously, it turns into Jade Liquor. It flows together to form the Flowery Pond. From here it may disperse to turn into essence or be guided downward to form sweet dew. Thus the mouth is known as the Flowery Pond. Use the sweet spring to rinse and swallow and thus moisturize your inner organs and enrich your entire body. As it flows along, it benefits the hundred channels, supports and nourishes the myriad spirits as well as the limbs, joints, hair, and whiskers. Complete this practice and you will attain life.

The *Zhongjing* (Central Scripture) says: Stillness means long life; agitation means early death. However, even if you manage to find stillness and do not nourish yourself properly, you will reduce your longevity; if you are agitated and yet manage to nourish yourself, you can extend your years. Having said this, it is easy to manage stillness but hard to control agitation. Thus, it is best to follow the appropriate ways of nourishing life at all times: then, when in stillness you are nourishing yourself and also when in a state of agitation.

Han Rong, *zi* Yuanchang (of the Later Han), says: Alcoholic drinks are the ultimate distilled flavor of the five grains. They can be of great benefit, but they can also diminish people's health. [7a] Thus all good things in life are hard to control and easy to overdo. You have to be very careful to do just what is right for nourishing your inner nature.

Shao Zhongzhan says: The five grains fill the flesh and body but do not add to longevity. The hundred medicines cure diseases and extend life but they do not delight the palate. Delighting the palate and filling the flesh is what ordinary people like. Tasting bitter foods and extending life is what Daoists value highly.

The *Huangdi neijing suwen* (Yellow Emperor's Inner Classic, Simple Questions) [ch. 1] says: The Yellow Emperor asked Qi Bo, "I have heard that people of old all reached an old age of a hundred full of vigor and without declining. In other words, their blood and *qi* were still at full throttle. People today, I note, having barely reached half that age are failing in their activities. Is it because the world changed over the generations? Is it that people have lost something?"

Qi Bo replied: Those among the people of high antiquity who knew Dao patterned themselves on yin and yang and lived in harmony with their rules and calculations. They practiced properly in their bedchamber relations, were moderate in their food and drink, had a regular schedule of sleep and waking, and did not engage in foolish activities. For this reason they could relish the spirit fully and live out their destiny as given by Heaven, going even beyond a hundred years.

People today are not like this at all. They take alcohol as nourishing fluid and think of foolishness as normal. [7b] Drunk to the gills, they stumble into the bedchamber, giving in to mad passions and duly exhaust their essence, even delighting as they waste their inherent perfection. They have no clue as to what it means to hold on to satisfaction; exerting their spirit with no sense of proper timing. They are all for gaining quick pleasures in their minds, flitting around wildly in the realm of yin and yang. The whole pattern of their lives, their rhythm of waking and sleeping is completely without moderation or regularity. Thus they can't even make it to fifty without going into decline.

Lord Lao says: A long human life lasts for a hundred years, but with proper moderation and preservation, one can extend that to a thousand. It is like the wax of a candle: use it sparingly and it will last long. Most people are full of great words while I speak little; they have many vexations while I hardly remember anything; they are aggressive and violent while I never get angry. I don't let my mind get entangled in human affairs; I don't pursue the work of service or employment. Serene and at peace, I rest in nonaction, my spirit and *qi* spontaneously satisfied.

This is the medicine of no-death. I know truly nothing in all under Heaven! Without ever speaking of the hidden mystery, Heaven knows people's feelings. Without ever speaking of the dark and sublime, spirit sees people's bodies. I may speak mentally but utter only little: demons can hear human voices as they violate the taboos. When they offend a thousand times, Earth will receive their bodies. If people do good in public, they are rewarded by good fortune and other people; [8a] if they do good in secret, they are rewarded by the demons and spirits. If people do evil in public, robbers will get even with them; if they do evil in secret, the demons and spirits will get them. Thus Heaven never cheats on people but follows their actions like a shadow; Earth never cheats on people but follows their actions like an echo.

Lord Lao says: If people cultivate goodness and accumulate virtue yet encounter bad luck and disasters, this is because they received the left-over evil from previous generations. Similarly if they violate the prohibitions and do nothing but evil yet encounter good fortune, this is because they have received the left-over merit from valiant ancestors.

The *Mingyi xubing lun* (Famous Physicians Explain Disease) says: The fact that people do not live out their full destiny but in many cases die young is because they do not love or cherish themselves. Instead they exhaust their intention with anger and competitiveness, strive for fame and go after profit, accumulate toxins and battle their spirit. On the inside they harm their bones and skeleton; on the outside they destroy their flesh and muscles. Their blood and *qi* dwindle to nothing while their channels and vessels are increasingly obstructed. Their flesh and structure empty and neglected, they only invite toxicity and disease. Their proper *qi* diminishes daily, while their wayward *qi* increases without stopping. They are no different from someone trying to capture a huge wave and pour it into raging fire, to tame a powerful peak to dam a water flow. To speak about it is easy, but is it not very pitiful indeed? [8b]

Pengzu says: Reaching Dao means being free from vexation. Just don't think of clothes and food, sounds and sights, victory and defeat, gain and loss, sounds and sights—then you won't exert your heart or push your body to extremes. Instead, always do your exercises and breathing practice and you can reach a thousand years. Also, if you want a life without limit, make sure to take superior medicinal supplements.

Zhong Changtong notes: People waste their lives by giving in to the six emotions and five senses. They have a mind and don't worry about it thinking; they have a mouth and don't worry about it talking; they have a body and don't worry about it being at rest. Only if they can keep these three calm can they move beyond ordinary life. Instead, they take great delight in them, but they don't really love or cherish themselves. They use their minds to plot, never realizing just how much they keep increasing their self-destructive behavior day by day. Also, the just do not realize how their being keeps on changing. The contrast to men like Pengzu and Laozi could not be bigger. How would they ever be the same as most people? No, they are of their own kind and differ from all others in longevity and lifestyle.

Chen Ji, aka Yuanfang says: The root cause of the hundred diseases and of untimely death in many cases lies with food and drink. The afflictions people suffer due to their indulgence in food and drink are worse than those caused by sights and sounds. [9a] Sights and sounds people can give up for years together, but one cannot do without food and drink for even a single day. As they increase their intake, so their maladies multiply; even if they see them as an affliction, they still remain urgent necessities.

Zhang Zhan says: Those who renounce all rank and power, even though they may avoid active engagement in evil, will still subject their essence and spirit to harm and their body will inevitably die. That is to say, even if they are not subject to the misfortune of worldly enticement, they are still being invaded by outside forces such as heat and cold. These wreak havoc to their bodies and they slide slowly towards internal harm and loss of blood.

Others, who are rich at first and later fall into poverty, even though they may avoid active engagement in evil, will be subject to burning skin and lessening muscles, thus leading to a state where compliance and avoidance are out of harmony. In other words, the effect of wealth and poverty on people is that of being subject to benefit and harm. It is like having a lot of power and influence: they lead to pain and disease and cause a general decline of the body.

To balance outside influences, move to overcome cold and be s till to overcome heat. If you can practice movement and stillness in proper intervals, you can live long. Eventually your essence and *qi* will always be clear and still—then you are at one with Dao.

The *Zhuangzi* [ch. 6] says: "The perfected of old slept without dreaming." Zhenzi comments: People who are not bothered by affairs during the day don't dream at night. Thus Master Zhang lived for over a hundred years, remaining erect and strong throughout.

He also notes: The way to nourish inner nature is to avoid long periods of walking, sitting, lying down, looking, or listening. [9b] Don't go heavy on food and drink; don't get greatly intoxicated; don't wallow in deep sorrow or give in to worry; don't drown in melancholy or deep thought. Doing all this is called establishing harmony. Who can establish harmony will live long.

The *Xianjing* (Immortals' Scripture) says: My life is my own; it does not depend on Heaven. However, ignorant people do not realize this fact which is at the core of all good living. Instead, they open the door to the hundred diseases and wind pathologies—by giving in to lascivious intentions and extreme emotions, linked with an inability to properly take care of themselves. Thus they waste their lives and squander their bodies. Soon they are like dried up, withered trees: encounter a gust of wind and they break into pieces. They are like steep, sliding cliffs: encounter a strong wave of water and they tumble down. Today, if you cannot take proper medicinal supplements, just make sure to love and cherish your essence and moderate your emotions. This way you will at least make it to one or two hundred.

Zhang Zhan, in the preface to the *Yangsheng yaoji*, notes: The essentials of nourishing life are: 1. Endowed with Spirit; 2. Caring for *Qi*; 3. Nourishing the Body; 4. Guiding and Stretching; 5. Speaking and Talking; 6. Eating and

Drinking; 7. The Bedchamber; 8. Rejecting Habits; 9. Medicinal Supplements; 10.Various Taboos. Anything beyond this is too much. The key ideas are contained right here. [10a]

The Gray Ox Daoist says: People should not desire to feel exhilaration, since exhilarated people don't live long. They should make sure not to overdo physical activity: never get talked into lifting anything heavy, digging into the earth, or doing anything else that is hard and creates fatigue without proper rest. This will only lead to muscles and bones tiring and being exhausted. Overall, it is easier to engage in some physical exertion than learning to avoid exhilaration. If you are constantly active with something from morning to night and don't plan proper rest periods, you'll get nervous and tense. Just make sure you are aware of your extreme point and take a good rest, then begin your activity anew. This in essence is the same principle as in the practice of healing exercises. Now, flowing water does not mold; a door hinge does not rust. This is so because they move a lot.

After a filling meal it is quite useless for the body to sit or lie down; much better to go out for a walk or work on a task at hand. Not doing that can lead to energetic blockages and indigestion, or cause paralysis in the extremities and dark spots in face and eyes, in general diminishing one's destiny.

Huangfu Long once asked the Master: "Can you summarize the key ways of how to apply the methods of mastering inner nature?" The Gray Ox Daoist replied: [10b] "The body always move.; your food always reduce. In moving, never reach extremes. In reducing, never get to naught. Eliminate fat and heavy things, control all salt and sour flavors. Diminish thoughts and worries, lessen joy and anger. Get out of being fast and rushing, watch out for sexual exhaustion. Do this always—and you'll see results!"

Pengzu says: People naturally receive *qi* so that, even if they do not know any specific long life techniques and just nurture it as best they can, they should reach a full 120 years. If they do not make it to this point, it is because they have caused harm to their *qi*. On the other hand, if they have reached even a minor level of understanding Dao, they can reach 240; if they in addition take a regular dose of medicinal supplements, they should make it to 480.

Along the same lines, Xi Kang says [in his *Yangsheng lun*]: Guiding and nourishing the *qi* and attaining life's underlying principle—at the most one can reach a thousand years, but at the least make it to a hundred.

Pengzu says: The method of nourishing life consists mainly in not harming oneself. That is really it. It means: stay warm in winter and cool in summer, but never stray from what is appropriate for each of the four seasons and what suits your body's needs.

Pengzu says: Heavy clothing and thick comforters that keep the body from strain and hardship lead to diseases caused by wind and cold. Spicy foods and fatty meats, gluttonous overeating and drop-dead intoxication [11a] lead to ailments due to rising and coagulating *qi*. Sexual attraction and beautiful women, a gaggle of bewitching concubines in the bedchamber, cause the misfortune of exhaustion and depletion. Lascivious voices and decadent songs that delude the mind and entice the ears cause the erroneous ways of dissipation and recklessness. Racing horses and exciting outings, going off to hunt in untamed country, cause the disaster of growing madness. Striving for military victory, exploiting local disorder and weakness, cause defeat due to pride and excess. Thus the sages' and wise men' warnings against uncontrolled and irrational behavior are the tools of long life, which are very much like water and fire: beware of losing control, lest benefit turns into disaster.

Pengzu says: People who do not have the right way of practice will take medicinal supplements and yet cause decline and harm, creating deficiencies in *qi* and blood, hollowness in muscles and bones, emptiness in marrow and brain, and overall illness in themselves. Then they are subject to harm from outside entities, such as wind and cold, wine and sex, that all reach out to them. If they had sustained fundamental inner fullness and solidity of *qi*, how could they ever get sick?

In general, all immortals agree:

Among sins, none is greater than lasciviousness.

Among transgressions, none is greater than greed.

Among bad behaviors, none is greater than slander.

These three are the carriers of disaster—

If minor, they endanger oneself;

If major, they cause destruction to one's entire clan. [11b]

If you want to extend your years and suffer little illness,

Be very careful about them!

Do not activate your essence, or your life is cut short and you die young.

Do not indulge greatly, or your bones and marrow start to dissolve.

Do not expose yourself to great cold, or your muscles and flesh are harmed.

Do not cough and spit, or you lose your rich inner juices.

Do not shout out loud, or you startle your precious souls.

Do not wallow in long bouts of crying, or you get depressed.

Do not get angry or enraged, or your spirit is unhappy.

Do not think and ponder a lot, or your volition gets blurred and confused.

If you follow all this, you will certainly live long!

Chapter Nine

Balancing Body, Food, and Sex

The succeeding five sections of the *Yangxing yanming lu* present specific methods of how best to enhance vitality, working in the areas of diet, daily hygiene, breathing, exercises, and sex. Much less relying on citations of earlier sources than the first section, their presentation is yet very close to materials also covered in the *Yangsheng yaoji* and the *Ishinpō*. While citing much the same sources—including also the *Zhubing yuanhou lun* and Sun Simiao's *Qianjin fang* works—the text yet provides its own unique slant to the topic.

More specifically, the second section on dietary measures (trl. Switkin 1987) focuses dominantly on moderation: eat natural and non preserved foods that are freshly cooked and not raw, grown locally and in season, paying particular attention to matching the proper flavors with the annual circulation of *qi*. Use medicinal supplements, but also in moderation; drink wine and enjoy banquets, but not to intoxication and not too often. Make sure that the meals enhance your health, paying attention to the needs of your body and its particular conditions.

Always leave a bit of room in the stomach, eating lightly especially at night, and balance the intake of food with movement—ideally a walk of a mile or so after a meal—so that digestion can work properly. In addition, there are certain foodstuffs and combinations (such as rabbit and ginger, scallions and honey) that have been linked with certain medical conditions and should be avoided completely. In other words, the section gives advice that echoes what other traditional longevity texts propose and what most modern physicians would agree with happily. It makes people aware of the importance of diet and guides them toward making educated choices and prudent life-style decisions.

Section three on "Miscellaneous Prescriptions" is aptly named, the central emphasis being on miscellaneous. The section is in no apparent order, placing classical advice against overdoing anything and deep emotional suggestions next to highly mundane taboos against taking baths or urinating in a certain way, then combining this with matters that we would classify as weird and superstitious. Its underlying theme is everyday conduct, not unlike a Farmers' Almanac outlining which activities are best undertaken when and in what manner to ensure greatest success and benefit to personal health and well-being.

It begins with a reiteration of the series of things to do "little," in this case physical and emotional exertion: no long standing, sitting, walking, or gazing; no excessive yearning, sadness, anger, or joy. Then it moves into a variety of themes. Maintaining a good cosmic connection, for example, involves avoiding strong winds and bright sunlight, pointing at the moon, or urinating while facing west, north, or while gazing at the celestial bodies. It also means making an effort to avoid harmful deeds and intentionally speak of good things—any words being observed by body gods residing in and around the mouth and thus immediately brought to the attention of the celestial authorities. By extension, it also means being respectful of Earth: not standing too close to a well, not pushing up on tiptoe near the Stove God, and not looking at a dead body unless first fortified by garlic against its pathogenic miasma.

On a more concrete level, daily practices concern such mundane things are taking a bath and washing one's hair, for which officials in ancient China got a day off once every ten days, a regulation also adopted in medieval monasteries (Kohn 2003, 117-18). As the text notes, baths should not be taken in mixed company or after a meal, and one should avoid standing around while wet and thus risk exposure to wind. Hair, too, should not be washed after a meal, rinsed with cold water, or spread to dry near a furnace, lest it catches fire.

Sleep is another area of regulation. The text insists that one should not eat or drink in bed and avoid singing or other stimulating activities before going to sleep. It stresses that it is best to place one's bedstead away from windows and beams, put the head toward east in spring and summer and toward west in fall and winter, lie down to rest on one side with the knees bent, and keep one's mouth closed while sleeping. It also notes that it is good to get up earlier in the lighter months and later when it is dark longer—a practice that again matches traditional monastic patterns and was still undertaken in the Baiyun guan 白雲觀 (White Cloud Temple) in Beijing when the Japanese Scholar Yoshioka Yoshitoyo stayed there in the 1940s (see Yoshioka 1979). In addition, the text here notes that one should not turn on a light after waking from a nightmare, but instead call the nightmare demon's name to exorcise the negative *qi*. Similarly after waking from sleep, one should not use cold water to wash or drink, lest harsh *qi* enters the body.

Beyond all this, the text provides distinctly Daoist suggestions by spelling out a healing mantra to be recited several times on a daily basis and by giving several visualization instructions—one involving seeing a red energy within oneself and allowing it to shine forth, the other using one's reflection in a mirror to enhance self-awareness and conscious spiritual empowerment. Many daily taboos outlined here echo things found in Daoist monastic manuals, but they also reflect quite a few items still in medical and Feng Shui use today. Their presentation in no apparent order—another feature the text has in common with Daoist lists of precepts, rules, and regulations (see Kohn 2004a)—makes their content appear more obscure than it really is.

The fourth section (trl. Jackowicz 2003) focuses on breathing exercises and ways of guiding the *qi*, summarized under the heading "Absorbing *Qi*." In addition to materials used already in Section 1, it also cites the *Yuanyang jing* 元陽經 (Scripture of Primordial Yang) and the *Fuqi jing* 服氣經 (Scripture of *Qi* Absorption). The former survives in truncated form the Daoist Canon (DZ 334), focusing on the life and practices of Daoist recluses as emulating those of Buddhists (Lagerwey in Schipper and Verellen 2004, 244-45); the latter may refer to any number of texts with *fuqi* in the title, notably those contained in ch. 59 of the *Yunji qiqian*. Their general tenor is that *qi* is the manifest form of Dao on earth and in the human body and by treating it correctly and enhancing its working, one can get closer to Dao. The ideal state to attain is "spirit pervasion" (*shentong* 神通), which means the emitting of a bright radiance and the attainment of supernatural powers. Perceiving fully with spirit instead of the senses, advanced longevity practitioners as much as Daoist immortals and enlightened Buddhists are omniscient and can penetrate all phenomena with equal ease—and the control and manipulation of *qi* is the prime way of getting there.

The practice is meditative in that it requires quietude of body and stillness of mind. It is also physical in that one should limit the intake of food and drink, place the body in a certain position (usually either sitting up straight or lying flat on one's back), then make one's hands into fists, thereby closing the Work Palace (*laogong* 勞宮) point in the center of the palm, through which *qi*—and with it the various kinds of souls—can easily leave the body.

Next *qi*-absorption begins with making the body fully present mentally as a network of energetic centers and passageways. Practitioners inhale deeply, mix the breath with saliva in the mouth, then swish the tongue around to enhance the saliva, and eventually swallow it down. They guide the *qi* consciously into the abdomen and from there move it throughout the body in different ways, like a cloud of subtle energy flowing everywhere both inside and outside. To enhance the awareness of *qi*, one may also hold the breath or "close in the *qi*" and perform self-massages to keep the *qi* moving in an even manner. Supplemented by the careful use of food, the method can also be used for healing purposes in that one may direct *qi* to areas that need release or attention.

Following this, in section five the text deals with healing exercises, beginning with a lengthy citation from the *Daoyin jing* (see ch. 5 above). It outlines several sets of practices that typically begin with alerting the body gods by clicking the teeth a certain number of times and practicing basic *qi*-absorption. This is followed by physical movements in different positions of the body, combined with deep breathing and the focused mental guiding of *qi*. Most exercises are done seated, kneeling, or standing, but some also work from a squat or from "lofty pose" (*junzuo* 峻坐), a wide-angled seat. The *Ishinpō* (ch. 27) and Sun Simiao's *Qianjin yifang* 千金翼方 describe it: "If you sit in the lotus posture when it is cold, you will warm up but then your legs will go to sleep. Sit lofty by opening the legs into a character *ba* 八 position [wide apart]. This will drive out the cold and alleviate the five kinds of piles" (Kohn 2008, 13, 145).

A typical exercise is: "Cross the arms above the head to cover the ears with the opposite hand, then lift up as high as you can. Release when you feel heat rising from below. Do twice seven repetitions. This will prevent deafness." The *Zhubing yuanhou lun*, in its chapter on "Seasonal Disorders," and Sun Simiao's *Qianjin yifang* (ch. 12) provide a more detailed description of this practice, adding that the right and left arms should be crossed over the head, allowing the hands to reach the opposite ear from above. Also, they should pull the hair at the same time to stimulate the skull and, in addition to deafness this will prevent the hair from turning white, create a glow in the face and youthfulness in the body (Mugitani 1987, 116). Another typical practice is rubbing the palms together to generate heat, then rubbing the face or even the entire body from top to bottom. The latter, called "dry wash" (*ganxi* 乾洗) in medieval sources, is still actively practiced in qigong today under the name "marrow washing."

Besides series of highly specific and detailed instructions, the text also mentions two specific exercises: Wolf Crouch and Owl Turn. The Wolf Crouch may be similar to the Tiger Catch described in Sun's *Qianjin fang*, which involves moving forward while turning the head back to look over one shoulder (Mugitani 1987, 114). As for the Owl Turn, the modern master Ni Hua-ching has an exercise called "The Immortal Imitating the Owl Turning Its Head," which involves sitting with the foot of one leg pressing into the thigh of the other leg, then leaning forward and turning to look over the extended leg (Ni 1989, 47).

Animal-based exercises such as these appear already in the *Zhuangzi*, which mentions the Bear Amble and the Bird Stretch, as well as in the early Han manuscripts. The most popular and best-known set, however, is the Five Animal Frolics (*wuqin xi* 五禽戲), outlined here for the first time in some technical detail and repeated in the late Tang work *Laojun Yangsheng jue* 老君養生訣 (Lord Lao's Instructions on Nourishing Life, DZ 821; Mugitani 1987, 119). They go back to the famous physician Hua Tuo 華佗 of the 2nd century. According to his biography in the *Sanguo zhi*, he once said to his disciple that he had developed a set of five animal-based exercises specifically to keep people moving and prevent aging, using the tiger, deer, bear, monkey, and bird for his model (Kohn 2008, 165). Developed and widely used over the millennia, the set is still very popular today, involving a variety of different practice, both standing and moving (Wang and Barrett 2006).

The last section of the text concentrates on sexual control and practices (trl. Wile 1992, 119-22). It refers to various sexual classics associated with divine ladies who taught their arts to the Yellow Emperor, notably the Plain Woman (Sunü 素女), the Mystery Woman (Xuannü 玄女), and the Colorful Woman (Cainü 彩女) (see Gulik 1961; Ishihara and Levy 1970; Reid 1989). It begins by emphasizing the importance of essence, the indeterminate yet powerfully concentrated form of *qi* that appears most clearly as sexual fluid (semen, blood) but also forms the core of more solid body parts: hair, brain, bones, teeth, and nails. Each person is given a certain amount of essence at birth and uses it over time in accordance with the cycle of sexual maturity. One essence is used up, the person dies. People lose it most actively lost during sex but they can also use sex to enhance and balance it—especially males whose ejaculation causes major loss, less so for females who lose their vitality through menstrual blood and most severely in child birth (see Furth 1999).

Celibacy in this context is not an option, since not using the vital fluids would cause them to stagnate and create health issues. Even monastic Daoists are guided to keep their essence movement, but they do it through internal circulation in solo practice—the exception being "duo cultivation," when practitioners energetically interact with a partner to enhance the flow of essence (see Winn 2006; Liu 2009). Thus the text strongly notes that neither men nor women like being alone and they both need each other.

In terms of specific practices, it reiterates certain standard taboos against sex during times of natural upheaval—eclipses, earthquakes, thunderstorm, extreme heat or cold—then notes that one can optimize energetic benefits by engaging in intercourse during the so-called royal days in each season, as defined by their cyclical names. Its other practice descriptions match the classic bedchamber arts (*fangzhong shu* 房中術) which taught men to have interrupted intercourse, ideally with as many women as possible, preferably young and healthy ones. They should bring their partners to orgasm so the women would emit their sexual essence but never have an ejaculation themselves, changing partners frequently to keep the energetic supply fresh. The core of the practice, however, is not the interruption or the partner change, but the internal circulation and personal energetic enhancement (see De Souza 2011), thus matching the various other methods of nourishing vitality.

Translation

Nourishing Inner Nature and Extending Life[1]

2. Dietary Prescriptions

[11b] The Perfected says: Though one may regularly take medicinal supplements, without knowing the arts of nourishing life, it is difficult to actually attain longevity. The Dao of nourishing inner nature is to avoid eating to satiation, followed by lying down or extended sitting day after day. These actions diminish longevity. Rather, one should exert the body somewhat but not to the point of fatigue or by forcing oneself to do what is utterly unattainable. After eating, go for a walk or leisurely stroll—that will assist cultivation. People say that flowing water does not mold; a door hinge does not rust. This is because they move and overexert themselves constantly. [12a]

On another note, it is better not to eat much at night; if you do, make sure to take a walk in the yard for several *li* [about a mile]. This is most excellent. Eating to satiation and then laying down causes the hundred diseases, including indigestion and energetic blockages. Eat little but often, never a lot all at once. Always feel a little hungry even when full, a little full even when hungry. And make sure to eat before you get really hungry and to drink before you get really thirsty: the problem being that once you notice you are hungry you'll be tempted to eat too much too fast; once you notice you are thirsty, you'll drink too much. The, of course, after the meal, go for a walk.

---

[1] Sections 2-6 of the *Yangxing yanming lu* (DZ 838).

After your walk, take some rice flour and rub it on your belly, massaging it for several hundred times. This will be of great benefit.

The Gray Ox Daoist notes similarly: When eating, don't ever fill yourself up beyond satiation. To prevent this, Daoists eat before they get hungry and never overdo; and they drink before they get thirsty.

After each meal, walk several hundred paces. This is a good start. If you can walk about five *li* after the evening meal and before you go to sleep, that will really help eliminate all sorts of ailments. Also, in taking food, it is best to eat hot food first, then warm food, and anything cold last. [12b] If after having hot or warm food there is nothing cold, then drink one or two swallows of cold water. This is truly amazing. Remember it well—it is the essential method of nourishing life. And please note that it is best to take a few subtle breaths before eating, consciously swallowing the *qi* in one or two gulps. This will make sure you remain free from disease.

The Perfected says: Hot food harms the bones; cold food harms the organs. Hot things burn the lips; cold things make the teeth ache. After taking any of these, you may feel hesitant or nervous. Still, in order to live long, eat good meals. There is nothing to much to talk about. Still, be aware that drinking a lot leads to obstructions in the channels and veins; getting intoxicated leads to the scattering of spirit. In the spring, increase spicy foods; in summer, sour; in the fall, bitter; and in winter, salty. These flavors support the five organs, enhance blood and *qi*, and eliminate the various diseases. However, do not indulge in excessive eating of any of the flavors, whether sour, salty, sweet, [spicy], or bitter.

Also, match the organs with the seasons: in spring, do not consume liver; in summer, do not have heart; in the fall, abstain from taking lungs; and in winter, do not eat kidneys. Try to avoid taking spleen throughout the year. In this way the five organs are perfectly matched with the annual rhythm of Heaven. Also, avoid eating swallows, which are devoured by dragons upon entering the water and are very inauspicious to kill.

[13a] Going to sleep immediately after eating a good meal leads to disease and causes back pain. Drinking alcohol is fine as long as it is not too much, otherwise you'll get hick-ups. That is not so good. Falling asleep drunk you won't be able to control the wind nor manage to use a fan, all of which will diminish people's marrow. If you don't match your diet to the seasons, you will cause harm to the five organs. Also when drunk, don't be tempted to eat vigorously lest you develop piles and ulcers. Being drunk and full at the same time at the very least will cause facial discoloring and dry coughs; at worst, it will seriously hurt the organs and channels and cause a shortened life.

Always when eating, preserve the warmth of the food. When taken warm, it is easy to digest and superior to eating anything cold. Also, cooked food in general is better than raw; eating a little is better than having a lot. After a satisfying meal, don't go out galloping a horse or your mind will turn silly. When drinking water, don't gulp it down suddenly, or you'll get *qi* ailments and urinary troubles. If you have fermented milk, don't also take vinegar, or you'll get bloody phlegm and acid blood. If, when eating hot food you find yourself perspiring, do not wash the face, or you'll lose your color and your complexion will be as gray as a worm. Once done with the hot food, do not rinse the mouth with vinegar or fermented sauces, or your mouth will reek and your teeth rot. [13b]

Try to avoid getting a horse's sweat, breath, or hair into the food, because they can cause injury. Do not eat poultry, rabbit, and dog in the same meal. Anything fermented, dried on the eaves, or canned in water is preserved. We call it "densely preserved": it diminishes life.

If ever you are hungry for a long time, don't eat your fill immediately or suffer from constipation. Similarly, eating a lot at night and going to sleep without covering yourself properly predisposes you to death from cholera. When you first come down with it, make sure to avoid raw fish which causes incessant diarrhea. And, of course, in normal times, when you eat raw fish, do not join it with fermented milk, which causes it to turn into worms. Similarly, when eating rabbit, do not have dried ginger; this causes cholera. And when eating meat in general, do not select the fatty parts from the top. Having been looked at intensely by everyone, it causes energetic blockages and leaky boils.

Then again, do not eat fresh fruit on an empty stomach; this causes heat above the diaphragm and abscesses on the bones. Copper lids on cooking vessels tend to cause condensation which drops into the food. If you eat it, you may develop sores and carbuncles. If you have an unresolved cold and eat hot food, you may get wicked wind. You may drink alcohol but if you wash your face with cold water before the fever is gone, you'll get sores on the face. [14a]

After a satisfying meal, don't wash your hair or risk getting a head wind. When eating buckwheat with pork, don't have more than three portions; otherwise you'll be subject to hot wind. When drying meat, do not put with glutinous millet or hulled rice in the same earthen jar, because eating this combination will block off the *qi.* Roast dried meat over an open fire but don't move the coals about; only move them after you have taken it out. Don't eat its intersecting strands of tendons lest you suffer from afflictions and eventually die.

Between a sheep's shoulder blades there is a cut which looks like pearls and is called "sheep's hanging tendons." Eat this and you will suffer from epilepsy. Damp foods tend to be vague and you cannot see a clear shape or shadow. Eat it and you will get stomach ulcers. After contracting violent bowel disease [diarrhea], do not drink wine, since it heats the area above the diaphragm. When recovering from the disease, do not eat raw jujubes or mutton. Raw vegetables at this junction would be injurious to the complexion and may harm the entire body. If you do not recover properly, death may result from too much heat above the diaphragm.

When eating deep-fried cakes or other fatty items, do not drink cold vinegar, fermented juices, or water. Otherwise you'd likely lose your voice or get a bad case of the hiccups. Fresh scallions mixed with honey are not good for you. By all means avoid dried meat in conjunction with water. [14b] It develops a movement on its own which may well kill you. When producing sun-dried meat, do not let it get scorched. Do not eat sheep's liver and do not add hot peppers—they can harm the heart. Eating melon with mutton can cause fever. Too much wine with meat is called debauchery or gluttony and can lead to depression and madness.

Not regularly taking medicinal supplements and instead indulging in the five grains—that is the sign of a mediocre practitioner. Worried about getting sick and nourishing on *qi* while preserving essence and visualizing the spirit—that shows a high master. Such a one will live as long as Heaven itself.

3. Miscellaneous Prescriptions and Taboos: Releasing Harm and Inviting Goodness

> Long gazing harms the blood; long resting harms the *qi*;
> Long standing harms the bones; long walking harms the tendons;
> Long sitting harms the flesh. In general,

> Yearning for strength and vigor harms the person;
> Melancholy, anger, grief, and pity harm the person;
> Excessive joy and pleasure harm the person;
> Unresolved wrath and anger harm the person;
> Constantly striving to fulfill wishes harms the person;
> Distress over afflictions harms the person;
> Imbalance in cold and heat harm the person;
> Lack of yin-yang exchange harms the person. [15a]

In all exchanges, rely on healing exercises and the various longevity arts. Just avoid all that harms your person and engage in the bedchamber arts: this is the way of no-death.

> Great joy makes the *qi* soar wildly; great sadness makes it stagnate.
> Using essence causes people's *qi* and strength to fade;
> Too much gazing causes people's eyes to go blind;
> Too much sleep causes people's mind to be troubled;
> Fondness for rich food causes people diarrhea.

Ordinary people only know how to desire the five flavors; they do not realize that one can also sip primordial *qi*. The sage, on the other hand, is well aware that the five flavors cause disease; therefore he does not desire them. He realizes that one can absorb primordial *qi* and accordingly closes his mouth and does not speak, as a result of which his essence and *qi* are spontaneously in good accord. Saliva not swallowed, the Ocean [of *Qi*] is not moistened; the Ocean not moistened, the body fluids dry up. Thus we know that absorbing primordial *qi* and drinking the sweet spring [of saliva] is the foundation of extending life.

Bathing without regularity is inauspicious; so is bathing in mixed company. Bathing and soon getting drunk and filling up, then going for a long walk will lead to great fatigue and the inability to engage in the bedchamber arts. [15b]

A cautious elder who has fallen ill should not lie down with his head toward the north. This causes his six spirits to be uneasy. Someone who tends toward depression and is very forgetful should not stand on the toes near a well. An important rule, valid both today and in ancient times, is that seeing a ten-foot earth wall is not an invitation to sit or lie on it.

Avoid being blown on by strong winds, which can lead to epilepsy. And make sure never to glare at the sun or moon in rage, which might cause loss of eyesight.

People tend to pull off their clothes when they sweat heavily. If not careful, this can lead to many afflictions, including wind-ailments on one side. Never, following a bath, expose your unprotected head to the wind. If unlucky, there is a great wind and you get cut by it and invaded by cold. On the other extreme, do not bring fire near your face, which might cause convulsions and insanity.

Always when perspiring do not tiptoe or hang your legs; if you do this for a long time you will get rheumatism; your feet feel very heavy, and your hip starts to ache.

Always when the feet are perspiring, do not put them into cold water, because this might cause rheumatism in the bones as well as arterial blockages. Also, do not hold off on urinating for a long period, lest your knees become cold and numb and you invite rheumatism into your joints.

Always when you sweat from eating hot food, do not expose yourself to the wind; this might create blockages and headaches, which in turn may lead to blurred vision and great sleepiness.

Always when ready to go to sleep, it is inappropriate to sing or chant. After getting up, do not talk a lot, which might diminish your *qi*. [16a]

Always when a flying bird drops into the midst of people, they should not consume it; neither should birds whose beaks are open or that have sores under their feathers.

Always when washing the hair with very hot water, then rinsing with cold water you will get a head wind.

Always when lying down, avoid having your head right next to a lighted furnace, which might cause the head to be heavy, the eyes to be red, and the nose to be dry.

Always after sleep, make sure not to place the head next to a lighted lamp, which might cause the six spirits to become uneasy. During the winter, warm the feet and let the head remain cool; in spring and fall, allow both head and the feet to stay relatively cool. This, then, is the basic method of the sages.

Always when just done crying don't eat immediately let you get ailments of *qi*. At night when lying down, do not cover the head. A married woman should not stand on her tiptoes or squat near the hearth: this is a great taboo.

Always when spitting, don't' spit far lest you develop a lung ailment which may cause the hands to be heavy, the back to ache, and a cough to start.

Always when waking up from a nightmare, do not light the lamp and shine it on the nightmare demon or you will die. Leave it dark and call out the demon's name, and good fortune will ensue. But make sure you do not get close to it or call out in great anxiety.

Always avoid sleeping with your mouth open, because over a longer time this will cause great thirst and loss of blood coloring. [16b]

Always when getting up in the morning, do not use cold water to open the eyes and wash the face; this may result in blurred vision, loss of sparkle, and tearing.

Always when walking along a country road in the heat of summer and come to a river, do not wash the face, lest you create dark skin. Waking up suddenly after a deep sleep, don't drink water and sleep some more lest you get rheumatism.

Always when you perspire while being sick don't drink cold water which diminishes the *qi* of heart and stomach and prevents recovery.

Always avoid seeing or smelling a rotting carcass on an empty stomach, lest its *qi* enter your nose and you get sick.

Always if you wish to look upon a dead body, first drink wine and chew garlic to ward off its toxic *qi.*

Always prevent little children from pointing their fingers at the moon. Sores behind the two ears are called lunar eclipse sores. Pound toads into powder and apply that to them for a cure; it will also prevent other kinds of sores.

Always prevent a pregnant woman from looking at foxes or smell other people lest she get overly swollen.

Always when sleeping, avoid places right under windows and beams, which might cause the six spirits to become uneasy.

Always when sleeping in the spring and in summer, have your head toward the east; in fall and in winter, toward the west. This is most beneficial. [17a]

Always when you are hungry, urinate squatting down; after eating, urinate standing up; this keeps you free from disease.

Always when going to sleep, lie on one side with the knees bent; this increases the *qi* and vigor. Also, change sides every so often.

Always speak softly and smile a lot, getting to a point where you speak very little; never make loud sounds.

In spring sleep after dark and get up early; in summer and fall sleep at dusk and get up early; in winter sleep early and get up late. Each brings benefit. People commonly say: "Getting up early is not before cockcrow; getting up late is not after sunrise." In winter, as Heaven and Earth seal the yang-*qi* in the organs, people should not exert themselves to the point of perspiration, which causes yang-*qi* to leak and brings injury to the person.

Fresh from the bath, do not stand around and chat with your body still damp and exposed to the wind; nor lie down with a damp head lest you get head wind, blurred vision, hair loss, facial swellings, toothache, and possibly deafness. Don't walk around in damp or sweaty clothes for a long time, lest you get sores and itches. [17b]

Lord Lao said: In the first month, go out into the courtyard at dawn, stand facing east, bow several times, and chant: "I, so-and-so, year after year have received the grace of the Great Dao. Oh, Mysterious Gate of Great Clarity, I pray that you let me recover the benefits of the year so-and so just past!"

Both men and women should repeat this three times for best effect. If done consistently, it will extend your years. NOTE: The *Sunü jing* contains methods to purify spirit. The *Huainanzi* speaks of rules in venerating the stove god. Either wish to create a harmony of the body with the numinous perfected and to preserve a life of perfection.

Immortals' scriptures and texts on secret essentials all note that one should constantly be aware of one's heart *qi*, envisioning it like a chicken egg with the color red on the inside and yellow on the outside. This will help to avoid evil influences and prolong life. To get rid of further evil influences and the hundred demons, be constantly aware of it [the heart *qi*] as a blazing fire, a resplendent Dipper. As you keep this light bright, the hundred demons do not dare approach, and you may freely go even into the middle of an epidemic. At night, before going to sleep, moreover, always actualize red *qi* on the outside and white *qi* on the inside, enveloping your entire body. This, too, will keep you free from evil influences and all kinds of specters.

Lord Lao said: In pursuing Dao, never commit the five offensive acts and six unlucky deeds. Committing these brings great misfortune. [18a] The five offensive acts are excreting or urinating facing 1) west, 2) north, 3) the sun, 4) the moon, and 5) while gazing at the sky and the stars. The six unlucky deed are: 1) getting up at night and exposing oneself, 2) getting up at dawn in a rage, 3) cursing in the direction of the stove god, 4) stepping on the hearth fire, 5) having sex during the daytime, and 6) robbing or cheating a teacher or elders.

Always, when getting up in the morning, if you continuously speak of good things, Heaven will bring you good fortune. Do not just talk about anything or go about singing and whistling: that invites misfortune, so be very careful to avoid it.

Other sources of misfortune are: singing while lying in bed, going to sleep on the belly, eating or drinking in bed, and banging on a dish with spoons or chopsticks.

The Ruler of Yin resides on the left of people's mouths. Any nasty or malicious [words] he immediately notes and reports to Heaven. Heaven then judges one's spirit and material souls. The Ruler of Death resides on the right side of people's mouths. He immediately notes any bad speech and reports it to the Ruler of Destiny. The Ruler of Destiny records it in the ledger of sins; once it is full, he orders the person killed. [18b] The two deities continuously inspect the mouth, looking for faults in people. How can you not be careful of your speech! The tongue is the body's front troop; it brings forth all good and evil. Thus Daoists have many taboos about it.

Among other things, they recommend taking Jade Spring to prolong life and eliminate diseases. Jade Spring is the saliva in the mouth. Rinse and swallow with Jade Spring seven times every day at the six hours, i.e., at cockcrow, daybreak, noon, mid- afternoon, dusk, and midnight. Each time, make sure there it fills the mouth completely before swallowing. This prolongs life, fortifies hair and blood, strengthens teeth and bones, and enhances nails and muscles. Add a thousand strokes when combing the hair and it will not turn white. Also, every morning and evening click your teeth and they will not rot. Limit nail cutting and exercise your muscles.

Also, frequently focus on your reflection in the mirror in a practice called "visualizing the body." It means visualizing the body together with its spirits. Just looking at yourself, admiring your face and complexion for pure amusement is not the thing—but it is better than never working with the reflection. [19a]

Always in the early morning of the following days collect goji berries and boil them into a concoction:[2] 1/1, 2/2, 3/3, 4/8, 5/1, 6/27, 7/11, 8/8, 9/21, 10/14, 11/11, and 12/13. Add it to your bath. It will make you glow and keep you free from disease well into ripe old age.

At the time of lunar eclipses, try to save lives by getting rid of evil spirits. If you save as many as ten thousand, you gain the same merit as Heaven. [NOTE: Heaven does not like killing and sages follow its model. Not liking to kill means supporting Heaven and Earth in their continuous nurturing. Thus it invites good fortune.] Good dreams—talk about them; bad dreams—be quiet. This, too, nourishes inner nature and prolongs life.

4. Absorbing Qi to Cure Diseases

[2.1a] The *Yuanyang jing* states: Always take in the *qi* through the nose, then hold it in the mouth and rinse with it until it is full. Allow it to envelope the tongue and the lips and teeth, then swallow it. If you can do a thousand such swallowings in one day and night, this is most excellent. Also, eat and drink little. If you eat and drink too much, the *qi* rebels and the hundred arteries close up. If the hundred arteries close up, the *qi* will not circulate. If the *qi* does not circulate, disease arises.

---

[2] Common in the north and west of China, goji berries are considered life-prolonging, constructive, and energy enhancing. They improve complexion and eyesight, help with wasting disease and pulmonary consumption, and benefit the kidneys and sexual organs. See Stuart 1976, 250.

The *Xuanshi* (Mysterious Instructions) says: The will is the commander of the *qi*. The *qi* is the plenitude of the body. Doing good enhances life; doing evil destroys the body.

Thus the method of circulating *qi* consists of eating little, moderating oneself, moving the body, and harmonizing the *qi*. When the blood begins to feel light, stop the practice. Do not overdo it, [1b] or you will lose your gains and have to go back to the beginning.

As for the formalities [of practice], when swallowing *qi*, sit up with a straight body, be upright in your form, and keep your mind and intention focused and concentrated. Firmly guard yourself inside and out, above and below. Completely enclose the spirit, encircle the physical form, open and enhance the Four Extremes, and nurture the Primordial Pass. Once all is full and sufficiently replete, all pathogenic [*qi*] will leave of itself.

Pengzu says: Always hold the breath and practice breathing from sunrise to noon. Kneeling, rub the eyes, massage the body, lick the lips, swallow the saliva, and work with the *qi*. Repeat ten times, then stand up and move around, laughing and speaking. If you are tired and exhausted and not at peace, use stretching exercises and holding the breath to treat your affliction. Visualize the body clearly: head, face, nine orifices, five organs, four limbs, even the tips of the hairs. All has to be present. Become aware of the *qi* as a cloud circulating in the body, rising up to the nose and mouth and descending to the tips of the ten fingers. This will lead to purity and harmony, and a perfect spirit.

There is no need for needles, herbs, moxa, or blood-letting. Rather, circulate the *qi* in order to expel the hundred ailments. Follow it wherever it is needed and develop clear awareness there. If your head hurts, become aware of your head; if your foot hurts, become aware of your foot, using harmonized *qi* to attack the pain. From one moment to the next, it will dissolve by itself. [2a] If the *qi* is internally cold or frozen, enclose it [by holding the breath] to cause sweating. When sweat emerges it regulates the body, and the cold will be dissolved.

Circulating and enclosing the *qi* are the essentials of healing the body. Still, you must first properly understand their principles. Also, it is important to be empty and open, not full and satiated. If the *qi* has convergences and clogs, it cannot be open and flowing but will develop a mass. It is like a wellspring which must be neither obstructed nor exhausted. If, therefore, you eat delicacies such as fresh fish, fresh vegetables, and rich meats, joy and anger, anxiety and frustration will never leave. Rather, circulating the *qi* makes people develop superior *qi*. Anyone wishing to learn this method of circulation of *qi* should always use a step-by-step approach.

Liu Jun'an states: "Take in life, expel death—then you can live forever." This means: breathing through the nose is life, exhaling through the mouth is death. Normal people don't know how to absorb their *qi* in this way. You should always, from morning to night, breathe slowly and gently, inhaling through the nose and exhaling through the mouth. This is called "expelling the old and inhaling the new."

The *Fuqi jing* (Scripture of *Qi* Absorption) has: Dao is *qi*. Guard the *qi*, and you can realize Dao. Realize Dao, and you can live forever. Spirit is essence. [2b] Guard the essence and the spirit will be bright. When the spirit is bright, you can live long. Essence is the flow of blood and arteries, the numinous spirit that protects the bones. When essence leaves, the bones wither. When the bones wither, there is death. For this reason, to practice Dao you must treasure your essence.

From midnight to noon is the time of living *qi*. From noon to midnight is the time of dying *qi*. Always practice during the time of living *qi*. Lie down straight, close your eyes, and curl your hands into fists. [NOTE: Curling your hands into fists is making fists like an infant would, with the four fingers enclosing the thumb.]

Hold the breath. Mentally count to 200 [heart beats], then expel the *qi* by exhaling through the mouth. As you breathe like this for an increasing number of days, you will find your body, spirit, and five organs are at peace. If you can hold the breath to the count of 250, your Flowery Canopy will be bright. [NOTE: The Flowery Canopy is the eyebrows.]

Your eyes and ears will be perceptive and clear, and your body will be light and free from disease; nothing pathogenic bothers you any more.

To circulate the *qi*, inhale through the nose and exhale through the mouth. Allow the breath to become subtle and draw it out longer. This is called the long breath. Its inhalation is just one, but its exhalation comes in six different forms. [3a] The one way to inhale is with the sound of *xi*, the six ways to exhale involve the sounds *chui, hu, xi, he, xu,* and *si*. Ordinary people breathe one *xi*, one *hu*, and originally that's all there was. If you want to practice the exhalation method of the long breath, use *chui* when you are cold and *hu* when you are warm. The sounds are most excellent in the curing of diseases. *Chui* will drive out wind; *hu* will drive out heat, *xi* will drive out afflictions, *he* will make the *qi* descend; *xu* will disperse blockages, and *si* will moderate stress. Since ordinary people are frequently given to extremes, they will use a lot of *xu* and *si*. *Xu* and *si* re the core of the long breath.

This is a method that men and women can equally use in visualization. The method comes from an immortal's scripture. To circulate the *qi*, first remove the hair from the nostrils. We call this the road to spirit pervasion.

At times of fresh dew, evil wind, fierce cold, and great heat, do not take in *qi* like this.

The *Mingyi xubing lun* says: The reason why diseases arise is because of the five exertions. Once these are present, they will affect the two organs of the heart and kidneys which will in turn be subject to pathogenic *qi*. Then organs and viscera will equally become diseased. [3b] The five exertions are through 1) will, 2) thinking, 3) mind, 4) worry, and 5) fatigue. They create six forms of extreme pressure in the body, specifically in 1) *qi*, 2) blood, 3) tendons, 4) bones, 5) essence, and 6) marrow. These six forms of extreme pressure in turn cause the seven injuries which transform into the seven pains. The seven pains create disease.

People today have much pathogenic and only little proper *qi*. They are confused and likely to forget things, always grievous and injured, do not enjoy their food and drink, and do not gain weight and robustness. Their facial complexion is without glossiness, their hair turns white and they wither away. When this becomes serious, the person is subject to great wind. He will be stooped and brittle, his tendons restricting the four limbs from agility and pulling together the hundred joints. There will be blockages of the diaphragm, numbing of the body, shortness of breath, and many aches in the waist and back. This condition arises because people marry early and overuse their sexual essence. Due to this, their *qi* and blood become insufficient, which causes the arrival of the labors and forms of stress.

Usually when disease arrives and does not leave it is a matter of the five organs. If this happens, you must first get to understand the root [of the disease]. Unless you know the root, there is nothing you can do. [4a] Thus, people with heart disease tend to have cold and heat in their bodies, and the two breaths *hu* and *chui* will eliminate that. People with lung problems tend to have a feeling of distension and fullness in their chest and back; the *xu* breath will take care of that. People with spleen problems tend to have and upward floating wind and a habitual itchy ache in their bodies; the *xi* breath will eliminate this. People with liver disease tend to have eye pain, worry, anxiety, and no joy; the *he* breath should take care of that.

In all the twelve methods of aligning the *qi* described above, always pull the *qi* in through the nose and expel it from the mouth. Use *qi*-sounds that sound like the words *chui, hu, xu, he, xi* and *si* when you expel it. If you suffer from any affliction, rely on the method and all the [diseases] will come to honor and respect you. Apply your mind while doing it and all diseases will be cured without fail. This is the central art of long life.

5. Exercises and Massages[3]

The *Daoyin jing* says: In the early morning, before you get up, first click your teeth for two sets of seven. Then close your eyes, make your hands into fists, move your mouth three times as if rinsing to fill it with saliva, then swallow and hold. Hold the breath until you reach your maximum. When you cannot hold it any longer, let it out very, very slowly. Do three repetitions, then stop. [4b]

After this, rise to do the Wolf Crouch and the Owl Turn, shake yourself to the right and left, and again hold the breath in until you reach your maximum. Do three repetitions, then get off the bed. Make your hands into fists and hold the breath in while stomping the heels three times, then raise one arm and lower the other, and again hold the breath in to your maximum. Do three repetitions. Next, interlace the fingers behind the head and twist to your right and left, holding the breath each time. Do three repetitions. Now, stand up to stretch from both feet, again interlace the fingers, revolve the palms, and press forward. Hold the breath. Repeat three times. Do this entire sequence every morning and evening, completing at least three repetitions, but if can do more, so much the better.

Also, at dawn, do the following. Rub the palms of both hands together until they generate heat, then press them firmly over the eyes. Repeat three times. Next, with your fingers stimulate the four corners of the eyes. This will give you bright vision.[4]

According to the classical texts, "making the hands into fists" is the method by which one controls the [body's] gates with the help of the spirit souls and closes its doors with the help of the material souls. It means that you join your spirit and materials souls in securing the gates and doors of the body, thereby stabilizing your essence, brightening your eyes, maintaining your years, and reversing any white hair you may have. If you do this, especially in the winter months, all kinds of pathogenic *qi* and the hundred toxins cannot harm you. [NOTE: To make a fist, bend the thumb and curl it under the four fingers. [5a] With prolonged, uninterrupted practice you will no longer need to open they eyes [to make sure]. There is also a theory which says that the practice will prevent people from encountering demons and sprites.]

---

[3] The majority of passages in this section are also found in chapter 27 of *Ishinpo*. They are largely identical, albeit, arranged in a different order and on occasion ascribed to a different text. See Mugitani 1987, 113-19.

[4] Here ends the citation from the *Daoyin jing* (see ch. 5 above). The last exercise on bright eyes is also found in the *Zhubing yuanhou lun*, under "Eye Diseases."

The *Yangsheng neijie* (Inner Explanations on Nourishing Life) says: 1) semen; 2) saliva; 3) tears; 4) mucus; 5) sweat; and 6) urine—these are what diminishes human life. However, the diminishing can be light or severe. If you can refrain from losing mucus and saliva throughout your life and instead practice rinsing and filling the mouth [with saliva] and swallowing it— steadily holding it as if you were sucking on a date pit—you can support your *qi* and vitalize your body fluids. This is the main essence of the practice. [NOTE: This refers to the gathering of saliva and fluids. There is no real sucking on a date pit]

Every morning, click the teeth thirty-six times or more, ideally up to 300. This makes the teeth firm and prevents toothache. Next, rub the tongue around the mouth in a rinsing motion until the mouth is filed with saliva, then swallow. Repeat three times before you stop. Now rub the palms of the hands together until they generate heat and press them firmly over the eyes. Do twice seven repetitions and stop. This will give you clear vision.

Also, every morning when you first get up:

1. Cross the arms above the head to cover the ears with the opposite hand, then lift as high as you can. Release when you feel heat rising from below. Do twice seven repetitions. This will prevent deafness. [5b] According to another variant, begin by clicking the teeth and rinsing the mouth with Jade Spring [saliva] to swallow three times. Contract the nose [to inhale slowly] and hold the breath in while stretching the right hand above the head and reaching to the left ear. Do twice seven repetitions.

2. Take the left hand, stretch it above the head and reach it over to the right ear. Again do twice seven repetitions. This will help extend the years without going deaf.

3. Pull the hair on both temples to lift up the area. Do one set of 7, then gather the hair in both hands and pull it upward as far as you can, lifting it with vigor. Do one set of seven. This will open the flow of blood and *qi* and prevent the hair from turning white.

According to another technique, rub your hands together until they generate heat, then rub the face from top to bottom, eliminating all pathogenic *qi*. This will help you maintain a radiant glow on your face. Yet another way is to rub the hands together for heat, then rub and pound the entire body from top to bottom. This is called "dry wash." It will help you overcome wind and cold, seasonally hot *qi*, and headaches, as well as driving out the hundred diseases in general. Also at night, when you are ready to lie down, always rub your whole body. This, too, is a form of "dry wash." This will help you avoid harm from wind and pathogenic *qi*.

Another set of exercises begins by sitting in lofty pose [legs spread wide].

1. Look up and support your head [from the back] with your left hand, then use the right hand to turn the head upward. Move the hands back and forth with vigor. Do three repetitions. [6a] Reverse. Support the head with the right hand and move the hands back and forth. Do three repetitions. This will help eliminate sleepiness and fatigue.

2. In the early morning, before the sun rises, face south and sit in lofty pose. Place your hands on the soft flesh under the cheek bones. Press [the knuckles] strongly into this area, moving the hands back and forth. Do three repetitions. This will help maintain a radiant complexion on the face.

3. In the early morning before you have combed and washed, sit in lofty pose and with your left hand press your right hand down on top of your left knee; lean forward and push strongly on that knee. Repeat three times.

4. With your right hand press your left hand down on top of your right knee; lean forward and push strongly on that knee. Repeat three times.

5. Interlace the hands, stretch them forward, and push strongly. Repeat three times.

6. Interlace the hands again, press them in toward the chest, allowing the elbows to move forward and pushing them strongly together. Repeat three times.

7. Pull the left shoulder back while curling the right shoulder forward. With the same strength it would take to draw a fifteen-pound bow, draw the bow with the right hand, constantly maintaining the level of exertion. Repeat and reverse.

8. Place your right hand on the floor while raising your left hand up to push strongly against the sky. Repeat and reverse.

7. Curl your hands into fists and punch forward right and left. Do three sets of seven on each side. [6b]

8. Curl the left hand into a fist and strongly grip the fingers while moving the hand up the back. Repeat three times, then do the same with the right hand. This will help eliminate labored *qi* from the back, shoulder blades, shoulders, and elbows. The more often you repeat the exercise, the better.

At dawn, once you have completely one whole cycle, you can go further by sitting up, placing a long pole under your armpits [to hold the back straight] and hanging your left leg off the bed. In this position, slowly lift the leg straight up, then strongly pull it toward you. Do five sets of seven repetitions, then repeat with the right leg. This will help alleviate aches and sluggishness in the leg *qi,* cold *qi* in the pelvis-kidney area, and all kinds of rheumatism and cold stiffness in the knees and legs. It will take care of all of these.[5] If you add three sets of this in the evening, the effect will be even better. But make sure you do not do the exercise when you have just eaten or need to urinate. Also, if you do not have a staff handy, modify the practice by supporting your hand on an object behind you while pulling in the leg. Make sure the leg never touches the ground.

Also, every morning and evening, with brush your hair up to a thousand times. This will help eliminate all wind from the head and prevent your hair from turning white.[6] Once done with the brushing, if you take salt granules and fresh sesame oil to rub on the top of the head you will benefit even more. It is like rubbing a spirit salve on yourself, very good, indeed. Then again, when you decide to wash and groom your hair, make sure to first click your teeth 160 times, then collect saliva and swallow. To purify further, rinse your mouth with water and scour the teeth with a salty twig. [7a]

Holding the clear, slightly sour liquid in your mouth, swirl it around as if rinsing and allow it to become somewhat hot. Then spit the salty solution into your hands hand use it to wash the eyes. Once done, close the eyes and wash the face with cold water, making sure that the water does not get into your eyes. This procedure will make the teeth firm and clean, the eyes bright and tearless, and forever prevent rotting teeth. After washing the face and rinsing the mouth, moreover, swallow one or two mouthfuls of cold water. This will make the heart bright and clean, and eliminate heat from the chest and breast.

The physician Hua Tuo from Qiao County was very good at nourishing life. He had two main disciples Wu Pu from Guangling and Fan A from Pengcheng who studied these arts with him. Once Hua told Pu: "The human body needs a certain amount of movement, but it should not be carried to extremes. If the body undergoes regular movement, the grain *qi* is assimilated properly into the blood, the meridian flow is open, and disease will stay away. It can be compared to a door hinge that never rusts. The immortals of old and certain Daoists and practitioners in the Han dynasty accordingly practiced the art of gymnastics. [7b]

"They did the bear stretch and the owl turn, pulling the pelvis and rotating the joints—thereby holding old age at bay. I myself have developed a system called the Five Animals' Frolic. They are: 1.tiger; 2. deer; 3. bear; 4. monkey; and 5. bird. To eliminate disease and benefit the limbs, regularly practice these exercises. If there is an area of discomfort in the body, do one

---

[5] The *Zhubing yuanhou lun* has the same sequence under "Cold Disorders" (Mugitani 1987, 117)

[6] This practice is also noted in *Zhubing yuanhou lun*, under "Hair Disorders."

of the Animal Frolics. Practice until sweat has arisen, then stop. Cover the body with powder, and soon you will notice how it becomes lighter and how your appetite is improving." Wu Pu followed this practice and even in his nineties enjoyed keen hearing, clear eyesight, and a full set of strong teeth, able to eat like a youngster.

The Tiger Frolic: Squat on the floor with all four limbs. Move forward for three steps and back for two. In each case, begin by lengthening one hip forward while raising the opposite leg back and up into the air. Then place the leg back into the squatting position, moving forward or back. Do seven sets.

The Deer Frolic: Squat on the floor with all four limbs. Extend the neck forward and look back over your shoulder, three times to left and twice to the right. Next, stretch the legs, extending and contracting them also in a rhythm of three and 2.

The Bear Frolic: Squat on the floor with your hands wrapped around the legs below knees. Look straight up, then lift your head while stomping down alternately with your feet, completing seven repetitions on each side. [8a] Return to a straight squat and lengthen the back with your hands pushing off the floor.

The Monkey Frolic: Holding on to a horizontal bar, hang straight down by the arms and stretch the entire body. Contact and extend for one set of seven repetitions. Next, drape the legs over the same bar, hang down and curl and release your arms to the right and left. Do seven repetitions.

The Bird Frolic: Stand up straight, place both hands on the floor, and lift up one leg at a time, letting it soar upward while stretching the shoulders and lifting the eyebrows. Do it with strength. Repeat for two sets of seven. Then sit down, extend the legs forward, and with your hands grab the heels of the feet. Do seven repetitions. Sit up straight, contract and extend the shoulders seven times each.

Practice the Five Animals' Frolic with vigor so that a healthy sweat begins to flow. Once sweaty, cover the body with powder. This aids the digestion of grains, increase overall *qi*, and eliminate the hundred diseases. If you do them persistently, moreover, you will extend your years.

According to yet another method, sit quietly before all meals and rub yourself down. Then interlace the fingers, stretch the shoulders and thighs, and thereby open up all the energy channels. This exercise is as invigorating as drinking an herbal concoction.

Also, if you kneel upright and exhale while looking up, all *qi* blockages due to a full stomach or alcohol imbibing will dissolve immediately. If you do this in summer, moreover, you will feel cool and not hot. [8b]

6. Sexual Control to Diminish and Increase [Life]

The Dao treasures [sexual] essence. Expand it, and give life to a new person; retain it, and give life to your own body. Giving life to your own body, you can pursue transcendence among the ranks of the immortals. Giving life to a new person, you gain merit and neglect your body. Gaining merit and neglecting your body, your get increasingly mired in desire. How much worse, then, if you foolishly expand your sexual essence and wastefully discard it, diminishing your life constantly? Without realizing just how much you are losing, you get tired and exhausted, and your destiny declines.

Heaven and Earth have yin and yang. Yin and yang are highly valued among people, and the more they value these forces, the more they can join with Dao. Just be careful not to waste them.

Pengzu says: The highest practitioners sleep alone in their bed; medium practitioners at least have separate blankets. Taking a thousand pills of supplements is nowhere near as good as sleeping alone.

Colors make the eyes go blind; sounds make the ears go deaf; flavors make the palate go numb [*Daode jing* 12]. If you can follow this path regularly and consistently, and appropriately restrain and intensify [your sexual activity], you can open all sorts of blockages in the body and as a result attain long life.

The day-taboo means not eating to fullness in the evening. [NOTE: If you eat to fullness at night and go to bed with a full stomach, you will lose one day of your life.] The month-taboo means not drinking to intoxication in the evening. [NOTE: If you drink to intoxication at night, you will lose one month of your life.] [9a] In the evening, one should stay away from the inner chamber. [NOTE: One interchange diminishes life by a whole year; even nourishing [vitality] cannot restore it.] The taboo to the end of life means protecting one's *qi* in the evening. [NOTE: Lying down in the evening, keep the mouth closed. Letting it open, you lose *qi* while letting pathogenic *qi* enter.]

The Colorful Woman asked Pengzu: "Should a man of sixty hold his essence and guard the One?"

Pengzu replied: No. A man should not be without a woman. Being without a woman, his intention gets agitated, and an agitated intention labors the spirit. Any laboring of the spirit reduces longevity. If he kept his thoughts perfect and upright and remained free from all thinking, it would be most excellent. However, you'll hardly find one like this in ten thousand.

On the other hand, holding essence by force is hard to do and easy to lose. It also leads to leakage of essence and makes the urine turbid, maybe even causing sex with ghosts. Also, wishing to prevent *qi* from getting aroused, their yang energy is weakened.

Those who want to have sex with women should first become aroused, getting [the penis] to stand erect. Then very slowly connect with her and gradually gain her yin *qi.* As you pull this into you, you quickly get even more erect. [9b] Once fully erect, have sex, always moving slow and relaxed. Feel when your essence is fully aroused, then stop.[7]

Hold your essence and slow your breath. Close your eyes, lie flat on your back, stretch the body, and guide the *qi.* Then move on to have sex with another woman: always once fully aroused, immediately change partners. By changing partners you can live long. If you have sex with only one woman, her yin *qi* gets feeble and is of little benefit.

The way of yang patterns itself on fire; the way of yin matches water. Water controls fire, yin extinguishes yang. Following this over a long period without stopping, the yin *qi* swallows the yang, while the yang transmutes and diminishes. The gain does not compensate for the loss.

On the other hand, having sex with twelve women without ejaculating causes one to maintain beauty and sexiness even in old age. Having sex with 93 women without ejaculating causes one to reach 10,000 years.

When essence lacks, one gets sick; when essence ends, one dies. Be constantly careful! Constantly alert!

Having lots of sex with only occasional ejaculation, the *qi* will always increase again without getting deficient or diminished. Having lots of sex with ejaculation, on the contrary, the essence will not increase again and approach exhaustion. [10a] Having lots of sex at home, it is best to have one arousal without ejaculation for each one with. If you cannot have lots of sex, simply count on having two ejaculations each month, thus allowing essence and *qi* to increase again naturally. However, this will take longer and be more subtle, and you won't be able to get arouse quite as rapidly as if you were having lots of sex without ejaculation. [NOTE: The Colorful Woman realized the Dao at a young age and knew how best to nourish her inner nature. At the age of 170 she still looked like she was only 15. The Shang rulers venerated her. It was around that time that she talked to Pengzu.]

Pengzu also said: Debauchery leading to failed longevity is not due to the doings of ghosts and spirits. It comes directly from using intention toward satisfying vulgar and depraved impulses. As essence gets aroused and there is the urge to ejaculate, they try to please their partner, exhausting their strength without gaining satisfaction. Not only do they not give rise to

---

[7] Following Douglas Wile and reading *zhi* (stop) instead of *zheng* (upright).

mutual vitality, but on the contrary they cause each other harm. In some cases this may lead to shock, emaciation, or diabetes; in others, it can cause insanity or malignant sores—all due to the loss of essence.

Should ejaculation happen, always guide the *qi* internally to supplement the area. If you don't do this, blood, arteries, marrow, and brain will diminish daily and even a slight invasion of wind and dampness will cause ailments and disease. [10b] This is because ordinary folk do not understand how best to supplement ejaculation losses.

Pengzu said: A man should not be without a woman, and a woman should not be without a man. Being alone and solitary yet thinking of sex diminishes longevity and gives rise to the hundred diseases. Demons and sprites pursue such people, enticing them into sex and causing them to lose their essence. Losing essence once this way is equal to a hundred times normally.

Should you wish to have children, hoping they are long-lived, wise, smart, prosperous, and noble, choosing the "lunar mansion" days for sex is most excellent. [NOTE: The "lunar mansion" days are recorded below.]

The Heavenly Elder [Tianlao, a minister of the Yellow Emperor] said: At birth people all contain have the five constant [phases] and their physical forms are pretty much the same. Still, there are distinctions of high and low, noble and humble—all due to their father and mother uniting their eight stars in an interchange of yin and yang. Should they not get the time right for their intercourse, their offspring will be merely average. Should they not match the lunar stations but get the time right, their offspring will be average to superior. Should they not match the lunar stations and miss the right time, their offspring will be common. Should they match the lunar stations, even if their offspring is not prosperous and noble, yet they benefit themselves, which is highly auspicious. [NOTE: The "eight stars" are the constellations Chamber, Threesome, Well, Demon, Willow, Stretch, Heart, and Dipper. [11a] When the moon is in these stars one may join yin and yang to produce offspring.]

The 2nd, 3rd, 5th, 9th, and 20th days of the lunar month are the so-called royal days of living *qi*. Having sex on these five days will never cause harm to blood and *qi*, ensuring continued freedom from disease. On any one of these royal days, after midnight and before cockcrow, slowly, gently, and playfully engage her Jade Spring and drink her Jade Sap. If one combines the *jiayin* and *yimao* days of spring, the *bingwu* and *dingwei* days of summer, the *gengshen* and *xinyou* days of winter with the lunar mansion days just listed, it is even more excellent.

To produce offspring, wait one, three, or five days after the woman's monthly flow. Pick the one among them that's a royal day, then use the time of living *qi* after midnight: spread you essence and you will have children— all male and long-lived, wise, and smart. Royal days, as said earlier, are those with the celestial stems *jia* and *yi* in the spring, *bing* and *ding* in the summer, *geng* and *xin* in the fall, and *ren* and *gui* in the winter.

Always, the key to nourishing vitality lies in cherishing essence. [11b] If you manage to ejaculate only twice a month, or once for each of the twenty-four nodes of the year, you will certainly reach a long life of 120. If you also take medicinal, you can live forever. What is distressing is that people do not understand this rule in their youth or, if they do, are unable to practice it sincerely. They get old first before they finally understand this, and by then it is too late. Sickness is hard to nurture [back to vitality]. However, although late, you can still protect yourself and lengthen your years. Yet practicing in this way in the full vigor of youth, you can grow the wings of immortals.

The *Xianjing* says: The way for a man and a woman to jointly become immortals is to deeply penetrate each other's energy without arousing essence. Visualize energy in the navel area, red in color and the size of a chicken egg. Very slowly move it in and out, stopping when essence gets aroused. Do this several ten times every morning and evening and you increase long life. To do this together, calm your intention and jointly practice the visualization.

Remember what Liu Jing said: In the spring, ejaculated once in three days; in the summer and fall, twice a month; in the winter close in essence and do not let it go. [12a] It is Heaven's way to store yang energy in the winter, and if people follow this, they can attain long life. One ejaculation in the winter matches a hundred in the spring.

Kuai Daoren noted: After the age of sixty completely avoid the bedroom. But if you can connect without ejaculation, you can still be with a woman. If you cannot control yourself, best stay away. Taking even a hundred different medicines is not as potent as this for attaining long life.

Daolin said: The source of destiny is the root of life. Its core certainly lies in this practice. You may take a great elixir, engage in breathing exercises and healing exercises, cultivate yourself in a myriad of ways, but you never get to understand the root of life. Think of a tree: it may have intricate branches and luxuriant leaves, yet without roots it cannot live long. The source of destiny is addressed in bedroom practice. Therefore the sages state: "To attain long life, start with what gives life." Bedroom practice can give life to a person and it can also kill him. It is just like water and fire: those who know how to use them enhance life; those who do not, may die. [12b]

Do not have sex while intoxicated or completely full: this can cause serious harm. Also, don't have sex while needing to urinate and holding it in: this can cause urinary problems, difficulty in urination, pain in the penis, and tightness in the abdomen. Having sex after being very angry causes boils.

Also, there should be no sex on the last and first days of the month, during lunar and solar eclipses, great wind and excessive rain, earthquakes, lightning, and thunder, great heat and cold, as well as the five days when spring, summer, fall, and winter are changing, being sent off and welcomed. During any of these times do not practice yin-yang. Other important taboos include the days that match those of one's birth year. [NOTE: When yin and yang are at odds, avoid all sex, since this may cause a diminishing of blood and *qi*, loss of proper and intake of pathogenic *qi*. It is very bad for your overall good *qi*. Avoid it carefully.]

Also, do not have sex after you've just washed your hair, are tired from traveling, or when feeling great joy or anger.

Pengzu said: Be very aware of changing emotions. Avoid great cold, heat, wind, rain, and snow, [13a] as well as eclipses of the sun and moon, earthquakes and thunderstorms. These are taboos of Heaven. Intoxication and satiety, joy and anger, depression and anxiety, worry and sorrow, terror and fear are the taboos of Humanity. Mountains and rivers, shrines and altars, the gods of Soil and Grain, wells and stoves are the taboos of Earth. In addition to these three kinds of taboos, there are also auspicious days: those called *jia* and *yi* in the spring, *bing* and *ding* in the summer, *geng* and *shen* in the autumn, and *ren* and *gui* in the winter. Throughout the year, days called *wu* and *ji* are royal. Use them to enhance long life or produce offspring; go against them and get sick yourself while causing bad luck and early death to your children. Just as Laozi said: Revert essence to nourish the brain and you will never grow old.

Or, as the *Zidu jing* has it: To ejaculate correctly, enter weak and withdraw strong. [NOTE: What does it mean to "enter weak and withdraw strong"? Insert the jade stalk between the zither strings and wheat teeth, then let it grow large and withdraw it. When it is weak again, reinsert. This is what is meant by "enter weak and withdraw strong." Continue in this fashion for 80 more moves to complete the full number of yang (81).] [13b]

Laozi said: Entering weak and withdrawing strong means that one knows the art of life. Entering strong and withdrawing weak means one will die even if blessed with a favorable destiny. This is just it.

Chapter Ten

The Medical Dimension

Another major Tang-dynasty compendium of longevity practices is the *Fuqi jingyi lun* 服氣精義論 (How to Absorb *Qi* and Penetrate [Ultimate] Meaning, YJQQ 57), which is regrouped in two different texts in the Daoist canon: a work of the same title that only contains sections 1 and 2 (DZ 830), and a text called *Xiusheng yangqi jue* 修生養氣訣 (Formulas on Cultivating Life and Nourishing *Qi*, DZ 277) which presents sections 3 through 9.[1]

The text, which outlines the different aspects of physical cultivation in nine steps, dates from the 730s and was written by the Highest Clarity patriarch Sima Chengzhen 司馬承禎 (647-735). A descendant of the imperial house of the Jin, he was well educated, then opted for a career in Daoism, at the time of high official status, and in 684 succeeded Pan Shizheng 潘師正 as patriarch of the leading school. Highly respected, he had audiences with several emperors and was officially installed on Mount Wangwu 王屋山 in northwest Henan.

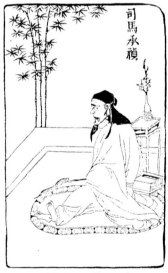

Fig. 18. Sima Chengzhen

---

[1] The text is translated and analyzed in Engelhardt 1987. For further discussions, see Engelhardt 1989; Baldrian-Hussein in Schipper and Verellen 2004, 373-74.

A prolific writer, he is best known for his work on "sitting in oblivion" (Kohn 2010b), but he also wrote on geography (Weiss 2012), swords and mirrors (Fukunaga 1973), numerology, and longevity practices.[2]

The dominant characteristic of his *Fuqi jingyi lun* is its pervasive emphasis on classical medical theory, centering on the five organs in their connection to the wider cosmos as well as to all different aspects of the body: parts, limbs, fluids, sounds, flavors, viscera, and so on. Relying on the medical classic *Huangdi neijing suwen*, he outlines typical symptoms and established remedies relating to the organs and their intricate network. He then provides healing methods that range from general awareness and moderation through herbal supplements, physical exercises, breath control, and swallowing *qi* to more religiously inspired ways, such as ingesting the Five Sprouts, merging energetically with the sun, taking talisman water, enhancing *qi* with pitch pipes, chants, and divine connection through prayer and worship.

Reading the nine sections of the text in reverse order, one should begin by establishing a clear diagnosis, analyzing one's physical condition with the help of medical theory and taking special care to spot latent diseases that may or may not erupt in the future. In a second step, one should treat these disease tendencies with various *qi*-absorption, guiding energy to the ailing area and chanting appropriate incantations. From here, one should move on to understand the five inner organs and learn to energize them to make sure they store ample *qi*. This is best done by taking care to live in moderation, avoiding excessive strain or emotions, carefully observing all cautions and taboos.

Moving into the more refined levels of practice, one next may replace ordinary food with herbal supplements, allowing the body to cleanse and refine itself as it opens up to subtler states. This, then, can be supplemented with "talisman water," i.e., the remnants of a burnt talisman taken with water. The last three steps involve healing exercises, swallowing and guiding *qi*, and ingesting the pure energies of the five directions, thus placing the adept into the larger cosmic context of Dao.

---

[2] For a discussion of Sima's life and works, see Kirkland 1986; Engelhardt 1987, 35-77; Kohn 2008, 147-50.

Translation

How to Absorb *Qi* [3]

1. The Five Sprouts

[2b] What keeps the body whole is being rooted in the organs and lungs [DZ: viscera]. What keeps the spirit at peace is being materialized in essence and *qi*. Although the body is endowed with the five spirits, once their images are set, the bone structure begins to decline and the *qi* diminishes. This leads to a general state of decay.

It is thus essential to take in cloud sprouts to enrich the body fluids, inhale misty radiances to nurture internal numen. Then the protective and defensive *qi* can preserve their purity and harmony; appearance and complexion can ward off withering and fading. Practice this over a long period and you will see just how amazing it is; you will accumulate good responses and connect to the gods, ascend to the Five Elders and be among the nine ranks of the perfected. What is outlined in the scriptural writings helps to see the pathways; what is emphasized in cultivation studies helps to find the best techniques.

Absorbing the Five Sprouts. Each day at clear dawn softly chant. [NOTE: The scriptural writings do not say which direction to face. [3a] Best face in the direction of each [sprout]. Sit up straight, make your hands into fists, close your eyes, click your teeth three times, then chant. For the central sprout, turn in the four cardinal directions.]

For the green sprout of the east: "I ingest the green sprout, drink it through the morning flower." This done, pass your tongue along the outside of the upper teeth, lick your lips, rinse your mouth, fill it, and swallow. Do this three times.

For the vermilion cinnabar of the south: "I ingest the vermilion cinnabar, drink it through the cinnabar lake." This done, pass your tongue along the outside of the lower teeth, lick your lips, rinse your mouth, fill it, and swallow. Do this three times.

---

[3] *Fuqi jingyi lun* (YJQQ 57). Variations in DZ 830 and 277 are given in brackets. Throughout, the DZ uses *qi* 炁 instead of *bi* 畢 for "conclude" at the end of chants; *yan* 咽 instead of *yan* 嚥 for "swallow" in practice instructions; *na* 納 in place of *nei* 内 for "take in" *qi* or breath; and *li* 理 rather than *zhi* 治 for "order" or "cure.".

For the lofty great mountain of the center: "I ingest essence and *qi,* drink it through the sweet spring." This done, pass your tongue over the back of the throat to collect the Jade Spring [saliva], lick your lips, rinse your mouth, fill it, and swallow. Do this three times.

For the radiant stone of the west: "I ingest the radiant stone, drink it through the numinous fluid." [3b] This done, pass your tongue over the inside of the upper teeth, lick your lips, rinse your mouth, fill it, and swallow. Do this three times.

For the mysterious sap of the north: "I ingest the mysterious sap, drink it through jade sweetness." This done, pass your tongue over the inside of the lower teeth, lick your lips, rinse your mouth, fill it, and swallow. Do this three times.

Conclude all repetitions, then take in *qi* through the nose as much as you can and very slowly release it again. Do this at least five times: this completes the perfect method. [NOTE: Your intention should match the direction in question. For this, best breathe in each direction according to the appropriate number. That is to say, nine times east, three times south, twelve times center, seven times west, and five times north.]

According to another version, first master enhancing the sweet spring of the center and chant: "White stones craggy: step carefully. Deep spring gushing: pure jade fluid. I drink it for long life: enhance longevity and destiny." [NOTE: Saying it like this deviates from the original text. Following it properly avoids trouble.][4]

This reflects techniques found in *Lingbao wufuxu.* The scriptures of Highest Clarity contain further variations on the cloud sprouts of the four directions. [4a] The method is highly secret. Do not pass it on lightly.

Whenever you absorb *qi,* always first practice the five sprouts to connect to the five organs. Then use the following basic correspondences for best results.

direction	color	internal	external	body match
east	green	liver	eyes	meridians
south	red	heart	tongue	blood
center	yellow	spleen	mouth	flesh
west	white	lungs	nose	skin
north	black	kidneys	ears	bones

---

[4] This note is not found in the DZ. The previous note is recorded as text there.

The lungs are the Flowery Canopy among the five organs. They come first because they are located above the heart and opposite the breast bone. They have six leaves, and their color is a silky, shiny pink. Their meridian issues at Little Rise 少商 [4b] [NOTE: This is located at the inside tip of the index finger of the left hand, in the low spot about two millimeters from the nail.][5]

The heart is located beneath the lungs and above the liver, opposite and one inch below Pigeon Tail 鳩尾 [CV-15]. Its color is a silky, shiny red. Its meridian issues at Central Pulse 中衝 [PC-9]. [NOTE: This is located at the inside tip of the middle finger of the left hand, at the low spot about two millimeters from the nail.]

The liver is located beneath the heart and behind the small of the back. It has four leaves on the right and three on the left. Its color is a silky, shiny violet. Its meridian starts at Great Trust 大敦 [Lv-1]. [NOTE: This is located on the third knuckle of the big toe on the left foot.]

The spleen rests right above the navel, close to and slightly in front of the stomach. Its color is a silky, shiny yellow. Its meridian begins at Hidden Whiteness 隐白 [Sp-1]. [NOTE: This is located at the tip of the big toe on the left foot, at the corner of the nail, like the tip of a scallion leaf.]

The left and right kidneys face the navel area and rest on the pelvis. Their color is a silky, shiny purple. The left kidney is Upright Kidney 正肾 [肾俞 = Bl-23]; it corresponds to the five organs. The right kidney is Gate of Destiny 命门 [GV-4]; here males store their semen and females harbor the ability to get pregnant. Their meridian begins at Bubbling Spring 涌泉 [K-1]. [NOTE: This is located at the central indentation in the sole of the left foot.]

[5a] To absorb the *qi* of the five sprouts, always think of them entering your organs and let their fluid connect easily to their related organs. You can also circulate them through the entire body system and thus cure various diseases.

For example: To ingest the green sprout, think of its *qi* entering the liver, then envision the green *qi* inside it as bountiful and life-giving while seeing its green fluid blending and permeating the organ. Keep your attention there for a long time, then move on to envision the *qi* in the Great Trust

---

[5] The acupuncture points mentioned in this section largely match those still in use today, except that they are placed on both hands or feet and not only on the left. However, the lung and heart / pericardium meridians *end* at these points rather than begin there. The point given for the lung meridian in the DZ is called Little Yang 少阳 and today is known as Little Shop 少商 (Lu-11).

point on the foot. Circulate it further so it moves into the liver meridian from where it can flow through all the channels of the body, upward connecting to the eyes. Like this, absorb the *qi* of all the directions.

The best time to do this is after the *chou* hour [1-3 a.m.]. Make sure you wash and rinse properly, don your cap and robe, then enter your special chamber. Light incense and sit up straight to face each direction. Calm all thinking and clear your mind. Then, with full attention, carry out the practice.

2. Absorbing Qi

Qi is the prime source of the embryo and the root of the body. As soon as the embryo takes birth, primordial essence begins to disperse; [5b] as soon as it moves, its fundamental substance starts to decay. Thus take in *qi* to stabilize essence; preserve *qi* to refine the body. If essence is full, spirit is complete; if the body is stable, destiny [life expectancy] is extended. If both your prime and your root are [DZ: sufficiently] firm, you can live forever. Just look at the ten thousand things: there is not one that has *qi* but no body; there is not one that has a body but no *qi*. In light of this, how could you, intent on preserving life, avoid to concentrate *qi* and strive for ultimate softness?

The Great Clarity Talisman for Guiding *Qi* [DZ: with illustration]: To absorb *qi* and give up grains, first write this talisman while facing the dominant direction and swallow it. Take one talisman each for seven days, and continue for three rounds of seven. After this, take three talismans all at once. Throughout, light the five kinds of incense to the right and left.

To absorb *qi*, always first heal all bodily symptoms and ailments. Let your organs and viscera connect to *qi* and your limbs be at peace. Even if there are no old symptoms, take some herbal supplements; if there are some ailments, drink them in proper dosage. [6a] If your body is sensitive to cold and heat, for example, use an anti-phlegm concoction. To thoroughly purge the stomach and intestines, a laxative is beneficial. To remove obstructions and hindrances [in breathing], use a cough remedy as discussed below.

Stop the medication once your breathing is completely even and do a hundred-day retreat. This helps to purify the body and discipline the will. During this period gradually lessen the amount of food you eat, staying away from sour and salty flavors. Continue to take moisturizing items, though, including herbs like China root fungus, steamed and dried sesame, etc. All this is [DZ: particularly] good when preparing to give up grains.

When you first absorb *qi*, do not suddenly give up supplements or food. Rather, diminish them day by day, allowing *qi* and fluids to increase gradually. [DZ: As you master the energetic rhythms], they flow everywhere through the body, and the organs are fully at peace. Then you can give up supplements and food. Always take mashed and steamed food [DZ: laxative and moisturizing supplements] to aid this process. Do not eat anything hard, rough, heavy, constipating, cold, or slimy. Over a long period [DZ: In the end], you will notice how the stomach and intestines feel empty yet whole. No longer hungry or thirsty, you can purge and stabilize, advance and withdraw as you wish. I cannot describe the effect here in detail.

In spring or fall, pick an auspicious day in the beginning of the month, after the 3rd and before the 8th day, to begin. Start by taking a Great Clarity Talisman for Guiding *Qi* every day. [6b] Once you have taken your third talisman, enter the oratory, face east, and receive the radiance of dawn. This is most excellent. Open a window in the eastern wall to allow the sun light to hit your face as you lie down. There should be no obstructions to the east in the chamber. Wait until after the *zi* hour [1 a.m.], then loosen your hair, brush it several hundred times, and spread it backwards. [NOTE: Do this when you first practice. Later there is no need to spread your hair.] Next, light some incense. [NOTE: Do not use *xunlu* wood.] Face east, sit up straight, clear your mind, and stabilize your thoughts. Click the teeth and do some healing exercises. [NOTE: Instructions below.]

Sit quietly to balance the breath, then lie down on your back with your head pointing west. [NOTE: The original texts all say that the head should point east. However, if that is the case, one is facing west, which is not effective for maintaining the breath and inhaling the *qi*.]

The mattress should be thick and warm. Cover yourself according to the prevailing temperature so that you are comfortable. All below hips and legs should be [DZ: particularly] warm [YJQQ: on the right and left]. If you want your pillow low, make it lower than the back. If you want it high, set it to be in one line with the body, so that trunk, head, and neck are on the same level.

[7a] Loosen your clothes and belt, allowing them to be loose and comfortable. Your hands should be about three inches from the body and curled into fists. Your feet should be about five or six inches apart. Begin with a slow exhalation, then balance your breath. Imagine the *qi* of the first rays of the sun in the east, gather the sun's radiance into a flowing brilliance of cinnabar [DZ: and purple] hues. Pull the radiance toward you until it rests clearly before your face. Breathing in through the nose [NOTE: Having removed the hairs in your nostrils, at the beginning of each exercise, press the

thumbs toward the right and left side of the nose, pushing them up and down. Ten times of this will make the nostrils open to the *qi.*] gently inhale and swallow. [NOTE: Once you have practiced this for a long time, you will no longer need to inhale the *qi* but can just visualize it and then swallow. Entering the body of itself, this kind of *qi* is even more amazing.]

Swallow it three times, then bring it into the lungs. Open the lips slightly and exhale the *qi* very slowly. The inhalation of [DZ: People's] *qi* can be slow or fast. Balance it in accordance with your inner nature but never pull it in abruptly to the maximum. This would make it coarse, and if the *qi* gets coarse, it diminishes.

Now, swallow the *qi* again three times. If your breath is longer, you can also increase the number of swallowings to 5, 6, or 7—the latter being optimal. [7b] Doing so you can feel the lungs expand [DZ: open] and fill greatly. Stop swallowing once you reach this level.

Next, hold the breath, visualizing the *qi* in the lungs. From here, feel it run along the shoulders and into the arms, all the way into the fists. Then see it moving down into the stomach and to the kidneys, through the legs to the soles of both feet. If you notice a slight tingling between skin and flesh, sort of like the crawling of tiny insects, you are doing it right.

Once you have reached this stage, practice subtle panting breaths for a short while. Allow the panting to even out, then pull the *qi* in as described above, [DZ: swallow it,] and guide it through the body. You may feel your palms and soles getting [YJQQ: moist and] warm. This is a sign of expanded balance and harmony.[NOTE: Always when absorbing *qi,* begin by visualizing it entering the belly and do not direct it first toward the four limbs, because once it gets into the four limbs, it cools down and creates obstructions in the five organs. For this reason, you must not direct it first toward the four limbs and only then let it enter the belly. In this way, you follow the natural flow of *qi.*]

After this, there is no more need to visualize the *qi* in the lungs, but you can pull it directly into the large and small intestines. Here it rumbles about, then eventually flows into the abdomen beneath the navel, giving you feeling of satiation and fullness in the intestines. Stop here, bend the knees, curl your hands into fists, and hold the breath in. [8a]Drum the stomach nine times, visualizing the *qi* spreading through the entire body. Hold the breath in as long as you can, then exhale every slowly. Be careful not to hold it too long. If you hyperventilate, breathe in very slowly, then exhale with care.

If you have a feeling of breadth and fullness in the belly, stop. Should the belly still feel full and distressed, hold the breath and drum it. End this, then stretch the legs out and with your hands massage your face and chest and below several ten times. Similarly rub the belly and around the navel several ten times. Spread the legs wide and point the toes upward, then bend and flex them a number of times. Release the fists, relax your frame, forget the mind, and let go of the body until your *qi*, breathing, joints, and nodes are balanced and even. Once done with this, stop and get up. If you are sweaty, rub your head, face, and neck with powder. Then sit up straight and lightly shake your joints and nodes, so the body is aligned and steady. When this is reached, get up and move about. Breathe naturally.

There are many similar recipes which I cannot present here in their entirety. It is best that you follow your inclination in selecting them.

Now [DZ: Generally], why is it that in *qi*-absorption you must first halt it at the lungs, [8b] then move it into the stomach, and only from there go to the kidneys? The reason is that the lungs are the root of *qi*. Since all *qi* inherently belongs to the lungs, *qi* connects to them. Also, the lungs are the leader of the organs and form the Flowery Canopy that covers them. The main pathway and source of breathing, they serve as the official of transmission and distribution, and all order and patterning comes from them. The gate of the material souls, they are the executive among the five organs and the ruler over the other four. They connect to the twelve meridians. The *qi* flow begins here, makes a full circuit, and returns: they are the executive among the five organs. For this reason, we first make the *qi* halt in the lungs and only then guide its flow elsewhere.

The stomach is the ocean of the five organs and six viscera. Water and grain enter into the stomach; it is the great ruler of the six viscera. All organs and viscera are endowed by it: the five flavors enter the stomach and from here each goes to its proper home to nurture it with the five *qi*. Thus any *qi* in the five organs and six viscera issues from the stomach and all transformation begins with the *qi* in the mouth.

The kidneys are the spring of vital *qi*. They are the foundation of the five organs and six viscera and the root of the twelve meridians. [9a] The left kidney is Kidney Proper; the right is the Gate of Destiny. Thus by making the *qi* reach the kidneys, we increase essence and fluids.

Heaven feeds people with the five *qi*; Earth feeds people with the five flavors. The five *qi* enter through the nose and are stored in the heart and lungs; the five flavors enter through the mouth and are stored in the belly [DZ: intestines] and stomach. Once the flavors have reached their storage area, they mix with the five *qi* to bring forth saliva and body fluids. As *qi* and fluids stimulate each other, spirit arises spontaneously. [NOTE: How can the five flavors arise solely from the five grains? The five flavors are a form of *qi* and thus best supplemented with herbs. Contained in herbs, they are much superior to those found in the five grains.]

Although I have only described the lungs and kidneys here, their *qi* naturally flows through all the organs. Thus every exhalation issues both from the heart and lungs; every inhalation reaches both the kidneys and liver. And in the pause between exhalation and inhalation the spleen receives the flavors. The principles of exhalation and inhalation match the essential features of spirit and *qi.*

The Highest Lord once asked, "In what space [DZ: joints] does people's destiny lie?" The answer was, "In the space between exhalation and inhalation." He said, "Excellent. We can call this Dao." [9b]

Now, for all *qi*-absorption use the time between midnight and noon, and especially between cock crow and sunrise. This is cosmic yin: the yang within yin. From sunrise to noon is cosmic yang: the yang within yang. From noon to sunset is cosmic yang: the yin within the yin. And from sunset to cock crow is cosmic yin: the yin within the yin. People always match this rhythm.

Also, in spring, *qi* flows in the meridians; in summer, in the flesh; in fall, in the skin; and in winter, in the bones. In addition, in the 1st and 2nd months, celestial *qi* first [DZ: fully] straightens, earthly *qi* first arises, and human *qi* rests in the liver. In the 3rd and 4th months, celestial *qi* is fully straight, earthly *qi* has fully [DZ: strongly] arisen, and human *qi* rests in the spleen. In the 5th and 6th months, celestial *qi* is full, earthly *qi* is at its height, and human *qi* rests in the head. In the 7th and 8th months, yin *qi* begins to kill, and human *qi* rests in the lungs. In the 9th and 10th months, yin *qi* freezes, earthly *qi* begins to close down, and human *qi* rests in the heart. In the 11th and 12th months, freezing [DZ: *qi*] continues, earthly *qi* harmonizes, and human *qi* rests in the kidneys. Thus the months of the four seasons all match the movement of *qi.* practice your visualization accordingly.

Also, for all *qi*-absorption it is good [DZ: best] to use times when the weather is bright and clear. Do not actively inhale external *qi* at any time when there is wind and rain, darkness and fog but rather go into your secluded chamber, hold the breath, and absorb internal *qi,* aided by various herbal supplements. [10a]

Now, in absorbing *qi* and giving up grain, in the first week [of ten days], essence and *qi* tend to be weak and malleable and your complexion is gray or yellow. In the second week, your movements are stumbling, your limbs and joints are numb, your bowels only move slowly and with great difficulty, and your urine is reddish and yellow. You may also have diarrhea for a while, first hard then liquid. In the third week, the body is emaciated and it is very hard to move. [NOTE: This phase of sluggishness and weakness occurs because the focused *qi* is first activated. If you take various herbal supplements it won't come to this.]

However, in the course of the fourth week, you will find your complexion clearing up and your mind [DZ: and will] full at peace. In the fifth week, your organs are in harmony and your essence and *qi* are nourished from within. In the sixth week, your body is just like it was before, and all its functions are working just fine. In the seventh week, you are euphoric, will and determination soaring high. In the eighth week, you are serene and relaxed, full of clear faith in the practice. In the ninth week, you begin to look radiant and luscious, your voice powerful and sonorous. In the tenth week, the proper *qi* has reached all parts of your body and its efficiency is at its utmost.

If you practice this cultivation without stopping, your years and destiny extend. After three years, you will be free from boils and ulcers, and your face and complexion will have a strong radiance. After six years, your bone marrow is strong and your intestines turn into sinews and muscles. You will know all about life and death. After nine years of practice, you can order about the demons and spirits; jade maidens will serve at your side. Your brain is vibrant, your sides are armored, and you cannot ever be harmed again. Now you are called perfected.

The Five Cinnabar Stanzas for the Numinous Mind.[6] [NOTE: Practice these for fifteen days and your mind will connect to all. Do it for five years and both your mind and body will connect to all.] [11a]

The Stanza of the East for Long Life: "The one *qi* joins Great Harmony; attain the one Dao and all that is great. Harmonize with it, and nothing is not harmonious; mystery principle joins mystery moment." Chant this ninety times, and if the *qi* is not balanced, persist in chanting until it is.

The Stanza of the South for Not Being Hungry: "Don't use intention to think of intention, nor pursue not thinking at all. Have intention but don't use it to think, this method you can keep." Chant this thirty times, and if you get hungry, persist in chanting until you feel full.

The Stanza of the Center for Not Being Hot: "Keep eating *qi* and joining *qi*, it won't take long and it is firmly joined. *Qi* returns to be original *qi*, fol-

---

6 This section, until "Absorbing *Qi* with the Earthly Branches" is not in the DZ.

low it as it comes, follow it as it goes." Chant this 120 times, and if you get very hot, persist in chanting until you feel cool. [11b]

The Stanza of the West for Not Being Cold: "Cultivate and straighten the will, then let it go; keep practicing but don't get attached to letting go. Have will but don't cultivate it, be whole in yourself without knowing." Chant this seventy times, and if you get very cold, persist in chanting until you feel warm.

The Stanza of the North for Not Being Thirsty: "Don't use your heart to bind your heart, go back to having no master and release all binds. Be in your heart, but don't see it as heart; be in perfection and guard perfection's source." Chant this fifty times, and if you get thirsty, persist in chanting until you are no longer thirsty.

The mastery of heat, cold, and so on is described like this in the original texts. However, if you link this practice with the system of the five organs, there is the potential for errors. Thus, only when you are thirsty chant the Stanza of the North; doing so, you activate its particular spirit. When your spirit is restless, chant the Stanza of the East; when you are cold, chant the Stanza of the West when you are hungry chant the Stanza of the South; when you are thirsty, chant the Stanza of the North; and when you are hot, chant the Stanza of the Center.

You can also use the five organs to practice to the same effect, gradually lessening the condition with the help of their system. [12a] You can chant at any time, early or late, but it is most efficacious if done before noon. Chant it several times to the five directions. After that, chant the following "Praise to the Great Dao":

The Great Dao is formless, matching things it got its name:
It makes Heaven, Earth and all things come to life through *qi.*
All receive new material being, but only people contain numen,
The five phases and three powers; fall kills, spring engenders.
This precious verse in four times nine lines: chant it to preserve essence.
Cultivate and honor Great Harmony—never declining nor increasing.

Taste it—there is no flavor; sniff it—there is no smell;
Look at it—there is no color; listen to it—there is no sound.
Sitting and lying—it is nowhere; walking and moving—it has no path.
Floating about the Great Void, still deep in the Yellow Court—
It moves and goes nowhere; stays and is not present.
No action, no doing, no seeing, no hearing.

Neither coagulating nor dispersing, neither separate nor together,
Neither huge nor tiny, neither heavy nor light,
Neither yellow nor white, neither red nor green—
Dao is lofty, yellow, and superior: its core radiant and bright.
The Highest Lord provides these verses, rules Gold Town.
If you can hear them, your destiny matches your star of perfection.

With these five numinous stanzas, you can connect to the *qi* of each of the
five organs. While you chant them, make sure to visualize each organ in its
respective position. If you have any problems as specified in their words—
cold, heat, hunger, or thirst—first chant the relevant stanza separately. Face
the appropriate direction, sit up straight, close your eyes, clear your spirit,
and with your mouth closed chant mentally. Then move the tongue to swish
around the mouth and raise saliva. Slowly and subtly pull in the *qi* and swallow it, in each case guiding the *qi* to the appropriate organ.

This method alone is good for deficient and depressed conditions; however, even if combined with talisman water and herbs, it will not work for
consumption and serious injuries.

Absorbing *Qi* Using the Earthly Branches. Start working with *qi* in the
early morning of a *jiazi* week. Begin by facing the *chen* direction [ESE],
swish the tongue around the upper and lower teeth to stimulate saliva, rinse
three times with it, then swallow. Next turn to *yin* [ENE], *zi* [N], *mou*
[WNW], *shen* [WSW], and *wu* [S]. [13a]

According to another version, begin on a *jiazi* day and continue for an
entire ten-day week by facing *mou* and *chen* to swallow the *qi*. On a *jiamou*
day face *mou* and *chen*, continuing this for the remainder of the week. This
method as based on the six *mou* is unique to one school. Infuse *mou* energy
into the spleen, it being the center of storage and provisions—you will never
feel hungry again. Use the overflow to open up the rest of the body and you
won't need any other techniques.

How to Absorb Three, Five, Seven, and Nine *Qi*. Very gently pull the *qi*
in through the nose three times, then expel the dead *qi* once through the
mouth. Use three *qi* for a long time, then move on to pulling in five *qi*, again
expelling the dead *qi* once through the mouth. Use five *qi* for a long time,
then move on to pulling in seven *qi*, again expelling the dead *qi* once through
the mouth. Use seven *qi* for a long time, then move on to pulling in nine *qi*,
again expelling the dead *qi* once through the mouth. Practice using nine *qi*
for a long time, then move on to doing three, five, seven, and nine *qi* in a

row, pulling in a total of twenty-four *qi*, again expelling the dead *qi* once through the mouth. Practice with twenty-four breaths for a long time. [13b]

To swallow *qi* in reverse order, begin with nine and reduce the number to 3; to work in sequence, start with nine and increase the number to nine times nine or 81 swallowings, each round accompanied by one expulsion. This gives you a proper rhythm. This technique is amazing since it works with lots of inhalations and only few exhalations. If you don't want to be limited in this way, gradually increase the numbers further, but make sure to mentally keep count. "Dead *qi*" is the *qi* of the four seasons and five phases that is drained and exhausted. Visualize it and expel it. For all further practice continue working according to the prescribed method.

How to Nourish the *Qi* of the Five Phases in the Five Organs. In spring, on the six *bing* days at the *si* hour [9-11 a.m.], eat the *qi* 120 times and guide it to the heart. This will make the heart dominate the lungs but without the lungs harming the liver: it accordingly nourishes the liver.

In summer, on the six *mu* days at the *wei* hour [1-3 p.m.], eat the *qi* 120 times to support the spleen. This will make the spleen dominate the kidneys but without the kidneys harming the heart. [14a]

In the third month of summer, on the six *geng* days at the *shen* hour [3-5 p.m.], eat the *qi* 120 times to support the lungs. This will make the lungs dominate the liver but without the liver harming the spleen.

In fall, on the six *ren* days at the *hai* hour [9-11 p.m.], eat the *qi* 120 times to support the kidneys. This will make the kidneys dominate the heart but without the heart harming the lungs.

In winter, on the six *jia* days at the *yin* hour [3-5 a.m.], eat the *qi* 120 times to support the liver. This will make the liver dominate the spleen but without the spleen harming the kidneys.

This method presents the essentials of how to eat the *qi* of the five phases. Since it is performed nine times in each season, there are altogether 1,080 times of eating *qi*. Nourish each individual organ; when you have gone through all, start again at the beginning, making sure they do not supersede one another. Perform it with care. [NOTE: This method is special to one school. For more details about the five organs, see the section on the Five Sprouts above.]

3. Healing Exercises

[14b] All limbs and bones, knuckles and joints are made to be moved. All arteries and meridians, protective and defensive *qi* fully match [DZ: are in] a

state of all-pervasiveness. Keeping them at leisure and prolonged rest, they lose their circulation and proper function. For this reason, it is best to practice healing exercises, which help [all aspects of the body] to attain harmony and richness. A moving hinge does not rust![7] That expresses it perfectly.

In people, blood, *qi*, essence, and spirit are the main means to create [DZ: nourish] life and round off inner nature and destiny. The meridians and channels are the best way to move blood and *qi*. The protective *qi* is the key to open fluids and blood, strengthen [DZ: enhance] sinews and bones, and benefit joints and orifices [DZ: partitions]. The defensive *qi* is what we use to warm muscles and flesh, fill the skin, and provide the pores with nourishment, ensuring that they open and close properly.

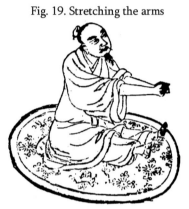

Fig. 19. Stretching the arms

In addition, the defensive *qi* enhances the circulation [DZ: cultivation] of floating *qi* in the arteries, while the protective *qi* guides the essential *qi* in the meridians. Yin and yang follow each other, inside and outside penetrate each other. It is all a never-ending jade-ring like circle.

The head is the seat of essential brightness [intelligence]. The back is the seat of the chest. The pelvis is the seat of the kidneys. The knees are the seat of the sinews. The bone marrow is the seat of the bones. [15a] Furthermore, the bones correspond to the eyes; the bone marrow matches the brain; the sinews are related to the joints; and the blood is linked with the heart. All the different kinds of *qi* belong to the lungs. Thus works the interrelated action of the four limbs and the eight major joints day and night. Thus you come to understand how the five labors diminish [your vitality] and the need to undertake [DZ: extend] proper movement and rest. The exercises of the Five Animals are particularly good for shaking and moving the joints.

In the human body, above and below depend on each; in the flow of *qi*, rise and fall change rhythmically. Among all the texts on healing exercises I have read recently, many have no clear order but the methods they present

---

[7] The image of the door hinge in connection with healing exercises is found first in the biography of Hua Tuo, the creator of the Five Animals' Frolic, in *Sanguo zhi* 29. See Despeux 1989, 242

all contain firm basic guidelines. If the five extremities are balanced and in harmony, practice according to a regular number of repetitions. If a certain area has deviations or disease, add to the number of repetitions that affect this area and practice with more vigor.

Generally, healing exercises should be undertaken between the *chou* and *mao* hours [3-7 a.m.], on days [DZ: at times] when the weather is clear and harmonious. To begin, loosen your hair and brush it in all four directions, touching the top of the head 365 times. Then either spread the hair back or tie it into a loose knot. Next, light incense, face east, and sit up straight. [15b] Make your hands into fists, close your eyes, and focus your thoughts on the spirit. Click the teeth thirty-six times, relax the body, and allow the breath to become even. Perform the following in the exact order provided.

First, hold the breath while interlacing the five fingers of the two hands. Reverse the palms and stretch both arms vigorously forward to full extension, pulling the shoulders and pushing against an imaginary resistance. Hold. Raise the arms, turn the palms out and stretch upward to full extension.

Next, from the shoulder lower the left arm and use it to lift the right elbow strongly, causing the left elbow and shoulder to be pressed back over the top of the head. Lower the left arm and press it downward with force [while still pressing the right arm upward]. Push the left hand toward the left, opening the right armpit and lifting the ribs. Now reverse. Lift the left arm back up, then lower the right and perform the sequence on the other side. After this, lower both arms, interlace the fingers behind the head, and lift the elbows, opening the chest and allowing the head to fall back. Alternating the arms and head back and forth, allow them to vigorously stretch in both directions. Keeping the fingers interlaced at the neck, lower the elbows slightly, then twist the torso to the right and left. To close, place the hands on the knees and subtly blow out the *qi*, allowing the breath to flow freely. Start again from the beginning. Complete a total of three cycles.[8]

4. Talisman Water

[16a] Talismans, written in cloud script and radiant stanzas, consist of spiritual, numinous characters. Their writing matches cosmic symbols, thus spirit and *qi* is present therein, and the individual characters are luminous. Embedding pure life, we use cinnabar ink for their absorption.

---

[8] The DZ edition (DZ 277) continues with three more pages of concrete exercises to perform. For a summary, see Kohn 2008, 153-55.

Water is *qi* made fluid, latent yang represented in moisture. Part of the realm of form, it yet endows everything. Water is the mother of *qi*: when water is clean, *qi* is pure. *Qi* is the foundation of the body: when *qi* is in harmony, the body is at peace. Although the constructive and protective energies in the body naturally provide internal fluids and the organs and viscera in the belly give off external moisture, it is yet possible to connect them to the stomach and intestines to increase the body's saliva and *qi*. One may also guide the numinous power of a talisman in this direction, usually supported by chants and other esoteric arts.

For this reason I have selected several efficacious methods of taking talismans in water for your use. Follow the instructions for bet activation. The talismans all come from original scriptures.[9]

To use the talisman, sit facing the direction of the moon working with the fullness of the sun. Light incense and write on paper in cinnabar ink. Hold the water mug in your left hand and the talisman in your right. [NOTE: Use a pint of water to take it, or maybe a little more or less as you like. Using purified well water is ideal, but you can also take spring water.] Then chant:

> Metal, wood, water, fire, earth—
> The *qi* of the five stars, the essence of the six *jia*, the three perfected:
> Come and devour my stale *qi*, enhance my yellow father and red child.
> Guard my inner center without deviation.
> [NOTE: Chant this three times in one breath.]

Afterwards, click the teeth three times [NOTE: while still holding the talisman and the water.] Then burn the talisman over the water and let the ashes drop into it. [NOTE: Don't let them scatter and get lost.] Face north, bow several times, and take it.

5. Taking Herbal Supplements

The five organs connect to constructive and protective energies; the six viscera work with the flavors of water and grains. [16b] By absorbing *qi*, the tendency is to create an excess of *qi* in the organs; by giving up grains, the tendency is to create an insufficiency of flavors in the viscera.

---

[9] The YJQQ text ends here. The method is translated from DZ 277.6ab. It continues with further methods with illustrations that are not included here. See Engelhardt 1987, 141-46.

The *Suwen* [ch. 2] says: "If no grain is taken for half a day, the *qi* weakens; for a whole day, it is minimal. For this reason, there are various medicinal herbs to replace the grain. They let the *qi* and flavor reach the organs and viscera, keeping them whole." [ch. 5] "Clear yang forms Heaven; turbid yin forms Earth. Clear yang exits through the upper orifices; turbid yin leaves through the lower ones. Clear yang rises to the pores; turbid yin moves to the five organs. Clear yang fills the four limbs; turbid yin fills [DZ: reverts to] the six viscera. Clear yang is *qi*; turbid yin is flavor. Flavor depends on the body; the body depends on *qi*; *qi* depends on essence. Essence consumes *qi*, just like the body consumes flavors. *Qi* is yang; flavor is yin. When yin is dominant, yang ails; when yang is dominant, yin ails. Harmonize *qi* to open them; harmonize flavors to fill them. Fully open, the body no longer gets exhausted; completely filled, it no longer gets tired."

It is thus good to take supplements based on grasses and trees, matching their nature and flavor to each organ or viscera. For example, there are compounds such as Organ Calming Pills and Qi-Straightening Salve. [17a] Even if someone starts out having no ailments or symptoms, with organs and viscera balanced and harmonious, he can still work with the Pills or Salve. Next, there are things like fungus and sesame as well as the various drugs based on cinnabar [DZ: other single-element drugs]. Someone who has an ailment in the organs can work with them as appropriate, increasing or lessening the dosage. Then there are people with various chronic diseases or serious infections. They need to seek the help of a physician to deal with these conditions that are not easily cured otherwise.

The recipe for Organ Calming Pills includes: China root fungus, cinnamon rind, and licorice root [NOTE: 1 pound each, roasted], plus ginseng root, juniper berries, yams, and ophiopogon [2 pounds each, core removed.] combined with asparagus root [4 pounds]. Pound these ingredients to a fine powder, then bind them with honey to form pills. They should be the size of *tong* tree seeds. [17b] Take thirty pills twice a day with liquid, such as juice made from pine needles, goji berries, and the like.

The recipe for Moisturizing *Qi* Salve includes: asparagus root, yellow essence, digitalis extract, and atractylis [5 pints each, boiled individually, then mixed], plus China root fungus, cinnamon rind [2 pounds each], yams, water plantain [5 pounds each], and licorice root [3 pounds]. Pound these ingredients very fine, then strain them through a silk sieve to make them extremely soft. Boil them together, then add three pints of decocted sesame and almonds as well as two pints of honey. Stir consistently until it becomes a thick stew, then continue stirring without stopping until it becomes a paste, the smoother and thicker, the better. Let it cool, pound it several thousand times, and fill it into sealed containers for hardening. [18a]

Take a little at a time for ingestion, using about a pill the size if a plum kernel every morning. Let it melt in the mouth before swallowing. Repeat 2-three times in the course of the day. It is best to produce this salve in the 8th or 9th month and use it by the 3rd month. If you make it in the 2nd or 3rd month, concoct it to an even thicker consistency so it does not spoil in the summer heat.[10]

6. Cautions and Taboos

[18a] The way *qi* works, it's hard to stabilize when you take it in [inhale] and easy to exhaust when you let it go [exhale]. Being hard to stabilize, you have to preserve it and make it whole; being easy to exhaust, you have to take care [DZ: make good use] of it and avoid leakage.

The perfected said: Studying Dao is like being concerned with breakfast—you never want to go without. Taking care of *qi* is like watching your face [reputation]—you never want it to be other than whole.

He also said: Someone who takes care of his *qi* as if he had suffered from an acute, life-threatening illness, in my experience, rarely gets old and depressed. Someone who is gregarious [DZ: and social], talking and laughing a lot, should restrain himself; [18b] someone who runs about and shouts a lot should slow down to find more balance. In all the different kinds of behavior, whether they engender enthusiasm or caution, make sure to avoid diminishing [of *qi*].

The way people's inner nature works, they share the same inherent structure with Heaven and Earth and mingle their *qi* with yin and yang. Thus their skin, bones, organs, and energies are all rhythmically regulated through inhalation and exhalation, advance and retreat, cold and heat, etc. They are all properly balanced by according with the two forces and the five phases.

Thus, we know that when Heaven and Earth are not at peace, yin and yang are in disorder. Then the organs and viscera are imbalanced, and the vessels and meridians get sick. If disorder enters from the outside, the hundred diseases arise through wind; if it enters from the inside, they come from

---

[10] The DZ edition continues with one more page of medicinal recipes. For a summary, see Engelhardt 1987, 165-70.

qi. Thus it is said: Being relaxed and serene, with perfect *qi* well settled and essence and spirit kept within—how would disease ever arise? This is so true!

Based on these words, you should understand the true nature of body and spirit and be able to keep them whole; discern the ailments arising from within and without and be able to guard against them.

The *Suwen* [ch. 27] says: "Heaven has its [lunar] stations and [planetary] orbits, Earth has its roads and rivers, and people have vessels and meridians. When the weather [as created by Heaven and Earth] is good, the roads and rivers are clear and smooth. When it gets cold, they freeze. [19a] When there is a deep freeze, they get blocked. When wind and rain arise, they surge and overflow."

Sometimes an empty pathology enters into the body's constitution: that is because water was subjected to wind. When the weather is warm and the sun is bright, people's blood becomes quick and liquid, and the defensive *qi* rises to the surface. When the weather is cold and the sun is hidden, people's blood gets congealed and blocked, and the defensive *qi* sinks inward. Blood and *qi* like warm and hate cold. Cold means obstruction and an inability to flow, whereas warmth means joy and easy movement.

When azure heaven's *qi* is clear and still, people's will and intention are well ordered. Going along with them, their yang *qi* stabilizes and pathogenic *qi* remains powerless. Such is the benefit of going along with the growth of the seasons. At new moon, people's blood and *qi* start to get concentrated and the defensive *qi* begins to move. At full moon, *qi* is replete and the flesh is strong. At end moon, *qi* is empty and the flesh is drained, the vessels and meridians are vacant, and the defensive *qi* leaves the body to fend for itself. For this reason it is essential to go along with the natural changes and adequately balance blood and *qi.*

For example, if at a certain time an empty, pathogenic energy attacks and the body is also empty, it encounters the empty *qi* of Heaven. [19b] The two kinds of emptiness stimulate each other, increasing their impact, which then moves right into the bones and harms the five organs. Thus it is said: You cannot bypass knowing the taboos of Heaven. . . .[11]

---

[11] The remainder of this section continues presenting measures of keeping *qi* under control by matching personal practice to the rhythm of the seasons, months, and days. It relies largely on the *Suwen,* citing it extensively, and repeats information that is standard in traditional Chinese medicine. See Engelhardt 1987, 172-75.

7. The Five Organs

[21a] As life manifests in this body, it takes material shape in the five organs; the body may decline, yet the organs' [essence] never perishes. As spirit turns into inner nature, it is endowed by the five organs; inner nature may deviate, but the *qi* is never destroyed.

In the same way, Heaven has the five planets: they advance and retreat to create the web and woof of the firmament. Earth has the five peaks: they stand still and stable to settle the directions and positions of the planet. *Qi* has the five phases: they interact and transform to determine the expansions and boundaries of the cosmos. People have the five organs: they enliven and nurture [the person] to provide a good place for essence and spirit.

organ	house of	root of	home of
heart	spirit	life	spirit
lungs	*qi*	*qi*	material souls
liver	blood	meridians	spirit souls
spleen	flesh	storage	constructive *qi*
kidneys	will	boundaries	essence

They are responsible for the functioning of the nine orifices, the movement of the four limbs, the solidity of the bones and flesh, and the functioning of vessels and meridians. [21b] None of them is not endowed at the source by the five organs, from where *qi* divides to flow into the hundred parts of the body. It is thus essential to match heat and cold to expand harmony; preserve essence and *qi* to increase longevity.

Now, the heart is the chief among all the organs. If the chief is bright, the circuits are open and all is well connected. Since all [organs] are the children of the heart, how can you not be aware of the pervasive order of spirit?

organ	position	fluids	sound	*qi*	body	expression
heart	exterior	sweat	belch	thunder	meridians	complexion
lungs	right	nasal	cough	heaven	skin	body hair
liver	left	tears	speak	earth	muscles	nails
spleen	executive	oral	laugh	grain	flesh	lips
kidneys	interior	saliva	sneeze	rain	bones	head hair

The chief among all twelve [organs and viscera] is the heart: it is the office of the lord and ruler: spirit brightness comes from here. [22b] The lungs are the office of the prime minister: order and structure come from here. The liver is the office of the military: planning and strategy come from here. The gall bladder is the office of justice: judgments and decisions come from here. The central belly is the office of the secretariat: joy and pleasure come from here. The chest is the gate of the Upper Heater. The spleen and stomach are the office of storage and provisions: the five flavors come from here. The large intestine is the office of transportation: change and transformation come from here. The small intestine is the office of reception and surplus: creativity and development come from here. The kidneys are the office of enforcement and action: skill and expertise come from here. The Triple Heater is the office of rivers and canals: water ways and passages come from here. The bladder is the office of districts and provinces: fords and fluids come from here. They all transform *qi*, each having their own area of specialization so make sure not to lose or neglect any one among them.

If the chief is bright and radiant, the inferiors are at peace and in harmony— nourish your vitality with this, and you will live long and never perish. If the chief is dark, the twelve offices are in peril, causing Dao to close in and block off, so nothing can get through. This greatly harms the body. If you nourish your vitality with this, you will certainly perish.

8. Treating Diseases with Qi-Absorption

[23a] Now, the effect of *qi* is both far-reaching and amazing. For example, as celestial *qi* descends, there are cold and heat and the changes of the four seasons. As earthly *qi* ascends, there are wind and clouds and the climatic differences of the eight directions. Combined from the two forces [yin-yang] and formed into one structure, the individual person is the great integration of body and *qi*. As we preserve these and make them our true home, spirit and numinous power become strong and vibrant. As we use them while [DZ: being able to] complying with the prohibitions, our work is most effective.

How powerful, then, is it to use our own mind to direct our *qi*, to apply our own body to combat our ailments? What disease could resist this and not be cured?

Thus take time to work on yourself, find ease and relaxation, and it will be easy for you to focus [on the *qi*] and work on whatever aches or ailments you may have and make them better. So, if you are serious about healing yourself, start after sunrise when the celestial *qi* is most harmonious and still. [23b] Sit up straight, facing the sun, close [DZ: lower] your eyes, make the hands into fists, and click the teeth nine times. Visualize the scarlet brilliance and purple rays of the sun, slowly pulling them into your body as you inhale, then swallow them. Envision this healing energy entering the afflicted organ or viscera. Should the affliction not be in an organ or viscera, but rather in the limbs, bones, muscles, or joints, still practice like this and first move the *qi* to the organ in charge.

Hold the breath in for as long as you can, then release and repeat. Do a total of nine swallowings, becoming increasingly aware of the *qi* in the organ. Then actively visualize that *qi* attack the afflicted area. Again, hold it there for as long as you can, then exhale slowly and subtly. Allow the breath to become stable, then swallow the *qi* again to work on the ailment. Also, be aware whether the afflicted area gets warm and damp. It if starts to sweat, this is an excellent sign.

Should the pain be in the four limbs, best treat it also with healing exercises, using them first, before working with *qi*. Should it be in the upper torso, rub and think of [DZ: pinch] it first, then flow the *qi* there. Should it be in the head, loosen the hair and comb the scalp with vigor for several hundred strokes, then shake the head to the left and right several ten times. Next, inhale deeply, interlace the hands on top of the head, then vigorously press down while pushing the head upward. [24a]

Next [while holding the breath], visualize the *qi* as it flows into your brain and all the way to the top of the head, then see it exit through the pores of skin and hair, letting it dissipate. Exhale, release the hands and move the *qi* evenly through the entire body. Repeat. Notice how the head and neck get sweaty and the afflicted area releases and opens up. This is the sign you were waiting for.

Should the ailment be in the organs and viscera, [DZ: then] lie down flat on your back, inhale, and guide the *qi* into the afflicted area. Do five or six swallowings, then hold the breath in once to work on the pain, releasing it consciously and intentionally. If the disease is long standing and there are lumps and hardened accumulations, you won't be able to cure it with *qi*; all you can expect is a [DZ: slight] awareness of opening and balancing. Also, there is nothing wrong with using medicinal herbs for the same healing purpose—the nature of herbs being quite efficacious.

Even if you use *qi* to work on the afflicted area and even if the *qi* is working and the affliction dissipates through the skin, it is best to consult the Hall of Light Chart to determine the acupuncture points most potent for healing this area, then [DZ: imagine and] guide *qi* to them. Once you know the points, you can further apply the pitch pipes in accordance with the twelve months, using them to massage the point and thus pull out the pathogenic *qi*. While you do that, mentally visualize its dominant *qi* moving in the appropriate direction. [24b]

Huangzhong is the pitch pipe of the 11th month: 9 inches long with a circumference of 9 mm, like all the others. Dalü: 12th month, 8"; Dacu: 1st month, 7"; Jiang jiachong: 2nd month, 7"; Jiang guxi: 3rd month, 7"; Jiang zhonglü: 4th month,. 6"; Jiang shengbin: 5th month, 6"; Jiang linzhong, 6th month, 6"; Jiang Yize: 7th month, 5"; Jiang nanlü: 8th month, 5"; Jiang wushe: 9th month, 4"; Jiang yingzhong: 10th month, 4". [25a]

All of these should be made from bamboo grown on the southern side of the mountain with round openings. If their nodes have grown branches, however, you cannot use them. They work best when hands and arms have no strength—but even though we speak of "hands and arms," this really applies to any ailing spot in the body. Begin by taking one hand and very slowly massage the painful area. Do this for a good long time, then stop. Next, close your eyes and direct your vision inward to visualize the five organs. Swallow the saliva three times. Click the teeth three times. Be in your heart and chant:

[I invoke] the Highest Lord, four mysteries, five phases, six courts,
three spirit souls, seven material souls, heavenly passes, earthly essences
divine talismans, constructive and defensive *qi*, celestial womb,
highest radiance, four limbs, hundred spirits, and nine orifices!
May the myriad numinous forces receive my registration
and the jade planets inscribe my name in the Jade City ledgers.
Jade maidens protect my body; jade lads guard my life.
Forever I match the two Luminants.
Like the flying immortals of Highest Clarity, I live with sun and moon.
My years matching Heaven, I transcend this world
Soar up to the immortals and attain the rightness of Great Peace.

Nasty winds causing pain, noxious demons, flying monsters,
water sprites filing sepulchral plaints, [25b] two *qi* vacillating,
maltreating my four limbs, making me rise and fall—

Against all of them, I invoke:
Lord of Taishan, Ding gods, dragons and tigers, radiant and majestic—
Come and kill the demons and all nasty, pathogenic influences!
Destroy and investigate all anonymous accusations,
the hundred forms of poison, all secret defamations against me

and let me once again have the radiance of sun and moon!
See who harms me and send the North Culmen to destroy them all.
Wherever there is trial, let there be light!
This I submit to your holiness.

Always during the time of living *qi* swallow the saliva twice seven times. Direct it toward the painful area in the body, face the dominant direction, and chant:

Mystery on the left, mystery on the right:
the two divinities join their perfection.
Yellow on the left, yellow on the right:
the six florescences accord with each other.

Wind *qi*, nasty ailments,
all secret influences in the four directions:
let jade fluid flow there to soak into them,
move up and down, open everywhere.

On the inside, chase out water and fire.
on the outside, eradicate all that's inauspicious.
Let me live forever as a flying immortal,
my body forever hale and strong.

Conclude this, then again swallow the saliva twice seven times. Should you need to urgently attend to an ailing area, swallow 31 times. Do this always and you will be completely free from disease.

9. The Indication of Diseases[12]

[26a] Life and life expectancy [fate] depend on bodily form and spirit; the harmony of *qi* rests with the organs and viscera. When body and spirit are properly cared for, life is complete and longevity ample. If the organs and viscera are clear and at rest, *qi* is at peace and one remains free from disease.

Still, even as we first receive essence and begin to coagulate in the womb, we each follow the different modes of the four seasons. Even as we

---

[12] Again, the text ends with several *Suwen* citations and summarizes basic medical knowledge as described in the classics. See Engelhardt 1987, 196-99. I only render the first part.

take birth in this body and establish ourselves in inner nature, we relate to the rhythms of the five constants [phases]. For this reason, there are potentially many disturbances and aggravations, increasing accumulations of passions and desires. Thus, whether one suffers from an ailment right from the beginning of life or contracts a disease as the body develops, always joy and anger, sadness and worry are the agents that create disease from the inside, while heat and cold, food and drink are those that bring it about from the outside.

During our age of great strength and vigor, we are content to just ward off turbid influences. When we reach our years of decline and decay, however, we rush to practice self-cultivation. Yin and yang being at odds with each other, body and *qi* develop mutual conflicts, [26b] and a variety of ailments begin to arise that lead to depletion and come with lots of different symptoms.

Someone who practices *qi*-absorption and has already cut off grains may yet find his body gradually declining, essence and *qi* no longer full and complete, spirit and spirit soul no longer quite as radiant. This may well be due to an old ailment rising up again, bringing forth new symptoms and even leading to signs of depletion. At this point find out where it comes from, then you can treat it effectively.

If *qi* and blood tend toward yin and yang and become lopsided, the *qi* is disturbed in the defensive channels while the blood flows in the meridians. If blood and *qi* are separate—one replete, the other empty—blood tends toward yin and *qi* toward yang, and there is madness and terror in the person. If blood tends toward yang and *qi* toward yin, there is dullness. If blood tends toward rising and *qi* toward sinking, there is annoyance and resentment and one gets angry easily. If blood tends toward sinking and *qi* toward rising, there is mental confusion and one forgets things a lot. If yang is empty, one feels cold outside; if yin is empty, one feels hot inside. If yang is in excess, one feels cold inside; [27a] if yin is in excess, one feels hot outside.

The way the five organs work, they all come out through the meridians and function through blood and *qi*. If blood and *qi* are not in harmony, the hundred diseases develop. If blood gives rise to excessive *qi*, the belly and intestines leak nourishment and insufficiency results. If the pathogenic energies of Heaven are stimulated, the five organs are harmed; if the inherent cold and warmth of water and grain are stimulated, the six viscera suffer. If the dampness of Earth is stimulated, skin, flesh, muscles, and channels are harmed. . . .

.

Chapter Eleven

Advanced Breathing

Yet another Tang systematization occurred in the area of breathing practices as a basic way of absorbing *qi*. This is mainly documented in the *Huanzhen xiansheng fu neiqi juefa* 幻真先生服內氣訣 (Master Huanzhen's Instructions on How to Absorb Internal *Qi*, DZ 828). Not known otherwise, Master Huanzhen seems to have lived in the 8th century and, as the preface of the text says, searched for ways of enhancing life through working with *qi*. He had not much luck with textual research but one day, in the Tianbao reign period (742-755), encountered a master from south China, connected to Mount Luofu 羅浮山, who taught him the basics in oral transmission (Maspero 1981, 461n3). These "instructions" (*jue* 訣) form the foundation of his main work. Other than that, he is also mentioned as the commentator of the *Taixi jing* 胎息經 (Scripture of Embryo Respiration, DZ 130), a short text of about 90 characters which focuses on the close connection of spirit and *qi* and gives instructions on deep meditation (trl. Huang and Wurmbrand 1987, 1:43-48).

Master Huanzhen's instructions were popular. They also appear in the Song encyclopedia *Yunji qiqian* (60.14a-25b) and in the Ming-dynasty longevity classic *Chifeng sui* 赤鳳髓 (Marrow of the Red Phoenix), a collection of longevity methods by Zhou Lüjing 周履靖, dated to 1578 (trl. Despeux 1988). This work consists of three sections: techniques of breathing and guiding *qi*, exercise sequences, and sleep exercises, including those associated with Master Huanzhen (Despeux 1988, 65-80).

In addition, the same techniques are also found in the *Songshan Taiwu xiansheng qijing* 嵩山太無先生氣經 (*Qi* Scripture of Master Great Nonbeing of Mount Song, DZ 824) which also appears under the title *Taiwu xiansheng fuqi fa* 太無先生服氣法 (Master Great Nonbeing's Method of *Qi* Absorption, YJQQ 59.8b-10a).[1] Its preface mentions the Dali period (766-779) as the time when the author supposedly met Master Wang of Mount Luofu to receive the instructions. The work is further mentioned in the *Tangshu* 唐書 (History of the Tang; 59.4b). A yet different dimension of the text appears in the 12th-century *Tongzhi* 通志 (Comprehensive Record): it names yet a different author and dates it slightly later, to the Dazhong period (847-859) of the 9th century (67.43a; see Maspero 1981, 507).

Whichever it is, as it stands today, the text presents breathing practices for *qi*-absorption in fifteen sections:

No.	Heading	Chinese	Actual Practice
1	Getting Ready	*jinqu* 進收	set up room, prepare body
	Cleansing *Qi*	*taoqi* 淘氣	calming meditation
2	Revolving *Qi*	*zhuanqi* 博氣	lift pelvis, drum, exhale old
3	Balancing *Qi*	*tiaoqi* 調氣	calm, steady breathing
4	Swallowing *Qi*	*yanqi* 嚥氣	swallow breath and saliva
5	Guiding *Qi*	*xingqi* 行氣	flow *qi* to head and organs
6	Refining *Qi*	*lianqi* 錬氣	regulate internal energy
7	Surrendering to *Qi*	*weiqi* 委氣	let it flow wherever it goes
8	Enclosing *Qi*	*biqi* 閉氣	hold breath, open blocks
9	Spreading *Qi*	*buqi* 布氣	external *qi* healing
10	The Six *Qi*	*liuqi* 六氣	exhale with six breaths
11	Balancing *Qi* & Fluids	*tiao qiye* 調氣液	adjust body temperature
12	Regulating Food & Drink	*shiyin tiaohu* 食飲調護	what to eat
13	Abstaining from Grain	*xiuliang* 休粮	how not to eat
14	Guarding Perfection	*shouzhen* 守真	sexual control
15	Absorbing *Qi* through Embryo Respiration	*fuqi taixi* 服氣胎息	daily routine for continued practice

Three among these sections are already found—almost verbatim—in the medieval *Daoyin jing* (see ch. 5 above): those on revolving *qi*, swallowing *qi*, and the six breaths. The remaining sections are added here, integrating methods of systematic breath holding and *qi*-guiding found in the *Yangxing yanming lu* (see ch. 9) as well as food and fasting regimens from the *Taiqing*

---

[1] For more on this text, see Maspero 1981, 460-61, 468-69; Lévi in Schipper and Verellen 2004, 370-71.

tiaoqi jing (see ch. 6). The new dimension here is the integration of practices, the systematic presentation, and the clarification of terminology.

The basic idea that the text begins with is that when people go to sleep at night, their *qi* is semi-enclosed in the body and the various digestive fumes of the evening meal are not processed fully. To remove these noxious vapors from the body and open the way for the circulation of pure, fresh *qi*, practitioners begin by setting up a quiet, clean, warm, and well ventilated room with a bed platform raised above the floor and equipped with a comfortable mattress. They practice during the hours of rising *qi* between midnight and noon, ideally around day break. They begin by exhaling vigorously to remove stale *qi* from the bowels, then meditate silently to calm their thoughts, click their teeth to alert the body gods, massage the face, and stretch their limbs.

From here, the more systematic practice begins. "Revolving *qi*" involves lying down on the back and raising the pelvis into what is commonly known as Bridge Pose, then drumming the belly and exhaling with *he* to release stale *qi* from the abdomen. "Balancing Qi" means breathing calmly, evenly, and steadily, inhaling through the nose and exhaling through the mouth. This calms the mind and steadies the body energies. "Swallowing *qi*" means keeping the primordial *qi* in the body by inhaling through the nose and mixing the breath with saliva, then consciously swallowing the mixture down while drumming the belly. Ideally the *qi* flows smoothly and softly along its prescribed path to enter the Ocean of *Qi* in the abdomen. However, to help the process along, adepts can also use their intention or support its flow by rubbing the relevant passageways.

"Guiding *Qi*," next, is a mental exercise that moves the *qi* around the body, guiding it both upward into the Niwan Palace, the upper elixir field in the center of the head, and downward into the five organs, the other elixir fields, and all the way through the legs to the soles of the feet. As adepts find themselves soaked with *qi*, they can also make it move faster or slower, actively pushing out blockages and obstructions, which they see leaving through the fingers and toes as they perform a long exhalation.

From here, adepts become more adept at working with *qi*. "Refining Qi" means keeping the *qi* in the body and allowing it to self-regulate in a closed environment. "Surrendering to Qi" takes the ego further out of the process: adepts let the *qi* flow wherever it goes, following it calmly and smoothly with a detached and serene mind. "Enclosing *Qi*" means holding the breath in—as opposed to "not breathing" (*buxi* 不息) which means holding the breath out—and consciously directing the *qi* into a an area that is felt blocked or obstructed, which may cause an ailment or a difficulty in destiny. "Spreading Qi" is a variant of this: it means directing the *qi* outward to assist others in their healing process. Further concentrated healing occurs next with the help of the Six Breaths, today known as the Six Healing Sounds (Chia and Chia 1993, 105). They are:

1. *Si* 嘶—hissing with lips wide and teeth together;
2. *He* 呵—guttural rasping with mouth wide open;
3. *Hu* 呼—blowing out the breath with rounded lips;
4. *Xu* 嘘—gently whistling with pursed lips;
5. *Chui* 吹—sharply expelling the air with lips almost closed;
6. *Xi* 嘻—sighing with mouth slightly open.
(Maspero 1981, 497-98; Despeux 2006, 40)

The Six Breaths can be practiced in various ways and—as the text spells out—for different sets of symptoms: the most common way is to create the sounds by exhaling in the way specified, usually while visualizing the related organ in its relevant color and/or seeing symptoms recede and obstructions clear. Another version of the practice may also involve the vocalization of the specific sounds, so that a stronger vibration is felt in the relevant organ. A yet different technique, practiced by advanced Daoists today, is non-vocal and non-sounding: practitioners create the breaths and their vibrations mentally, directing them into the organs in an entirely meditative way.

The text from here moves on to several supporting techniques that involve food and sex. "Balancing *Qi* and Fluids" involves using breathing methods to regulate the internal temperature of the body, relieving dryness and coolness in the mouth. "Regulating Food and Drink" recommends certain types of food as well as proper ways of cooking, flavoring, and aiding the digestion. "Abstaining from Grain" introduces techniques of fasting, insisting that by becoming adept at the various breathing methods the appetite for food gradually diminishes and it will be easy to replace food with the ingestion and swallowing of *qi*. "Guarding Perfection" emphasizes the importance of essence and sexual fluids and warns practitioners against wasting valuable life powers through sexual activities. The final section, on "Embryo Respiration," recoups the basics, outlining the essential aspects of the practice and enhancing the importance of remaining aware of *qi* and connected to Dao.

Translation

How to Absorb Internal *Qi*[2]

Preface

[1a] The bodily form depends on *qi*; *qi* relies on the bodily form. When *qi* is complete, the body is whole; when *qi* is exhausted, the body dies. For this reason, none among the practitioners of nourishing life fail to refine the bodily form and nourish the *qi* when working to preserve life. There has never been a case of someone having a bodily form and not having *qi*, or of having *qi* and not having a bodily form. In other words, bodily form and *qi* need each other for mutual completion. Isn't this splendid?

I myself have pursued utmost Dao and searched the scriptures for instructions, personally worked to control *qi* and guard perfection for over thirty years. Yet, all I have heard and seen in this time has not fully satisfied my heart.

Then, in the Tianbao years [742-755], I came into contact with the Perfected of Mt. Luofu. The master at the time was on his way back from the Northern Peak and stayed over in a local rest house. There we met. I thought him a rather strange person, yet when I approached and spoke to him, I found he was really a master of Dao far beyond the ordinary.

I humbly entreated him to explain some ways of expelling and taking in [*qi*], one or two key commands of self-cultivation. [1b] Really, the ultimate pattern of exceptional grace can never be expressed in words or phrases and the utmost core of Dao is never contained in scriptures and writings: it is always transmitted by word of mouth.

The many methods of *qi*-absorption—the Two Luminants, Five Sprouts, Six Stems, etc.—all involve external *qi*. External *qi* requires strength and solidity; it is not easy to absorb for ordinary followers. But then there is also internal *qi*, described in terms of embryo respiration. This exists naturally deep within the body and cannot be obtained by an external quest. Without encountering a perfected, without receiving oral instructions, one labors for it in vain and can never get close.

---

[2] *Huanzhen xiansheng fu neiqi juefa* (DZ 828).

The record I have compiled here is thus entirely based on the oral instructions of the perfected, setting them down clearly and in proper order. It is not reflective of any form of ignorant or silly self-delusion.

The master always used to say, "My life is my own; it does not depend on Heaven" [*Baopuzi* 16]. And, "I share the same one *qi* with Heaven and Earth; I am patterned on them. How can life and death be just me?" [*Xisheng jing* 26]. These statements really contain the essence of his true and perfect teaching! As long as you cultivate and venerate Dao, bow to him repeatedly and continue to honor him deeply. [2a]

Having been fortunate to receive these instructions, moreover, be sure to pass them on with good care. Do not reveal them wantonly or let them get lost!

1. Getting Ready

[1a] Whenever you want to absorb *qi*, first prepare a high, dry, quiet, and empty place. The room must not be too wide, and your work needs to be protected from wind. Always have room to burn incense to the left and right. NOTE: But do not let it steam up and pollute the room.

The mattress should be thick and soft and allow your legs to be a little bit raised. NOTE: The *Zhen'gao* says, "The bed should be high so that the demons' blowing cannot reach you." That is to say, demons and spirits are skilled at using earth *qi*, blowing it at people. To prevent this, the bed should be about three feet high.

The cover should modulate cold and dampness, and ideally create some warmth in winter. The pillow should be over two inches high so your head is level with your back.

Every day after midnight when the time of living *qi* begins or around the fifth watch when you first wake up, begin by blowing out all stale and bad *qi* from the belly. Do one set of nine repetitions. Exhale very subtly so that you yourself cannot hear your expression. At the fifth watch, the *qi* of Heaven is in perfect harmony and your belly is empty—this allows for optimal practice. [1b]

Start by closing your eyes, then click the teeth thirty-six times to alert the gods in the body. After this, use your fingers to rub the sides of your eyes in big and small moves. Then press the right and left sides of the nose, pushing toward the ears. From here, massage the entire face and eyes. This is what the perfected do when they get up in the morning. Increase the amount of your practice in accordance with how much time you have.

Next, use healing exercises to open up your nodes [of *qi*] and joints [of bone]. For this, swish your tongue over the upper lip to collect the inner and outer fluids of the mouth. Wait until the mouth is well filled, then swallow it. Make the *qi* descend into the belly and visualize the god of the stomach receiving it. Do this three times, then stop. This is called "rinsing and swallowing numinous juices to moisten the five organs." Your face will develop a rosy glow, but the method benefits the entire body.

After this, sit steady and immobile, relax the spirit, and make the mind like a withered tree, emptying the self as if you were discarding clothes. Turn your vision inward, revert your hearing, and let go of the myriad thoughts and concerns.

After this cleanse the *qi*. To do so, close your eyes and make your hands into fists, only opening when the *qi* begins to disperse. The reason why we make the hands into fists is to close the passes and block off all sprites and pathogenic *qi*. [2a]

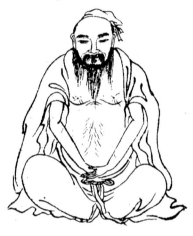

Fig. 20: Sitting steady and immobile

Anyone just starting to learn how to absorb *qi*, who finds his or her *qi* pathways not yet open, should not make fists. Instead, wait a hundred days or even half a year, and only make fists when you feel the *qi* is moving openly and smoothly through the body and a slight coating of sweat covers your palms. The *Huangting jing* [Nei 15] says: [3]

> Close and block the Three Passes, make firm fists.
> Rinse and swallow golden fluid, take in jade radiance.
> Get so you don't need food: the Three Deathbringers perish.
> For long periods naturally practice this and meet with great success.

---

[3] The last line of this stanza is not found in the *Huangting jing*. Instead, it reads: "Keep mind and intention always at peace, and reach joy and success." For a searchable online version of the original, see http://www.xiulian.com/XMZHF/013htj.htm.

2. Revolving Qi

The Instructions say: The five organs in people each have their proper *qi*. At night, during sleep, the breath is shut in, so that after waking up in the morning when getting ready to absorb *qi*, you first need to revolve the *qi*. This is to allow complete digestion of the evening meal and to eliminate old *qi*. Only after doing this can you balance the *qi* for proper absorption.

To revolve *qi*, first close your eyes and make your hands into fists. Lie down on your back while looking up, then bend the arms so that the two fists are placed between the nipples. Place the feet on the mat to raise the knees and lift the back and buttocks. Hold the breath in, then drum the Ocean of *Qi*, causing the *qi* to revolve from the inside out. Exhale with *he*. Do one or two sets of nine repetitions. This is called revolving *qi*. [2b] After this, go on to balancing *qi*.

3. Balancing Qi

The Instructions say: The nose is the gate of Heaven; the mouth is the doorway of Earth. Thus, it is best to inhale through the nose and exhale through the mouth. Do not do this wrong. If you do it wrong, the *qi* will go into reverse mode and causes ailments. Whenever you inhale and exhale, thus be very careful.

Also, when you do the balancing, make sure that you breathe so softly that your ears cannot hear it. Do five, seven, or nine rounds to achieve complete evenness of breath. This is called balancing *qi*. After this, go on to swallowing it or, if it is night time, enclose it, i.e., do not exhale through the mouth.

4. Swallowing Qi

The Instructions say: The most marvelous part of absorbing *qi* is swallowing it. Ordinary people swallow external *qi*, thinking that internal *qi* cannot be distinguished and separated clearly. How can they be so deluded? Masters of breathing do it quite easily and appropriately. [3a] Make no mistake about it.

Now, people all come to life in this physical body because they are endowed with the primordial *qi* of Heaven and Earth. The body naturally isolates primordial *qi* and uses it properly. Every time when people swallow and breathe in or out, their internal *qi* mingles with external *qi*, and the *qi* from the Ocean of *Qi* naturally follows the exhalation and rises all the way into the throat.

What you have to do is to wait until the very end of the exhalation, then abruptly close the mouth, drum the abdomen, and swallow the *qi* back down. This causes a gurgling sound like water dripping. In men, the *qi* descends on the left side of the body, in women on the right. It passes the twenty-four articulations [of the esophagus], going drip-drip like water. If you can hear this clearly, the internal and external *qi* look after each other perfectly and will isolate as appropriate. Use your intention to send the *qi* along and with your hands massage its passageways, making it go quickly into the Ocean of *Qi*. The Ocean of *Qi* is located three inches beneath the navel; it is also called the lower elixir field.

When you first begin your practice of *qi*-absorption, the Upper Heater may not yet be open. In that case, use your hands to massage its area and thereby make the *qi* descend all the faster. [3b] Once it flows through nicely, there is no more need for massages. Instead, you may get to a point where you just close your mouth and swallow the *qi* three times consecutively. Swallowing dry is called "cloud practice." Rinsing the mouth once and swallowing of *qi* mixed with saliva is called "rain activity."

When you first begin to absorb *qi*, and the *qi* is not flowing quite through yet, practice every swallow separately and do not try to do three consecutive swallowings. Wait until the *qi* is open and clear, and only then very gradually add to it until you get to a small level of attainment. After about one year it will all be open and clear, and in three years you will reach complete attainment. Then you can absorb it with ease.

All those who are new to the practice, as long as the *qi* does not go through yet in one swallow or does not go quite far enough, have to practice carefully one swallowing at a time. Definitely wait until you hear the gurgling, dripping sound which indicates that the *qi* is going straight down to the Ocean of *Qi*.

5. Guiding Qi

The Instructions say: Near the back of the lower elixir field, there are two caverns that connect the spine and the meridians all the way up to the Niwan Palace in the head. Niwan is the name of the key passage in the brain. Every time you swallow in three consecutive gulps, quickly visualize the internal *qi* being received in the lower elixir field, using your intention to send it there. [4a] Then make it enter the two caverns at the back of the elixir field and imagine that you see it in two strands moving up and entering the Niwan Palace.

From here it smokes and steams into all the body's palaces, like a dense forest spreading downward, all the way through hair, face, head, neck, and shoulders into the hands and fingers. Once there, it also moves down through the chest and into the middle elixir field, the spirit in the Heart Palace. From here, the *qi* drips further into the five organs and continues to flow into the lower elixir field. Allow it to continue down along the legs, so that it reaches the Three Mile point [on the leg; Stomach 36], moving through the thighs, knees, calves, and heels to get all the way to Bubbling Spring [at the center of the soles; Kidney 1]. This is what we call isolating the *qi* and managing it to the best advantage.

We drum it like thunder and lightning and moisten it like wind and rain. Just as Earth has springs and wells that without thunder and lightning drumming on them would not be able to moisten the myriad beings, unless people revert and purify their stale and bad *qi,* they cannot be at peace. Then, even if they have fluids and saliva, they are not fit to properly rinse and swallow *qi.* Yet even if they manage to let the *qi* moisten and drip into their five organs, creating radiance and color within, they yet cannot properly revert essence to nourish the brain. [4b] Without a proper exchange and harmonization of [*qi*], they cannot enrich and raise it. Absorbing internal *qi* without proper breathing, moreover, they cannot direct or use it. Thus we know that the method of reverting and moisturizing and the principle of consecutive application are patterned on Heaven and modeled on Earth.

Now, imagine that inside your body the stale and bad *qi* has clustered into blockages, that the pathogenic *qi* has created blood contusions. As these are opened and cleared away by the proper *qi,* they all leave through the fingers and the tips of the toes. This is called dispersing *qi.* To do so, open the palms of the hands and do not make the hands into fists. Do this one time and for one cycle, freeing yourself from ailments, then again do another round of balancing *qi* by applying the hands as described earlier. If applying the hands is difficult again, drum and swallow once more like before. Enclose the *qi* and drum and swallow for thirty-six breaths. This is called a small attainment.

If you have not cut off grains at this point, just go this far and still take small meals. This will open and expand the belly, making it vacant and tranquil. No question whether you are sitting or lying down, if ever your belly feels empty, just swallow the *qi.* In one day, from morning to night, you can do ten rounds, i.e., a total of 360 swallowings. Absorb *qi* like this over longer periods, reaching 360 swallowings: this is also called a small attainment. [5a]

Once you get to doing 1,200 swallowings a day, this is called a great attainment. We also call this great embryo respiration. Another method we call a great attainment is to enclose the *qi* [hold the breath] for the count of 1,200. Your complexion will may not have an essential radiance yet, but then there are still other practices to do: refining *qi*, enclosing *qi*, surrendering to *qi*, spreading *qi*, and more—all presented in some detail below.

6. Refining Qi

The Instructions say: To absorb *qi* and refine the bodily form, enter the chamber at first light, loosen your clothes, untie your hair, and lie down face up, with palms open and hands not made into fists. Comb the hair and make it spread out on the mat, then balance and swallow the *qi*. After swallowing, enclose it and hold it for as long as you can. Then calm your mind, cut off all thoughts, and follow the *qi* wherever it flows, regulating it all in its sealed environment.

Now exhale, expel the breath, and balance your breathing. Wait until the *qi* is even, then begin refining it. Do this ten times and stop. People who are new at absorbing *qi* may not be completely open. In that case, with leisure and very gradually increase the number from one to ten. [5b] Wait until the passages are fully open, then increase the number some more, going from ten to twenty and even fifty repetitions. When the *qi* flows freely all around the body, sweat will appear. Once you reach this stage, you have found its proper effect.

With a calm will and harmonious *qi*, you may then lie down without getting up, thus blocking off wind and reversing the aging process. This is a good way of extending one's years. Just make sure you do it at a pure and auspicious time. If the *qi* is murky and confused, go to sleep and do not practice. You will always be able to freely move your four limbs and there will be no afflictions or depression. Also, you do not have to do this every day. Just pick a pure and auspicious time. And it does not matter if you do it for five or ten days. As the *Huangting jing* [Nei 1] says:

> Thousand disasters dissolved, hundred diseases leave.
> No need to fear tigers, wolves, or other murdering beasts.
> This is how you stop old age and come to live forever.

7. Surrendering to Qi

The Instructions say: The method of surrendering to *qi* allows the *qi* in the entire body to become harmonious and even, and the spirit in all aspects of the person harmonized and radiant. [6a] It can be practiced in any posture, whether walking, standing, sitting, or lying down. Just make sure that the doors and windows allow the influx of harmonious *qi.* Whether lying down on a bed or sitting up, you easily enter a state where there is no spirit, no conscious awareness. Deep and serene, you allow the mind to become one with the Great Void. Once there, balance and enclose the *qi* ten to twenty times, in all cases flowing easily along with it and not letting it get into a struggle with your intention.

After quite some time, the *qi* will emerge from the hundred pores of the body and you won't need to exhale any longer, not even as much as two tenths of your normal rate. Keep balancing it and repeating the practice until you can do this for more than ten breaths. That is best. Again, you can do this in all postures, whether walking, standing, sitting, or lying down. Practice it diligently, and the hundred nodes will be open and pervasive, your facial complexion radiant and glossy, spirit auspicious and *qi* pure. You will always look and feel as if you had just stepped out of a refreshing bath, only doing the practice again in times of slight deviation. You should always feel clear and deeply at peace. As the *Huangting jing* [Nei 23] says: " Highly pursue nonaction, all the souls at peace, Clear and pure [HTJ: still], spirits come to talk to me." [6b]

8. Enclosing Qi

The Instructions say: If all of a sudden there is a hang-up in your cultivation of long life or you unexpectedly encounter a disease or affliction, quickly go to your secret chamber and practice the methods of absorbing *qi* while opening your hands and feet. After this, balance the *qi* and swallow it. Think actively of the place of your suffering, enclose the *qi* and imagine it dripping in there, all the while using your intention to attack the ailment. Exhale as soon as the *qi* reaches its extreme. Once done, swallow it again in close succession and attack the ailment as described. Do it fast, then stop.

Balanced the *qi* again, then repeat the practice and attack the ailment some more. Do this twenty to fifty times, until you notice sweat emerging from the afflicted area. Stop only when it is thoroughly soaked. If the pain has not diminished yet, repeat the practice every day at midnight or at the fifth watch when day breaks. Do it systematically, using your intention to attack the ailment.

For example, if the ailment is located in the head, face, hands, or feet, or wherever else it may be, just attack it there. There will be none that is not cured. Thus we know that the mind commands the *qi.* It can also command the *qi* effectively to release through the hands which affords a most amazing relief. Its effects and powers are beyond belief. [7a]

9. Spreading Qi

The Instructions say: Any time you want to spread the *qi* to heal someone else's ailment, first obtain the *qi* from the direction associated with the organ of the patient's suffering. Spread this *qi* and infuse it into the patient's body. Make the sick person face the direction of origin and have him or her rest the mind and clear all thoughts. Then begin spreading *qi.* After completion, tell him or her to swallow *qi.* All demons and robbers will flee naturally, and all pathogenic *qi* will be eliminated.

10. The Six Breaths

The Instructions say: The Six Breaths are *xu, he, si, chui, hu,* and *xi.* Of these breaths, the first five belong to one each of the five organs, while the sixth is related to the Triple Heater.

1. *Si* belongs to the lungs, which govern the nose. If you are too hot or too cold, or if you are very tired, inhale and exhale with *si.* The lungs also control skin, subcutaneous layers, and abscesses. If you have a condition of this type, use *si* to effect an immediate cure. [7b]

2. *He* belongs to the heart, which governs the mouth and tongue. If you suffer from a dry mouth or rough tongue, blocked *qi* that does not flow, or another affliction in this area, use *he* to expel it. If you are very hot, open the mouth wide; if you are a little warm, open the mouth slightly. While doing so, create the attention to expel the disease and you will be easily cured.

3. *Hu* belongs to the spleen which governs the Central Palace. If heat and cold are just slightly out of balance, if the belly, stomach, and intestines are distended with *qi,* or if you feel depressed and the *qi* does not flow right, cure this with the *hu* breath.

4. *Chui* belongs to the kidneys which govern the ears. If the hips and belly are chilled and the sexual organs are weak, use *chui* for relief.

5. *Xu* belongs to the liver which governs the eyes. Treatises note that if the liver is in excess, the eyes will be red. If you have any condition of this sort, use *xu* to control it.

6. *Xi* belongs to the Triple Heater. If the Triple Heater is unwell, it can be cured with this breath.

Although each of these breaths has its own area that it will provide relief, [8a] yet if any among the five organs or the Triple Heater are too cold or too hot, overworked or exhausted, or suffer from imbalances due to wind and other pathogenic influences, all these symptoms can be regulated by going back to the heart. And since the heart matches the *he* breath, using this breath can cure all manner of ailments. It is not necessary to employ all six.

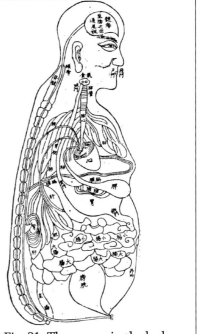

Fig. 21. The organs in the body

11. Balancing Qi and Fluids

The Instructions say: People commonly eat the five flavors, and the five flavors each belong to one of the organs. Each organ, moreover, has stale *qi*, which will be emitted with the breath through the mouth. Now, the Six Breaths, including also that of the Triple Heater, all emerge through this gate of the body and the host of defilements will be expelled with them, combining to form stale *qi*. Thus, after every period of sleep, upon waking up, emit the *qi* like steam and smoke from the mouth, breathing so softly that even you cannot hear it yourself. Inspect and examine it carefully until you know when you have done enough.

Generally, if the inside of the mouth feels burning and dry, there is a slight pain in the mouth, the tongue is rough and swollen, there is not enough saliva when swallowing, or if the throat hurts upon swallowing so that you have trouble eating, you have a condition of extreme heat. In that case, open the mouth very wide and exhale with *he*. After every swallowing, close the mouth tightly, then release the *qi* with *he*. Do this 10-20 times, then beat the heavenly drum seven or nine times. [8b]

Next, move the tongue around the Flowery Pond [mouth], then swallow the saliva. Again exhale with *he*, then swallow again. This will cause the heat to retract and eventually stop completely. Make sure to wait until pure water and sweet spring arise in the mouth. This is a sign that the heat is in retreat and the organs are cooling.

If the saliva and fluid in the mouth are cold and insipid and you have no sense of taste, or if you have overdone *he* and your chest and head are stuffy, so that you cannot taste your food and receive no water when eating and drinking, then you have a cold condition. For that, use the *chui* breath to warm up. With this method of warming and creating heat you can regulate until the mouth is nice and warm and the chest is comfortable. Once you feel that, stop. As the *Huangting jing* [Wai A:6-7] says: "The clear water from the Jade Pond drips to the Numinous Root. All who cultivate this will live long." It also [Nei 3] says: "Rinse with and swallow the numinous fluid, and no disasters dare approach."

12. Regulating Food and Drink

The Instructions say: Any food taken after working with *qi* has to be well measured and in proper order. If you eat too much, you create excess in the body; if you eat too little, you bring forth deficiency. In all cases you need to find the right place to stop any excesses and only then you can absorb *qi* in the right amounts on a more permanent basis. [9a]

Every morning at day break eat a little tepid, watery rice or sesame gruel. These are very effective in controlling your spleen *qi* and allow you to have sufficient juices and body fluids. At noon it is best to have some noodles, rice cakes, or dumplings, but be careful they are tepid and not too hot, lest their ingestion disturbs your proper *qi*. Cooked stews with scallions and leeks are also good. Grains should be millet, rice, sorghum, or wheat: they all benefit people.

People practicing *qi*-absorption best match their food and drink with the changing patterns of the four seasons. Also, these and other foodstuffs should not be taken every single day. Rather, eat them depending on your personal inclination as time goes along.

Game with white fat is very good to eat, however not during days of fasting and retreat. On the thirty-six days matching the divine bird spirits, avoid all birds or beasts that resemble them in any form. Dates, chestnuts, and the like you can eat as long as they are cooked or make into dumplings.

Whatever you choose, be careful not to eat to full satiation. If you are full, you will harm the heart, and the *qi* will have a harder time flowing properly.

Generally all hot noodles, turnips, root vegetables, peppers, ginger, and stews should be strictly avoided. Salty, sour, and pungent foods are best taken in very small amounts and carefully regulated. [9b] After every meal, moreover, exhale with *he* a few times to eliminate all poisonous and stale *qi* through the mouth and make sure that there is no residual harm.

People practicing *qi*-absorption should keep their stomach and intestines vacant and clean. For this, all things raw, cold, sour, smooth, gooey, greasy, old, hard, rotten, or decayed, or again anything else that is hard to digest must not be taken. If by accident you eat one of the above or a similar item, even if only one mouthful, you will feel a slight pain or unease where it touches. Thus be very careful about it.

Only eat soft foods as convenient. Before each meal, first swallow the *qi* three or five times, then proceed to eating food. It is also excellent to take three or five fresh peppercorns as part of the meal. After you finish eating, again take three corns—they will aid the digestion and pull the *qi* downward, opening the Triple Heater and benefiting the five organs. They also eliminate stale waste, dissolve food remnants, and enhance proper *qi.*

Practicing *qi*-absorption over prolonged periods, you will be able to avoid all things cold, frozen, hot, or damp. Your eyes bright, your hair growing, you will be able to absorb your *qi* in ways that cannot be described. The *Taiqing diaoqi jing* (Great Clarity Scripture on Balancing *Qi*) has yet a different advice regarding the taking of peppercorns. When you take them, they will pull the *qi* downward and it will emerge [as gas]. Be careful that you don't hold it back—holding it back may cause disease. [10a]

Also, every time you have an empty stomach, drink one or two cups of clear liquor as your disposition allows. This is most excellent. It helps you stay warm in winter and cool in summer, enhances proper *qi*, and systematically gets rid of all pathogenic influences. This practice is not particularly subtle, but be careful not to overdo it. If you overdo the drinking, you will get sleepy and even drunk. Once drunk, you harm your spirit and reduce your longevity.

Should you encounter some venerable and noble people, don't restrain yourself but go ahead and drink with them as the situation requires, but every so often exhale with *he* three or five times. If you further open your mouth wide and exhale with *he* several tens of times, you will completely eliminate all toxins from yeast and dregs. Whenever you balance and absorb *qi*, always drink one or two pints, taking them very slowly. Don't be too forward with the wine, lest you lose all sense of the taste for the food. Yet don't be too withdrawing, either. Just be like always.

Also, avoid getting in contact with new births, corpses, the six domestic animals, and any other kind of defiled and unclean *qi.* Nor should you go even close to their door or move about in their immediate neighborhood. This is very inauspicious for your proper *qi.* Should you unintentionally en-counter one of the above listed defilements, quickly enclose the *qi,* detach the mind, close your eyes, and hurriedly pass it by. Then find one or two cups of wine and rinse with it for a thorough cleansing. Notice how the *qi* enters your belly. [10b]

If this does not calm it down, practice balancing the *qi* to force out the stale *qi.* Then swallow and inhale fresh, new *qi,* consciously sending it through the body and helping it along with a hands-on massage. After this, take a peppercorn and drink one or two cups of wine to get the bad *qi* to dis-perse. Should it not disperse readily, do not force it with extreme measures but let it leave easily and without pain. It won't disperse probably because there is an obstruction in the Upper Heater. The best way to deal with it is by balancing the *qi* all the way, guiding it through the body to be harmonious and even. Also, eating oily, fatty, or pungent foods will do a lot of harm to your proper *qi*—so curb their intake with conscious intent. Always make sure you understand what may harm you, then you can make your actions compliant.

Practicing *qi* absorption for one year, you will open up the *qi.* Practic-ing for two years, you will open up the blood. Three years of practice will complete the effort and your primordial *qi* will be concentrated and firm, and even if accidentally you come into contact with something contrary, it cannot do you any harm. Every day do a thousand swallowings or more. This will reverse the aging process and let you recover youth. All this comes gradually with practice. The *qi* transforms and balances the saliva, blood, essence, bone marrow, and muscles.

In one year the practice will completely renew your *qi.* In two years, it will renew your blood. In three years, it will reach to your meridians. In four years, it will renew your flesh. [11a] In five years, it will get to your bone marrow. In six years, it will renew your muscles. In seven years, it will revi-talize your bones. In eight years, it will renew your hair. And in nine years it will reach to your whole body. All the 36,000 gods will remain in the body, transform into immortal lads, and be called perfected. Practice with diligence and do not get lazy. Your nodes and joints will function smoothly, and the five organs will be strong and firm. As the *Huangting jing* [Nei 19] says:

"Thousand by thousand, hundred by hundred—just follow the path. One by one, ten by ten—like piling up a mountain."

In this manner, your internal *qi* does not leave and external *qi* does not enter, heat and cold cannot invade you, knives and weapons will do you no harm. You come to ascend and soar into the transformations, reaching a life as long as the Three Luminants.

13. Abstaining from Grain

The Instructions say: Should you wish to abstain from all grain, just use the above method and diligently practice it. After three years, proper *qi* will flow freely through you: your marrow is solid, your bones are full, the hundred body gods maintain their positions, and the Three Deathbringers are driven out completely. Once you reach this stage, you gradually will have no more desire to smell the five flavors and will come to think more and more of not eating at all. Then, if you want to stop eating, you just stop: it is not difficult at all. [11b]

Should you notice an empty feeling in your stomach, just swallow the *qi*, be it morning or evening, and without worrying about limits or restraints. With prolonged practice you naturally know how much and how often to practice. There is not need to trouble with specific guidelines, nor should you use medicinal or other supplements.

Generally people who take medicinal supplements don't know how to absorb *qi*. Petty and picky, they make medicinal supplements their main concern, worrying about them to the end of their days, yet their bodies never get firm on the essential level. They never reach full attainment and do not take the same care as superior practitioners. The *Huangting jing* [Nei 30] says:

> The fruits of the hundred grains are the essence of the Earth.
> The attraction of the five flavors are enticements for the demons.
> Smells disturb the radiant spirits, diminish embryo *qi*.
> Three spirit souls confused, material souls troubled:[4]
> How like this can you reverse aging and go back to infancy?
> Why not eat *qi* instead, the essence of Great Harmony?
> To bypass all death and enter the Yellow Pavilions above?

This is just it!

---

[4] This line is supplied from the *Huangting jing*.

14. Guarding Perfection

The Instructions say: Most people of the world are given over to passions and
desires, harming their vitality and cutting their life-expectancy short. That
holds true for antiquity as much as for today. [12a] Never preventing their
decline early on, people inevitably invite endless regrets. Only as they get
closer to the end [of life], they finally start to feel sorry for themselves and
begin to take care of their lives. Only after they have become mired in sin
and stiffness do they finally start to think how they can possibly pursue
goodness; only after they are full of disease do they finally start to go after
medicines. Yet, Heaven's network being already set up, how can they ever be
saved?

For this reason, wise and superior practitioners concern themselves
with destiny well before they see the end [of life], ward off misfortune well
before anything goes astray, and manage disease well before it begins to
manifest. They shake their clothes and open themselves to the world, cultivate their minds and recover their connection to Dao.

Now, Dao is *qi*, and *qi* is the master of the human mind. The master of
qi in turn is essence, and essence is the root of all life [*Daode jing* 16]. Love
your essence and value your *qi*—and your life is forever stable. As the
Huangting jing [Wai 1:26-27, 29, 19] says:

> The square inch [heart]—keep it diligently firm.
> Concentrate spirit, reverse the aging process, recover strength and valor.
> Nurture now your jade stalk, make it very strong—
> Quickly firm your essence and maintain yourself!

It also [Nei 21] says:

> For long life, be very careful about bedchamber urgency:
> How it pushes death and makes the spirits weep.
> If you let the ocean leak, the hundred rivers slant.
> Leaves fall from the tree: it withers, gone its verdant greenness.

Now, there is no way to reach long life and eternal vision [*Daode jing* 59]
without loving essence and preserving *qi*. [12b] Ordinary people know nothing of the way of the female elixir and sexual control. Even though they may
try to work with their *qi*, they yet never get to the point of dissolving desire
and thus cannot avoid getting caught up in it. Thus it is said:

People always lose Dao; Dao never loses people.
People never really know life; life never leaves people. [*Xisheng jing* 32]

Masters of self-cultivation and nourishing [vitality] thus protect themselves well.

15. Qi-Absorption through Embryo Respiration

The Instructions say: Essence is *qi*, *qi* is Dao. First click the teeth thirty-six times. Turn the head to right and left. Stretch the neck forward like a turtle. Then to begin embryo respiration, fill the throat and swallow the *qi*. Repeat three times.

Keep the mouth closed, let the tongue move about inside and out, rubbing the gums to produce saliva. Let it fill the mouth and mentally flow it upward to the center of the head, then swallow it. This supplements the Niwan Palace above. The Niwan is the center of the head. Below it, the *qi* moistens the five organs. As Laozi said: "Sweet rain moistens the myriad beings." In the same way, embryo fluid moistens the five organs. [13a]

Never stop doing this night and day, and you will become a perfected. Above reach to the spirit immortals, below attain long life without limit. If you have any disease or trouble in your body, just imagine the *qi* going there, and any ailing spots will be healed. Perfect *qi* will drive out all old and stale influences, reaching above and soaking below. Just be aware of your body gods clear and bright, and the *qi* will naturally be harmonious and pervade all. Thus the sages tend to say:

People are in *qi*, *qi* is in people.
People never leave *qi*, *qi* never leaves people.
People obtain *qi* and come to life.
People lose *qi* and get to die.

All the principles of life and death rest entirely with *qi*. Thus keep harmonizing and strengthening your *qi*, never getting close to death. To do so, every day between midnight and the fifth watch, stretch out your lefts, make your hands into fists, and place them about five inches to the side of your body. Rest your head on a pillow no higher than two inches. Close your eyes and swallow the *qi* as outlined above. Afterwards wash [your face] and comb [your hair], then warm a cup of wine and drink it. This will benefit your embryo respiration and moisten your six viscera. This is the secret method of the immortals from Mount Emei. I cannot explain it here in more detail. [13b] Lord Lao said:

> Numinous fungus and jade radiance all reside in your belly.
> Famous mountains and great marshes offer drugs to take.

Thus you closely connect to Dao. My way is easy to do, anyone can practice it [*Daode jing* 70]. Get up early, stretch out the legs, swallow and breathe evenly. Then interlace the hands behind the head, pull the head forward while pushing the neck back. Repeat three times and stop. Interlace the hands and stretch them forward. Repeat three sets of two exercises. Next, twist right and left. Repeat three sets of two repetitions. Continue with swallowing the saliva 20 times. Pay attention to all four limbs: if anything does not feel good, rinse the mouth three times with your tongue and again swallow the saliva 20 times. This makes the *qi* flow to the sick spots and helps them get well.

Even for ten thousand [pieces of] gold, do not pass this on unless the right person appears—you lay yourself open to continuous misfortune for three generations.

Chapter Twelve

Internal Alchemy

Internal alchemy (neidan 內丹) has been the dominant form of Daoist practice since the Song dynasty. It combines numerous techniques and intricate philosophical concepts into a complex system, geared to allow adepts to refine accessible, tangible body energies into highly spiritual forms while awakening and activating subtle powers and connecting to ultimate reality. Perceiving the body as an intricate network of energy channels and centers, pervaded by flowing subtle vibrations, they utilize sexual energy as the starting point of their exploration and soon come to see themselves as layered levels of body-mind dimensions that grow increasingly finer and eventually merge with the divine (see Skar and Pregadio 2000; Kohn and Wang 2009).

Typically passing through three major stages—refining essence (*jing* 精) into energy (*qi* 氣), energy into spirit (*shen* 神), and spirit into the formless purity and vast emptiness of Dao—adepts strive to identify, control, modify, and transform subtle energies as they are present in the human body and mind. One effect of this transformation is the attainment of long life, just as basic longevity practices form the foundation of more advanced alchemical practices. While the Daoist canon contains many scriptures and manuals on internal alchemy, only few of them discuss methods for nourishing vitality or can be connected directly to the *yangsheng* tradition.

One of them is the *Wai riyong miaojing* 外日用妙經 (Wondrous Scripture of Exterior Daily Practice, DZ 646), a short text that extols the importance of moderation, virtue, and concern for others, laying the ethical foundation for spiritual advancement. Inscribed in stone in 1352, and erected by the Mongolian governor of Zhouzhi in Shaanxi at the ancient Louguan temple, the text reflects the teachings of the school of Complete Perfection (Quanzhen 全真) (see Cedzich in Schipper and Verellen 2004, 1187-88). This

251

school—founded in the 1170s, elevated under the Mongols, and still the dominant Daoist organization in mainland China—uses a monastic setting adapted from Chan Buddhism, requires strict morality and asceticism, and focuses largely on internal alchemy cultivation (see Yao 2000; Eskildsen 2004; Komjathy 2007).

Another work of internal alchemy connected to nourishing life is a short description of a seated exercise sequence known as the Eight Brocades (*baduan jin* 八段錦)—not to be confused with the standing Eight Brocades popular today, which go back to the Ming dynasty and probably originated in a martial arts environment. This is found in the *Xiuzhen shishu* 修真十書 (Ten Books on Cultivating Perfection, DZ 263), an extensive compendium that dates from the 13th century and collects materials associated with the Bai Yuchan 白玉蟾 school of internal alchemy.[1] The text consists of two parts, a general description of the exercises in short phrases and a more detailed commentary; it is followed by an illustration of each Brocade.

The practice begins with a seated meditation, during which adepts close their eyes, focus inward, and eliminate all extraneous thoughts. They click their teeth and snap their fingers against the back of their heads to wake up the gods inside the body. Next, they turn the neck to loosen up the throat muscles, so they can swallow the *qi* more easily. Then they collect the *qi* by moving the tongue around the mouth and let it circulates around the body in accordance with the "firing times," i.e., following a set pattern of yin-yang interchange that facilitates the optimal potency of *qi*. To activate the lower body, where the *qi* is to center and turn into the wheel of fire, adepts next massage the kidney area, the so-called Gate of Essence while holding their breath and visualizing a radiant fire descend from the heart.

In the second half of the sequence, adepts first roll their shoulders to cause the *qi* to move upward from the abdomen, then twist the torso to allow it to flow smoothly along the spine toward the head. As the *qi* fills the chest area, they eliminate its fire from the body by focusing on the heart, exhaling with *he*, and raising their hands palms up above their heads. The last Brocade consists of a seated forward bend, while adepts hook their hands around their

---

[1] See Boltz 1987, 234-37; Schipper and Verellen 2004, 946. The text is also contained in the *Chifeng sui* of the 16th century (Despeux 1988, 112-17). An English translation, with different sequencing and a mixture of text and commentary, is found in Yang 1988, 40-51.

feet and stimulate Bubbling Spring in the center of the soles (Kohn 2008, 180-83).

Having thus balanced the fundamental *qi*-powers of fire and water, adepts return to a meditative posture and once more swallow breath and saliva, letting the mixture descend into the abdomen, where it harmonizes the various qi channels and continues to purify the person. The effect is an overall cleansing and liberation from negative forces and natural extremes, aiding good health and the extension of one's years. Within the context of internal alchemy, moreover, the practice serves to prepare adepts for a meditation called "burning the body" (fenshen 焚身). This is a more intense practice to eliminate illnesses, psychological obstructions, and demonic influences. It involves swallowing *qi* in the form of a mixture of breath and saliva and guiding it into the lower elixir field where, in conjunction with the fire of the heart, it turns into a wheel of fire that gradually expands and burns throughout the body to cleanse it in readiness for advanced practice (Baldrian-Hussein 1984, 162).

The main contribution of internal alchemy to the longevity tradition is its vision of the body in increasingly subtle terms of energetic awareness, expressed in the literature in various levels of symbolism. As a result, there are texts and charts that depict the body with a vibrant internal landscape, populated not only by deities but by alchemical furnaces and cauldrons, metals and other elixir ingredients plus cosmic animals, stars, mountains, rivers, and fields as well as abstract patterns, such as the trigrams of the *Yijing* 易經 (Book of Changes). Yin and yang energies, at the root of the alchemical endeavor, thus are felt as kidney-water and heart-fire in internal *qi*-circulation; as the dragon and tiger dancing around each other in a vibrant mating ritual; as true lead and mercury combining in the alchemical cauldron; or as the trigrams for fire and water, Li ☲ and Kan ☵, intermingling and combining so that their central line mutates, changing them into Heaven and Earth, Qian ☰ and Kun ☷.

One text that illustrates the richness of this new internal body vision without becoming too obscure is the *Yin zhenjun huandan gezhu* 尹真君還丹歌註 (Perfected Lord Yin's Songs on Reverting the Elixir, with Commentary; DZ 134). It consists of a poem in 28 lines ascribed to the medieval master alchemist Yin Changsheng 尹長生, best known due to his association with the famous *Zhouyi Cantong qi* 周易參同契 (Tally to the Book of Changes, DZ 999-1008), a rather obscure but frequently cited alchemical classic (see Pregadio 2000; 2006).

While the poem is cited by the Daoist master Peng Xiao 彭曉 during the Five Dynasties (907-960), the commentary is allegedly by Chen Tuan 陳摶, physiognomist, Daoist master, philosopher, and internal alchemist who, after his ascension in 989, continued to appear to inspired seekers in trances to reveal various later techniques, including healing exercises for the twenty-four solar phases of the year and some major Buddhist practices of the Huangbo school that made it to Japan (see Kohn 2001b; Russell 1990). The text here describes the basic body set-up of internal alchemy, including the first union of the two main ingredients, to eventually culminate in the creation of the elixir (Baldrian-Hussein in Schipper and Verellen 2004, 843; Kohn 2001b, 127-38).

Translation

Daily Moderation [2]

Respect Heaven and Earth; honor the sun and the moon;
Fear the law of the land; follow on the way of the kings;
Obey your father and mother.
To superiors be honest and withdrawing;
To inferiors, be harmonious and kind.
All good things do, all bad things eschew;
From perfect people learn; debauched people avoid.

High knowledge is dangerous; deep knowledge is enriching.
Be calm and always at peace, restrained and always content.
Be cautious without worrying, patient without shame.

Give up all excesses and devote yourself to perfect harmony.
Conceal others' flaws, praise their virtues.
Practice skillful means and teach your neighborhood.
Befriend the wise and good; keep away from sounds and sights.
In poverty, stick to your lot; in wealth, give to charity.
In action, be even and deliberate; in repose, rely on others.

---

[2] *Taishang Laojun wai riyong miaojing* (DZ 646)

Always battle your ego; never give in to jealousy and hate
Reduce stinginess and greed, give up cunning and craftiness
Those oppressed help to liberate, those hoarding try to change.
Never break your promises, always speak the truth.
Think of the poor and orphaned, aid the homeless and indigent.
Save those in danger and trouble, accumulate hidden merits!

Always practice compassion, never kill any beings.
Listen to words of loyalty; be free from a scheming heart.
Follow these rules to ascend to the beyond!

The Eight Brocades [3]

The First Brocade

Click the teeth thirty-six times to assemble the gods. Then place both hands on
your head and beat the heavenly drum
twenty-four times.

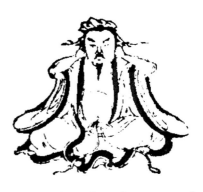

   NOTE: Close your eyes and sit [cross-
legged] with mind darkened.

   Make your hands into fists, calm
your thoughts and spirit. [4] Click your
teeth thirty-six times and hold your
Kunlun [head] in both hands.

   Interlace the hands behind the skull and hold them there for a count of
nine breaths, breathing so softly that your ears will not hear it. Also, for all
the following exercises, do not allow the breath to be audible. Beat the heavenly drum on the right and left, so it can be heard twenty-four times.

   Lift the hands so that the palms cover the ears. Place the index over the
middle finger and let them snap against the back of the skull. Do this twenty-
four times on the right and left.

---

   [3] "Chongli Baduan jin," in *Xiuzhen shishu* 19.1a-6b.

The Second Brocade

Move the Heavenly Pillar to the right and the left, twenty-four times on each side. Softly move the Heavenly Pillar.

NOTE: Shake the head to the right and left, turning it slightly to look over each shoulder and upper arm. Do this twenty-four times.

Beforehand, make sure your hands are made into fists.

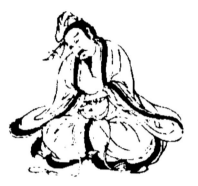

The Third Brocade

Move the tongue around the mouth to the right and left, reaching upward to the gums. Repeat thirty-six times. Swallow the saliva in three gulps like a hard object. After that you can circulate the *qi* in accordance with the firing regimen.

NOTE: Use the red dragon to stir up the water torrent. The red dragon is the tongue. Move the tongue around the mouth and teeth, reaching as far as the right and left inner cheeks.

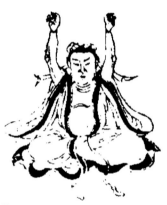

Wait until the saliva fluid arises, then swallow. Rinse the mouth thirty-six times. Another version says to drum, then rinse.

As the divine fluid fills the mouth, swallow the one mouthful in three gulps. The saliva used for rinsing is divided and swallowed in three gulps, making a rippling, gurgling sound. Then, as the dragon circulates, the tiger comes galloping naturally. The dragon is the fluids; the tiger is the *qi*.

The Fourth Brocade

Massage the hall of the kidneys with both hands, rubbing them thirty-six times. The more you do of this, the more marvelous the results.

NOTE: Hold the breath and rub your hands together until they develop heat. Inhale pure breath through the nose and hold it briefly. Rub the hands together to make them very warm.

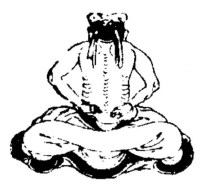

Release the breath very softly through the nose and massage the ulterior Gate of Essence on the back. The Gate of Essence is the outer kidneys on the back of the waist. Use the palms of the hands for their massage, then bring them forward and make them into fists. Complete this, then hold the breath for the count of one.

That is to say: once again hold the breath as before. Imagine a fire burning at the wheel of the navel. With the mouth closed, inhale through the nose and imagine using the fire of the heart to descend [the qi] to the lower elixir field. If you feel this as very hot, move on to the following instructions.

The Fifth Brocade

Rotate the torso at the single pass like an axle to the right and left. Repeat thirty-six times.

NOTE: Turn the central pulley [torso] to the right and left. With the head raised, move and roll the shoulders thirty-six times.

Imagine the *qi* leaving the elixir field to move upward.

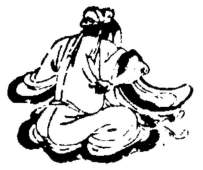

It goes through the Double Pass [in mid-spine] and enters the Skull Door [7th cervical vertebra]. Inhale pure breath through the nose and let it leisurely move up to highest perfection.

The Sixth Brocade

Rotate the torso at the double pass like a pulley to the right and left. Repeat this thirty-six times.

   NOTE: Again, turn the central pulley [torso] to the right and left.

The Seventh Brocade

Rub both hands and exhale with *he*. Repeat five times. Interlace the fingers, palms facing out, and raise the arms above the head to support Heaven. Then press the hands against the top of the head. Repeat nine times.

   NOTE: Interlace the fingers and lift them up to open space. Interlace the fingers. Do either three or nine repetitions.

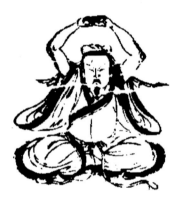

The Eighth Brocade

Rub both hands and exhale with he. Repeat five times. With both hands formed into hooks bend forward and press the soles of the feet. Repeat this twelve times. Next again pull the legs in to sit cross-legged with back straight.

   NOTE: Extend both feet parallel. With both hands reach forward to press the center of the feet. Repeat twelve times. Gather the feet toward the body and sit upright.

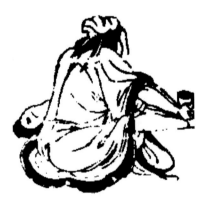

Meditation Practice

Wait now as the water reverts to rise. Wait until the saliva fluid in the mouth arises as it has not arisen before. Once again quickly use the procedure which consists of moving the tongue around the mouth to produce saliva as described earlier.

Once more rinse and once again swallow the saliva in three gulps. Once this is done, you will have swallowed the divine fluid altogether nine times. This means to rinse once again thirty-six times as before. Divide the mouthful of saliva into three gulps. Thus you get to nine swallowings.

As you swallow it down with a rippling, gurgling sound, the hundred meridians will naturally be harmonized and the river chariot [at the base of the spine] will create the perfect circulation [of *qi*].

Roll the shoulders and move and the body twenty-four times, then once again turn the pulley [torso] twenty-four times. Thereby you now develop a fire that burns the entire body. [3b] Imagine the fire in the elixir field naturally going up and down to burn the entire body. As you imagine this, the mouth and nose should hold the breath for a short while.

Doing this, wayward [*qi*] and demonic forces will no longer dare to approach you. Dream and waking will never be confused. Heat and cold can no longer penetrate you. And all kinds of calamities and ailments will stay away. If you practice this method between midnight and noon, the inner transformations will create a perfect union of Qian [Heaven] and Kun [Earth], establish the internal circulation in its proper stages, and make the eight trigrams revolve properly. The method is most excellent, indeed.

Reverting Cinnabar [5]

[1a] *The proper qi of the north is the River Chariot*

The north is the Black Emperor. He is the Ultimate Worthy. Among people, this corresponds to the yin of the lower prime [elixir field]. Its proper *qi* belongs to the phase water; in people this is the blood. As concerns the River Chariot [mercury], the *qi* of the north in its flow returns to the south. When fire refines water, dust is created. Transforming further, this becomes the water chariot. It is the essence of the lower prime.

---

[5] From *Yin Zhenjun huandan gezhu* (DZ 134).

The north with its color black and its phase water corresponds to the kidneys within human beings. The kidneys are the root of life: they divide into the essence of the sun and the moon, the energies of emptiness and non-being. The ruler of the kidneys transforms to become the human embryo.

The first position, in the east, is called Gold Dust

The east is the Green Emperor. He presides over the liver. The first position [*jia* and *yi*] is brought about through the phase water from the north and the phase fire from the south. [1b] Fire is born through wood. Nourished by water, wood grows intensely into green lushness. Therefore the songs speak of the first position. In human beings wood presides over the elixir field.

As to the production of gold dust, the rivers of the empire carry a fair amount of mud. Examples are the Han, the Yangzi, and the rivers of Jialing. All these bring forth gold dust. Workers rinse the gold particles out of the mud and refine it to yellow gold.

The same method is used in the refinement [of *qi*] in the human body. In the upper elixir field, there is a chamber known as the Jade Spring Cavern. In this cavern one finds a Jade Spring River, also called the Pure Clear Source. The effort to isolate it is called the great work. Spirit water knows no limit or shore. Collect it and guide it to the lower elixir field. As the days pass it will naturally coagulate and form grains of dust.

Both forces embrace and nourish each other: they belong to one structure

The two forces are yin and yang. Heaven is yang; Earth is yin. Left is yang; right is yin. [2a] Yin and yang are husband and wife. Within the human body, the upper elixir field is yang, the lower is yin.

As to embracing and nourishing, the four seasons continue to revolve, the five phases and Heaven and Earth mingle and interact. Thus the myriad beings come to life. When the sun embraces the moon, there naturally is radiant brightness. When the moon embraces the sun, stars and constellations appear. Husband and wife unite in harmony and create sons and daughters.

We now use the same method to isolate the spirit water of the upper elixir field. This is the great work. Refining it carefully, we guide it to the Jade Chamber in the lower prime. Thus embracing all, it revolves.

The red bird harmonizes and nurtures them; they bring forth the Golden Flower

The red bird is the phase fire. On earth it corresponds to the south and to the second position [*bing* and *ding*]. In the sky, it relates to the planet Mars. On earth it is fire, in human beings it is the heart. This fire is produced and destroyed by people themselves.

It greatly encompasses Heaven and Earth, minutely reaches into the smallest nook and cranny. Control it and it will cease; let it go and it will run wild. In the scriptures it is called the bright fire.

To harmonize means to refine. [2b] For instance one takes clay and fires it to produce pottery: it won't decay even after ten million years. Or one takes wood and burns it to charcoal: it remains in the earth for ten million years.

To harmonize, human beings isolate the water from the Jade Spring in the upper elixir field. With the fire of the heart they refine it until it enters the lower elixir field. Here they secure it behind the Jade Prison Pass. Once locked in, it is further treated with yin alchemy. Naturally a new spirit soul and a separate sun and moon arise. After nourishing them for a long time, their color turns bright and they form a new entity: the Golden Pond.

The *Dadan jue* (Great Elixir Formula) says: "Metal is the father, wood the mother. They are true lead and mercury. Lead embraces the five colors, it belongs to water and the north. There is metal [gold] in the water. This gold turns solid. It is then called the Golden Flower."

The Golden Flower is brought forth: the treasure of Heaven and Earth

The Golden Flower is like the gold dust found in the waters of the Han and the Jiang. It is brought forth naturally. [3a] One isolates elixir from the water found in the Chamber of Essence [kidneys] in the abdomen. After a few days the essence in this water turns to gold dust. Naturally it forms into a solid pearl. This process is called: the fire emerges from the water.

According to another method, one revolves the abdominal essence [semen, menstrual blood] by means of the fire of the heart. Settling in the upper prime, it coagulates into a pearl which is found in the Niwan Palace. This method is called: the water emerges from the fire.

Thus the *Huangting jing*. [Wai A:6-7] says "The clear water from the Jade Pond drips to the Numinous Root. All who cultivate this will live long."

Who among people is able to comprehend these words has found the true way of perfection

Whoever is able is not an ordinary person, because most people do not have any faith in Dao. Dao is called emptiness and nonbeing. The *Scripture*

[*Daode jing* 1] says: "Great Dao is not the ordinary way." Dao is like utter void and emptiness, it has nothing to depend or rely on.

The *Explanation* adds: "Like fish that live in water do not see it as water, so people living in Dao do not see it as Dao. [3b] In the same way dragons do not see the rocks and mountains they live in as rocks and mountains, nor demons see the earth as earth.

How could these words be wrong? The true way of perfection refers to the flower of essence in human beings. Many men lose this essence by wasting it on women who accordingly give birth to sons and daughters. They in turn closely resemble their parents in countenance, appearance, and temperament. Their fundamental dispositions are alike.

On the other hand, a seeker keeps his essence in his own body. He isolates the water of the upper prime and refines it in the lower elixir field. Soon it turns into elixir. This is called a valuable treasure.

The *Yinfu jing* (Scripture of the Hidden Talisman) says: "Yin and yang form a reciprocal oscillation and transformations are in complete accord."[6] Who among people is able to comprehend these words has completed the true Dao of Perfection.

At midnight call forth the tiger; in the early morning, the dragon.
Dragon and tiger bring each other forth; they are naturally joined
These two lines have to do with the two stems [of time calculation]. Midnight and tiger belong to yin. Yin in turn belongs to the female; the female has the disposition of water. Thus it is associated with the north and the third position [*ren* and *gui*]. This is the position of water.

The Yellow Emperor explains: "[The position of water] is called black. Lead can subdue mercury and turn it into dust." [4a] People who work on attaining the way of perfection enter this yin into the elixir field of yang. They practice it between midnight and noon [in accordance with the third position].

The dragon belongs to the phase wood. Wood is associated with the east. He further explains: "It is mercury. Mercury belongs to the phase fire." It is also known as mercury or as basic mercury. With the help of a drug that can subdue and control fire one can turn it into a treasure among men. Within the human body this is the flower of essence.

---

[6] DZ 31; translated in Komjathy 2008, 8:16

Chapter Thirteen

Women's Practice

After the arising of internal alchemy, with its emphasis on sexual energies, special cultivation practices for women began to develop. Helped by their greater independence and increased literacy, these practices are hinted at in early texts, then spelled out in some detail in materials on "women's alchemy" (*nüdan*), dating from the late Qing, i.e., 18th to 19th centuries. Much of this literature has been discussed and translated, [1] so here we limit the presentation to two short texts: an early poem and a later instruction manual.

The early poem is the *Dadao ge* 大道歌 (Song of the Great Dao) by the prominent Daoist woman poet Cao Wenyi 曹文逸 (fl. 1119-1125). Originally called Cao Daochong 曹道沖, she is has a biography in the Yuan-dynasty collection *Lishi zhenxian tidao tongjian houji* 歷世珍仙體道通鑒後記 (Supplement to the Comprehensive Mirror of Perfected Immortals and Those Who Have Embodied the Dao, DZ 298; 6.1b-3a). According to this, she was so famous that even Emperor Huizong called her to the capital and gave her the formal title "Perfected of Literary Withdrawal" (Wenyi zhenren 文逸真人).

Brief notes in Song bibliographies attest to her quality as an author and mention that she wrote commentaries to various Daoist texts, including one on the *Xisheng jing* and one, in two scrolls, on the *Daode jing* (Loon 1984, 104, 106). The latter remains in fragments and is cited in a Southern Song collection, the *Daode jing jizhu* 道德經集註 (Collected Commentaries to the *Daode jing*, DZ 707). Lady Cao is the sole woman among twenty commentators, described in the introduction as "Cao Daochong, master of stillness and humane virtue and the perfection of Dao."

---

[1] For studies, see Despeux 1990; Despeux and Kohn 2003; Valussi 2008; 2009 and Neswald 2009. For translations, see Wile 1992, 192-219.

Cao Wenyi was later venerated by several Qing-dynasty lineages of women's internal alchemy. This is evident in her appearances in spirit-writing séances and in various inscriptions preserved in the Baiyun guan. One group in particular honors her as patroness, the Lineage of Clarity and Stillness (Qingjing pai 清靜派), founded originally by Sun Buer 孫不二 (1119-1182), the sole woman among the Seven Perfected, leading disciples of the main founder of the Complete Perfection school.[2]

The *Dadao ge* is central to the program of this women's lineage. It has survived in two different versions, a short stanza cited in the *Changsheng quanjing* 長生全經 (Complete Scripture of Long Life, DZ 1466) of the Southern Song, and a more extensive opus found in the *Qunxian yaoyu zuanji* 群仙要語纂集 (Collection of Essential Sayings by the Host of Immortals, DZ 1257) by Dong Jingchun 董瑾醇 of the early Ming.

The first version consists of only one stanza that describes the fundamental vision of inner alchemical transformation. It says:

> Spirit is inner nature; *qi* is destiny.
> So that the spirit does not gallop far away, let the *qi* be firm.
> Originally the two are mutual and close,
> How could they ever be dispersed—the primordial stem of destiny.
> (13a)

This focuses on the cultivation of "inner nature" and "destiny" (*xingming* 性命), identified with spirit and *qi* (*shenqi* 神氣). Closely interrelated, the two signify the psychological and physiological aspects of human beings, inner nature referring to the mental, meditational dimensions of personality, while destiny indicates the more bodily aspects (see Lu 2009). Closely connected, both have to be developed equally until a level is reached that is often described in terms of "clarity and stillness." This level of equilibrium is reflected in the notion of the "stem of destiny," the fundamental way of being in the world, i.e., a state where the mind has been freed from desires and is completely absorbed in Dao (Despeux and Kohn 2003, 134).

---

[2] Sun Buer is another important paragon of women's practice, but she is more a model for immortality seekers and those striving to leave the world than for practitioners of longevity. For more on her, see Boltz 1987, 64-68; Cleary 1989; Despeux 1990; Despeux and Kohn 2003, 140-49.

While this version of the poem is commonly attributed to Cao Wenyi, an earlier citation of the same verse under the title *Lingyuan pian* 靈源篇 (The Numinous Source) appears in the *Daoshu* (16.1a) from the mid-12th century. Here the poem is not associated with Cao Wenyi but with He Xiangu 何仙姑, the single woman among the famous Eight Immortals, allegedly born under the Tang.[3] Like Cao Wenyi, she realized oneness with Dao and became an inspiration for women's successful cultivation.

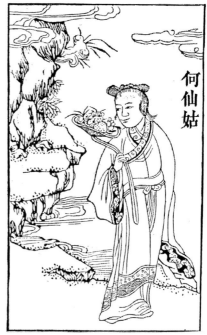

The longer and more elaborate version of the poem focuses to a large extent on longevity practices as a major stepping stone toward oneness with Dao. It begins by admonishing women to concentrate the mind and practice deep breathing, so that the stem of destiny is activated.

Fig. 23: He Xiangu, the lady immortal

Once accomplished, the body is strengthened and radiates with long life, while the mind becomes luminous and spirit begins to work like a numinous mirror, containing and reflecting all, yet evaluating and classifying nothing. Continuing to let go of plans, schemes, sensory amusements, and the outward trappings of worldly success, women find inner serenity, peace, and an ease that eventually grows into a sense of oneness with the Great Ultimate, the state of the universe at creation. This in turn causes a feeling of inner openness, of floating in the paradises of Huaxu and the Pure Land, as well as a vision of the body as consisting not so much of flesh and bones but of palaces and chambers where universal spirit and the gods come to reside.

Very practical throughout, it is obvious that the poem is not just for hermits working in isolation but for women in spiritual communities and lay followers who obey moral precepts and enter times of retreat. It concludes by reiterating the fleeting pleasures to be gained from worldly fame and profit and encouraging its audience to forsake them thoroughly. Practitioners can

---

[3] Studies of He Xiangu appear in Grant 1995 and Wu 2011, 131-43.

turn away from these pleasures by extinguishing the negative aspects of their lifelong habits, inner tendencies, and acquired skills—even poetry, the main claim to fame of the author. They do so gently and gradually yet relentlessly and with great persistence, always actively supported by Dao.

The second text comes from the *Nüdan tiyao* 女丹提要(Descriptive Notes on Women's Alchemy), a collection of materials on women's practice by Fu Jinquan 傅金銓, aka Jiyizi 濟一子 (1765-1845). A native of Jiangxi, he undertook extensive travels through southern China in a quest for spiritual practices, then settled in Sichuan in 1817, where he ran a local spirit-writing community and engaged in various internal practices (Despeux and Kohn 2003, 206). He was an avid collector and collator of texts, including also the *Nü jindan fayao* 女金丹法要 (Essential Methods for Women's Golden Alchemy), collated in 1813. Like other men of the time, he felt that women should be able to pursue personal cultivation but under proper guidance and supervision. As he says in the preface to the latter work:

> Since early times perfected women have been many, but their methods of refinement have not been recorded in books. In this era few have heard of them. Women practice for three years, while men need nine years [to reach perfection]. Even though as a daily practice it is quite easy, finding a master is very difficult. Men can go and seek a fortune [and a master with affinity] for a thousand li, but for women, leaving the inner chamber by just half a step is very difficult. There are thousands of chapters of alchemical treatises, but they do not list or include female practice. So I have put together this book. (1a; Valussi 2009, 145)

The *Nüdan tiyao* today appears as part of the *Nüdan hebian* 女丹合編 (Combined Collection on Women's Alchemy), an extensive collection by He Longxiang 賀龍驤, dated to 1906 (see Valussi 2008). The passage selected here begins after the initial poem attributed to Lü Dongbin, leader of the Eight Immortals and popular divine manifestation during spirit-writing séances.[4] It focuses on three features of destiny and explains the internal geography of women's bodies, centered on the navel area, known as the Gate of Destiny (*mingmen* 命門)—commonly located just below the navel and associated with sexual energies (Neswald 2009, 139).

Near it are the Yellow Court (*Huangting* 黄庭), described generally as the center of the torso in early literature and identified in later alchemical

---

[4] For studies of Lü Dongbin, see Ang 1993; Baldrian-Hussein 1985; 1986; Katz 2000; Mori 2002.

texts as the lower elixir field, the Dark Towers (*youque* 幽闕), the poetic name for the kidneys, as well as the Prime of the Passes (*guanyuan* 關元) and the Ocean of *Qi* (*qihai* 氣海). The passes are major energy gates along the spite through which essences rise up in alchemical transformation. They are Tail Gate (*weilü* 尾閭) at the coccyx; Narrow Strait (*jiaji* 夾脊) in the mid-back; and Jade Pillow (*yuzhen* 玉枕) at the back of the skull, but their core lies in the center of the torso. The Ocean of *Qi*, also the name of an acupuncture point on the Conception Vessel that runs along the front of the torso (VC-6), is often identified with the lower elixir field, but here is more subtle than that. In addition, this area of the body is also known as the Earth Palace (*kungong* 坤宮), and the text emphasizes that practice activates the phase earth, raising its energy to the chest area, in women the seat of vitality and original *qi* (Neswald 2009, 38).

This center in women is called the Milk Chamber (*rushi* 乳室) in the text, but more commonly described as the *Qi* Cavity (*qixue* 氣穴). Located between the breasts, the *Nü jindan* 女金丹 (Women's Golden Elixir), another text collected by Fu Jinquan and reprinted in the *Nüdan hebian* describes it:

> The *Qi* Cavity is where the monthly flow originates. It is found at the breasts, more precisely, in the area between them, about 1.3 inches from each. It is not identical with the nipples. In men, destiny resides in the lower elixir field; this is their *Qi* Cavity. In women, it resides in the breasts; this is their *Qi* Cavity (2.21a; Despeux and Kohn 2003, 191; see also Neswald 2009, 39; Valussi 2009, 155)

The goal of the practice is to reverse the tendency of the body to allow pure *qi* to descend from the breasts into the abdomen where it becomes blood and exits the body through the vagina. To do so, women use a mixture of meditation, massages, and herbal supplements. They have to act at the time of the "monthly messenger" (*yuexin* 月信) (Despeux 1990, 253-56). About two-and-a-half days before the onset of menstruation, this "messenger" signals the impending transformation of yang *qi* into yin blood. It comes with a group of well-known symptoms, such as leg pains, headaches, loss of appetite, mood swings, depression, or hyperactivity.

Women at this time can extract pure yin-*qi* from the yang-*qi* contained in their *Qi* Cavity, just as men at this "time of vibrancy" can extract pure yang-*qi* from their seminal essence. The imagery used to describe this process is based on the *Yijing*: women pull the yin from the trigram Li (fire), while men take the yang from the trigram Kan (water) (Despeux and Kohn 2003, 227).

In women, the three elixir fields are called "destinies," the topic of our selection. They are different from those in men, where they are located in the head, the chest, and the abdomen. Here they are the elixir field (Ocean of *Qi*), the Fetal Prime (womb), and the Blood Prime (*Qi* Cavity).

In girls, essence concentrates in the Yang Cavity in the head; it does not descend to form the menses and retains a pure, white color. In mature women, essence collects in the Yellow Chamber and forms breasts, emerging on occasion as breast milk. Every month, it descends into the elixir field, where it is transformed and expelled as menses. A central feature of the alchemical enterprise is to make it return upward and revert to a purer state. The text here notes that women after the age of forty-nine no longer have this process but can still revitalize their system and enhance long life by following the instructions.

The practice is summarily known as "decapitating the red dragon" (*duan honglong* 斷紅龍), leading—as the text describes—over several month to a lightening in the color of the monthly flow, then to its complete cessation, matching the goal of Daoists to return to the state of primordial nonbeing. In modern biomedical terms, this has to do with hormonal changes and neuro-endocrinology, notably the disruption of the pulsating release of LH at the hypothalamus which inhibits positive estrogen feedback, an increased production of hypothalamic β-endorphins, and the release of the hormone ocytocine (see Requena 2012). It also increases the output of melatonin, well known for its age-retarding properties, due to its antioxidant action, inhibition of platelet aggregation, and heart protection. The practice thus contributes actively to the nourishing of women's vitality at all stages of life.

Translation

Song of the Great Dao [5]

[4b] I am telling all you ladies straight:
The stem of destiny grows from perfect breathing
That irradiates the body and provides long life—empty or not empty—
The numinous mirror that contains Heaven and all beings.

The Great Ultimate opens to the wondrous, you attain the One.
Once you have the One, hold on to it, make sure you do not lose it.
Your inner palaces and chambers void and relaxed, spirit naturally stays.
Your numinous center decocts and smelts all hardened blood and fluids.

Sorrow now, now joy, then thoughts and worry,
Easy now, now working hard—the body gets worm-eaten and worn-out.
Harm in the morning, neglect at night—you never know your error.
Losing essence and confusing spirit, they have nothing to hang on.

Slowly, subtly you grind yourself down, step by step get weaker
Until you use up and exhaust primordial harmony, and the gods all leave.
The only thing to do is meditate in action, meditate while sitting,
But only sages can do this, ordinary folk cannot

Young shoots, soft and tender: go and cherish them. [5a]
Root consciousness dark and confused: change comes easily enough.
Stumble and don't know why: get rid of thorns and brambles.
I've never heard of a beautiful bride going out to tend the fields.

After nine years, the work is complete, the firing time sufficient.
Then you can go along with all in no-mind, your spirit changing swiftly.
The mind of no-mind: that's the perfect mind—
Move and rest equally forgotten, far removed from all desires.
Merge all forces to join in the One , then forget the One,

---

[5] *Dadao ge*, from *Qunxian youyu zuanji* (DZ 1257).

And you'll be able to emerge and go along with primordial changes.
Penetrate metal, pierce through stone—none with difficulty,
Sit and cast off all, stand and forget all—just be all at once!

Spirit is inner nature; *qi* is destiny.
If spirit never runs amok, *qi* is naturally stable.
Originally which among the two is closer to myself?
Losing either, how can I find my root?

This path, easy to know, is not easy to practice.
Forget in practice why you practice: the path is soon complete.
Don't just hold your breath and make that your main routine.
Count the breath following a plan, well, that's not quite it either.

Try hard to go easy, release all outside grime and labor,
But inside your mind is tied in knots—how is that any different?
Just regard the embryo residing in the womb
And let go of all mind, release all plans and schemes.

Concentrate your *qi*, making it very soft, and spirit stays forever. [5b]
Your perfect breath, going in and out, naturally lengthens.
Continuously expand, let it wind around, recover your prime destiny.
No need to draw from the numinous spring—it always flows of itself.

36,000 marks a great achievement.
Yin and yang lined up right in its midst.
Steaming through joints and channels, transforming bones and muscles:
Everywhere bright and radiant, no parts are unopened.

The Three Deathbringers leave through gates of yin
As a myriad heads of state arrive to pay the Red Emperor obeisance.
Ask the perfect where they hail from:
Originally from the Prime, they now reside in your Numinous Terrace.

In the old days, clouds and mist deeply shrouded all.
Today we meet in openness; the eyes of Dao are clear.
This is not just one morning or even just one night—
It's my original perfection, not just a mere technique.
My years are cold, solid, strong—just like stone and metal.

I fight to repel the shadow demons, increase my wisdom's power.
Coming from emptiness and serenity, essence is once more concentrated—
It is truly like in Huaxu Palace, the Land of Pure and Tranquil.

What, then, to do first to set up the foundation?
Make ultimate nonbeing my home: nothing is not done.
All projections and images in my thoughts go out completely;
All sprites and specters in my dreams are utterly tied up.

Neither agitated nor yet still: that's the great essential.
Neither square nor yet round: that's the utmost Dao. [6a]

Primordial harmony refined within lets you attain perfection.
Breathing used without never yields such results.
Primordial *qi* won't stay, the gods won't be at peace:
A worm-eaten tree with no roots, its branches and leaves wither.

Stop talking about snot and mucus, essence, blood, and stuff.
Once you get to the root and reach the source, it's all the same.
This thing—how can you add to its stable placement?
Yet it changes with time, following your intention and your mind.

In the body, stimulated by heat, it turns to sweat.
In the eyes, stimulated by sadness, it turns to tears.
In the kidneys, stimulated by thought, it turns to semen.
In the nose, stimulated by wind, it turns to snot.

Flowing and circulating this way and that, it soaks through the whole body.
Reaching the head, don't let it leave through spirit water.
Spirit water is hard to explain, cognizing it is subtle,
But it all comes directly from perfected *qi*.

Just know how to be serene and relaxed, free from thoughts and worries.
Fast and retreat to calm your mind, control all speech and talking.
Fill with the taste of buttery liquor, the sap of pure sweet dew:
Hunger and thirst dissolve completely in perfect simplicity.
Time comes you've fully reached the good, naturally wander free and easy,
Unlike the early days of refinement and concoction, full of toil and effort.
Yet even during times of toil, you don't really toil hard—

Leisurely and relaxed: that's how you nurture primordial spirit. [6b]

But what to do if the mind cannot find relaxation?
Get to this point, you need to let go of all grasping, just be whole in yourself.
If I think of myself as toiling hard, hardship just increases.
So live on fruit, dress in leaves, be still and solitary.

The mind knows the great Dao, yet cannot practice it.
Names and traces and self-identity: these are great afflictions.
Much better to find a leisurely place and do the great work,
Then strife starts to feel like peace, and you reach great stability.

Body and spirit described as two are had to make one whole.
So if you can't perfect your destiny, start work on inner nature.
Unless you let go of pursuing fame and going after profit,
You'll never manage to release emotions and be free from all affairs.

Intensely radiant among men—why focus on obstructions?
Containing all teachings in yourself—who'd control and push you?
Voice and value that lift Heaven—what good could they do?
Riding horses, writing verses—enough to make you noble?

Fancy clothes, delicious foods—forever without meaning.
Collecting jades, piling up gold—what do they do for salvation?
Practical expertise, literary skills, and even poetry—
All they can do is block your path of cultivation.

Like thin fleeting mist or hazy smoke,
Resting on falling petals, moving with willow catkins,
Misty and obscure, dark and vague, neither of Heaven nor of Earth—
These things arrive, yet never get to make any real rain or dew. [7a]
Fame or self—which is dearer to you?[6]
Half your life, for years and months, you run after them in circles.
Much better to cultivate refinement, work on *qi* and spirit.
As long as they remain unsettled, in vain you toil and labor.

---

[6] This echoes *Daode jing* 44: "Which means more to you, you or your renown?
Which brings more to you, you or what you own?" (Bynner 1944, 73)

How pitiful! Despite your good foundation,
Your inner palaces of gold and halls of jade are devoid of a true master.

Work diligently to become this master in yourself and remain so forever.
Set yourself up in emptiness and leisure—the realm of uselessness.
Nonbeing contains amazing reality, but getting hold of it is hard—
To release and nurture the inner child, first take care of its mother.

Seal and contain excellence and analysis, hide brightness and intelligence.
Just gather and collect essence and spirit, look like a fool or simpleton.
With strong mind and single will keep advancing forward:
The great Dao will be with you, never you to fail.

The Three Destiny Centers [7]

The subtle nature of destiny is hard to explain. It ebbs and flows constantly in thousands of changes and tens of thousands of transformations.

In human beings, the navel area is called the Gate of Destiny. Inside it lays the Yellow Court; beyond it stand the Dark Towers. Above it is the Prime of all Passes; below it is the Ocean of *Qi*. To its left is the Sun; to its right is the Moon—all shining brightly.

Similarly the three destiny centers radiate in different colors: yellow signals the elixir field; white, the Fetal Prime; and purple, the Blood Prime.

The Blood Prime is the Milk Chamber. Located in the middle, about 1.2 inches from each breast, it is not the two nipples. In men, destiny resides in the Elixir Field, the perfect soil of the elixir of life. In women, destiny resides in the Milk Chamber, the wood essence of mother *qi*.

The Fetal Prime contracts in the abdomen, while the Blood Prime brings forth blood, and the Elixir Field produces the elixir.

The great work commences in the hours between midnight and noon. In your mind, see the empty hollow of the Milk Chamber. Breathe slowly and softly, exhaling easily while inhaling deeply. Wait until the monthly messenger arrives, then guide the *qi* up from the Elixir Field to the Milk Chamber. The monthly messenger arrives before the monthly flow. What exactly is it? The word "messenger" contains the character for "person" on its

---

[7] From *Nüdan tiyao.*

outside, showing someone who has not yet returned home. This means that the messenger arrives first.

On the day when this messenger arrives, you will recognize it clearly. You might feel achy in your hips or legs, your head or eyes might be restless, or you may have no appetite for food and drink. When the messenger arrives with these indications, blood is being produced in the body. To transform it into *qi*, on these days before noon concentrate your mind with effort.

On the other hand, once your monthly flow has started, the red dragon with its yin essence can no longer be caught. It moves about in confusion and meanders wildly, killing people left and right.

There is nothing else but wait out the flow. During the two days following it test the area with a white cloth. If the color is yellow or golden, this shows that the flow has started to disperse.

With a clear mind make the effort to transport it upward and cut if off completely. Do this for several months in a row, and your monthly flow will change: first to yellow, then to white, and eventually to nothing at all.

Looking at this, realize that it is just like the path of return to nothingness.

In women, blood plays the role of the kidneys [in men], therefore they have an open orifice. After you reach forty-nine years of age, your loins dry up and your blood stagnates. You can no longer bear children.

If you nourish your vitality for a very long time, however, you can still give rise to the Blood Prime. This will feel as if you were with child—it reveals the wonder of reality being brought forth from the midst of nonbeing.

See how it happens, then cut it off once, and your life arises anew. From this point onward, work with concentration on both your inner nature and destiny, following the same procedures as the men.

Should wind arise in your navel area, thunder sound, and lightning hit, this signals the transformation of the numinous power of blood. By the same token, should clouds stream along, fog roll in, flowers bloom, and birds fly about, this signals the rise of the Prime of Earth. Who can ever understand its wonder?

Bibliography

Andersen, Poul. 1980. *The Method of Holding the Three Ones*. London: Curzon Press.

Anderson, Eugene N. 1988. *The Food of China*. New Haven: Yale University Press.

Ang, Isabelle. 1993. "Le culte de Lü Dongbin des origines jusqu'au debut du XIV siecle." Ph.D. Diss., Université de Paris VII.

Arthur, Shawn. 2006a. "Ancient Daoist Diets for Health and Longevity." Ph. D. Diss., Boston University, Boston.

_____. 2006b. "Life Without Grains: *Bigu* and the Daoist Body." In *Daoist Body Cultivation*, edited by Livia Kohn, 91-122. Magdalena, NM: Three Pines Press.

_____. 2009. "Eating Your Way to Immortality: Early Daoist Self-Cultivation Diets." *Journal of Daoist Studies* 2:32-63.

Bailey, Ronald. 2005. *Liberation Biology: The Scientific and Moral Case for the Biotech Revolution*. Amherst: Prometheus.

Balasz, Etienne. 1948. "Entre revolt nihilistique et evasion mystique." *Asiatische Studien/Etudes Asiatiques* 1/2: 2755.

Baldrian-Hussein, Farzeen. 1984. *Procédés secrets du joyau magique*. Paris: Les Deux Océans.

_____. 1985. "Yüeh-yang and Lü Tung-pin's *Chin-yüan ch'un*: A Sung Alchemical Poem." In *Religion und Philosophie in Ostasien: Festschrift für Hans Steininger*, edited by. G. Naundorf, K.H. Pohl, and H. H. Schmidt, 19-31. Würzburg: Königshausen and Neumann.

_____. 1986. "Lü Tung-pin in Northern Sung Literature." *Cahiers d'Extrême-Asie* 2: 133-70.

_____. 2004. "The *Book of the Yellow Court*: A Lost Song Commentary of the 12th Century." *Cahiers d'Extrême-Asie* 14:187-226.

Barrett, Timothy H. 1980. "On the Transmission of the *Shen tzu* and of the *Yang-sheng yao-chi*." *Journal of the Royal Asiatic Society* 2: 168-76.

_____. 1996. *Taoism Under the T'ang: Religion and Empire During the Golden Age of Chinese History*. London: Wellsweep Press.

Benecke, Mark. 2002. *The Dream of Eternal Life: Biomedicine, Aging, and Immortality*. New York: Columbia University Press.

Bentov, Itchak. 1977. *Stalking the Wild Pendulum: On the Mechanics of Consciousness*. New York: E. P. Dutton.

Berk, William R. 1986 [1895]. *Chinese Healing Arts: Internal Kung-Fu*. Burbank, Calif.: Unique Publications.

Bohm, David. 1951. *Quantum Theory*. New York: Prentice-Hall.

Bokenkamp, Stephen R. 1997. *Early Daoist Scriptures*. With a contribution by Peter Nickerson. Berkeley: University of California Press.

_____. 2007. *Ancestors and Anxiety: Daoism and the Birth of Rebirth in China*. Berkeley: University of California Press.

Boltz, Judith M. 1987. *A Survey of Taoist Literature: Tenth to Seventeenth Centuries*. Berkeley: University of California, China Research Monograph 32.

Bova, Ben. 1998. *Immortality: How Science is Extending Your Life Span—and Challenging the World*. New York: Avon Books.

Bynner, Witter. 1944. *The Way of Life According to Lao tsu*. New York: Perigree.

Cahill, Suzanne. 1993. *Transcendence and Divine Passion: The Queen Mother of the West in Medieval China*. Stanford: Stanford University Press.

_____. 2006. *Divine Traces of the Daoist Sisterhood*. Magdalena, NM: Three Pines Press.

Campany, Robert F. 2002. *To Live As Long As Heaven and Earth: A Translation and Study of Ge Hong's Traditions of Divine Transcendents*. Berkeley: University of California Press.

_____. 2005. "Living Off the Books: Fifty Ways to Dodge *Ming* in Early Medieval China." In *The Magnitude of Ming: Command, Allotment, and Fate in Chinese Culture*, edited by Christopher Lupke. Honolulu: University of Hawai'i Press.

Carlson, Ed, and Livia Kohn, 2012. *Core Health: The Quantum Way to Inner Power*. St. Petersburg, FL: Energy Essentials.

Cedzich, Ursula-Angelika. 2001. "Corpse Deliverance, Substitute Bodies, Name Change, and Feigned Death: Aspects of Metamorphosis and Immortality in Early Medieval China." *Journal of Chinese Religions* 29: 1-68.

Chan, Alan K. L. 1991. *Two Visions of the Way: A Study of the Wang Pi and the Ho-shang-kung Commentaries on the Laozi*. Albany: State University of New York Press.

Chia, Mantak, and Maneewan Chia. 1993. *Awaken Healing Light of the Tao*. Huntington, NY: Healing Tao Books.

Chopra, Deepak. 1993. *Ageless Body, Timeless Mind: The Quantum Alternative to Growing Old*. New York: Harmony Books.

Cleary, Thomas. 1989. *Immortal Sisters: Secrets of Taoist Women*. Boston: Shambhala.

Cohen, Kenneth S. 1997. *The Way of Qigong: The Art and Science of Chinese Energy Healing*. New York: Ballantine.

Couzin, Jennifer. 2005. "How Much Can Human Life Span Be Extended?" *Science* 309:71-83.

Craze, Richard, and Roni Jay. 2001. *Cooking for Long Life: The Tao of Food*. New York: Sterling Publishing.

De Souza, Eduardo. 2011. "Health and Sexuality: Daoist Practice and Reichian Therapy." In *Living Authentically: Daoist Contributions to Modern Psychology*, edited by Livia Kohn, 194-218. Dunedin, FL: Three Pines Press.

Despeux, Catherine. 1987. *Préscriptions d'acuponcture valant mille onces d'or*. Paris: Guy Trédaniel.

_____. 1988. *La moélle du phénix rouge: Santé et longue vie dans la Chine du seiziéme siècle*. Paris: Editions Trédaniel.

_____. 1989. "Gymnastics: The Ancient Tradition." In *Taoist Meditation and Longevity Techniques*, edited by Livia Kohn, 223-61. Ann Arbor: University of Michigan, Center for Chinese Studies Publications.

_____. 1990. *Immortelles de la Chine ancienne. Taoïsme et alchimie feminine*. Paris: Pardes.

_____. 2004. "La gymnastique *daoyin* dans la Chine ancienne." *Etudes chinoises* 23:45-86.

_____. 2006. "The Six Healing Breaths." In *Daoist Body Cultivation*, edited by Livia Kohn, 37-67. Magdalena, NM: Three Pines Press.

_____. 2007. "Food Prohibitions in China." *The Lantern* 4.1:22-32.

_____, and Frederic Obringer, eds. 1997. *La maladie dans la Chine médiévale: La toux*. Paris: Editions L`Harmattan.

_____, and Livia Kohn. 2003. *Women in Daoism*. Cambridge, Mass.: Three Pines Press.

DeWoskin, Kenneth J. 1983. *Doctors, Diviners, and Magicians of Ancient China*. New York: Columbia University Press.

Eberhard, Wolfram. 1971. "Fatalism in the Life of the Common Man in Non-Communist China." In *Moral and Social Values of the Chinese*, edited by Wolfram Eberhard, 177-89. Taipei: Chengwen.

Engelhardt, Ute. 1987. *Die klassische Tradition der Qi-Übungen. Eine Darstellung anhand des Tang-zeitlichen Textes Fuqi jingyi lun von Sima Chengzhen*. Wiesbaden: Franz Steiner.

_____. 1989. "*Qi* for Life: Longevity in the Tang." In *Taoist Meditation and Longevity Techniques*, edited by Livia Kohn, 263-94. Ann Arbor: University of Michigan, Center for Chinese Studies Publications.

_____. 1996. "Zur Bedeutung der Atmung im Qigong." *Chinesische Medizin* 1/1996: 17-23.

_____. 1998. "Neue archäologische Funde zur Leitbahntheorie." *Chinesische Medizin* 3/1998: 93-100.

_____. 2000. "Longevity Techniques and Chinese Medicine." In *Daoism Handbook*, edited by Livia Kohn, 74-108. Leiden: E. Brill.

_____, and Carl-Hermann Hempen. 1997. *Chinesische Diätetik*. Munich: Urban & Schwarzenberg.

Erkes, Eduard. 1958. *Ho-Shang-Kung's Commentary of Lao Tse*. Ascona: Artibus Asiae.

Eskildsen, Stephen. 1998. *Asceticism in Early Taoist Religion*. Albany: State University of New York Press.

_____. 2004. *The Teachings and Practices of the Early Quanzhen Taoist Masters*. Albany: State University of New York Press.

Ettinger, Robert C.W. 1964. *Prospect of Immortality*. Garden City, NJ: Doubleday.

Farquhar, Judith. 2002. *Appetites: Food and Sex in Post-socialist China*. Durham, NC: Duke University Press.

Feher, Michael, ed. 1989. *Fragments for a History of the Human Body*. New York: Urzone.

Feinstein, David, Donna Eden, and Gary Craig. 2005. *The Promise of Energy Psychology*. New York: Penguin.

Flanigan, Richard J., and Kate Flanigan Sawyer. 2007. *Longevity Made Simple: How to Add 20 Good Years to Your Life*. Denver: Williams Clark.

Foucault, Michel. 1973. *The Birth of the Clinic*. London: Tavistock.

Fukunaga Mitsuji 福永光司. 1973. "Dōkyō ni okeru kagami to ken" 道教における鏡 と検. *Tōhō gakuhō* 東方學報 45: 59-120.

Furth, Charlotte. 1999. *A Flourishing Yin: Gender in China's Medical History, 960-1665*. Berkeley: University of California Press.

Gallo, Fred, ed. 2004. *Energy Psychology in Psychotherapy*. New York: Norton..

Gerber, Richard. 1988. *Vibrational Medicine: New Choices for Healing Ourselves*. Santa Fe: Bear and Company.

Graham, A. C. 1960. *The Book of Lieh-tzu*. London: A. Murray.

_____. 1981. *Chuang-tzu: The Seven Inner Chapters and Other Writings from the Book of Chuang-tzu*. London: Allan & Unwin.

_____. 1986. *Chuang-tzu: The Inner Chapters*. London: Allan & Unwin.

Grant, Beata. 1995. "Patterns of Female Religious Experience in Qing Dynasty Popular Literature." *Journal of Chinese Religions* 23:29-58.

Greatrex, Roger. 1987. *The Bowu zhi: An Annotated Translation*. Stockholm: Föreningen för Orientaliska Studier.

Gribbin, John. 1984. *In Search of Schrödinger's Cat*. Toronto: Bantam Books.

Gulik, Robert H. van. 1961. *Sexual Life in Ancient China*. Leiden: E. Brill.

Hall, Stephen S. 2003. *Merchants of Immortality: Chasing the Dream of Human Life Extension*. Boston: Houghton Mifflin.

Harper, Donald. 1994. "Resurrection in Warring States Popular Religion." *Taoist Resources* 5.2: 13-28.

_____. 1998. *Early Chinese Medical Manuscripts: The Mawangdui Medical Manuscripts*. London: Wellcome Asian Medical Monographs.

Harrington, Alan. 1977. *The Immortalist*. Millbrae, Calif.: Celestial Arts.

Hendrischke, Barbara. 2000. "Early Daoist Movements." In *Daoism Handbook*, edited by Livia Kohn, 134-64. Leiden: E. Brill.

Henricks, Robert. 1983. *Philosophy and Argumentation in Third Century China: The Essays of Hsi K'ang*. Princeton: Princeton University Press.

Holzman, Donald. 1956. "Les sept sages de la fort des bambus et la societe de leur temps." *T'oung Pao* 44: 31746.

_____. 1957. *La vie et la pensee de Hi K'ang*. Leiden: E. Brill.

Homann, Rolf. 1971. *Die wichtigsten Körpergottheiten im Huang-t'ing-ching*. Göppingen: Alfred Kümmerle.

Hsia, Emil C. H., Ilza Veith, and Robert H. Geertsma. 1986. *The Essentials of Medicine in Ancient China and Japan: Yasuyori Tamba's Ishinpō*. 2 vols. Leiden: E. Brill.

Huang Yongfeng 黄永锋. 2007. *Daojiao yinshi yangsheng zhiyao* 道教饮食养生指要. Beijing: Zongjiao wenhua chubanshe.

＿＿＿. 2008. *Daojiao yinshi chishu zhexue yanjiu* 道教服食技术哲学研究. Beijing: Dongfang.

Huang, Hsing-Tsung. 2000. *Fermentation and Food Science*. In *Science and Civilisation in China*, vol. VI, part 5. Cambridge: Cambridge University Press.

Huang, Jane, and Michael Wurmbrand. 1987. *The Primordial Breath: Ancient Chinese Ways of Prolonging Life Through Breath*. 2 vols. Torrance, Cal.: Original Books.

Ikai Yoshio 豬飼祥夫. 2004. "Kōryō Chōkasan kanken Insho yakuchūkō" 江陵張家山漢簡引書釋註. Draft paper. Used by permission of the author.

Ishida, Hidemi. 1989. "Body and Mind: The Chinese Perspective." In *Taoist Meditation and Longevity Techniques*, edited by Livia Kohn, 41-70. Ann Arbor: University of Michigan, Center for Chinese Studies Publications.

Ishihara, Akira, and Howard S. Levy. 1970. *The Tao of Sex*. New York: Harper & Row.

Jackowicz, Stephen. 2006. "'ion, Digestion, and Regestation: The Complexities of the Absorption of *Qi*." In *Daoist Body Cultivation*, edited by Livia Kohn, 68-90. Magdalena, NM: Three Pines Press.

Kalinowski, Marc. 1985. "La transmission du dispositif des Neuf Palais sous les Six-dynasties." In *Tantric and Taoist Studies*, edited by Michel Strickmann, 3:773-811. Brussels: Institut Belge des Hautes Etudes Chinoises.

Kaltenmark, Max. 1953. *Le Lie-sien tchouan*. Peking: Université de Paris Publications.

Kaptchuk, Ted J. 2000. *The Web that Has No Weaver: Understanding Chinese Medicine*. New York: Congdon & Weed.

Katz, Paul R. 2000. *Images of the Immortal: The Cult of Lü Dongbin at the Palace of Eternal Joy*. Honolulu: University of Hawaii Press.

Keightley, David N. 1978. "The Religious Commitment: Shang Theology and the Genesis of Chinese Political Culture." *History of Religions* 17: 211-25.

Kendall, Donald E. 2002. *Dao of Chinese Medicine: Understanding an Ancient Healing Art*. New York: Oxford University Press.

Ki, Sunu. 1985. *The Canon of Acupuncture: Huangti Nei Ching Ling Shu*. Los Angeles: Yuin University Press.

Kirkland, J. Russell. 1986. "Taoists of the High T'ang: An Inquiry into the Perceived Significance of Eminent Taoists in Medieval Chinese Society." Ph.D. Diss., Indiana University, Bloomington.

Kleeman, Terry. 1998. *Great Perfection: Religion and Ethnicity in a Chinese Millenarian Kingdom*. Honolulu: University of Hawaii Press.

Klein, Bruce J., and Sebastian Sethe, eds. 2004. *The Scientific Conquest of Death*. Buenos Aires: Libros EnRed.

Knaul, Livia. 1985a. "The Winged Life: Kuo Hsiang's Mystical Philosophy." *Journal of Chinese Studies* 2.1:17-41.

_____. 1985b. "Kuo Hsiang and the *Chuang-tzu*." *Journal of Chinese Philosophy* 12.4:429-47.

Kobayashi, Masayoshi. 1992. "The Celestial Masters Under the Eastern Jin and Liu-Song Dynasties." *Taoist Resources* 3.2: 17-45.

Kohn, Livia, ed. 1989. *Taoist Meditation and Longevity Techniques*. Ann Arbor: University of Michigan, Center for Chinese Studies Publications.

_____. 1991. "Taoist Visions of the Body." *Journal of Chinese Philosophy* 18: 227-52.

_____. 1992. *Early Chinese Mysticism: Philosophy and Soteriology in the Taoist Tradition*. Princeton: Princeton University Press.

_____. 1993. *The Taoist Experience: An Anthology*. Albany: State University of New York Press.

_____. 1995a. "Kôshin: A Taoist Cult in Japan. Part II: Historical Development." *Japanese Religions* 20.1: 34-55.

_____. 1995b. *Laughing at the Tao: Debates among Buddhists and Taoists in Medieval China*. Princeton: Princeton University Press.

_____. 1998. "Counting Good Deeds and Days of Life: The Quantification of Fate in Medieval China." *Asiatische Studien/Etudes Asiatiques* 52: 833-70.

_____. 2001a. *Daoism and Chinese Culture*. Cambridge: Three Pines Press.

_____. 2001b. *Chen Tuan: Discussions and Translations*. Cambridge: Three Pines Press, E-Dao Series.

_____. 2002. "Quiet Sitting with Master Yinshi: Medicine and Religion in Modern China." In *Living with the Dao: Conceptual Issues in Daoist Practice*, edited by Livia Kohn, 157-72. Cambridge, Mass.: Three Pines Press, E-Dao Series.

_____. 2003. *Monastic Life in Medieval Daoism: A Cross-Cultural Perspective*. Honolulu: University of Hawaii Press.

_____. 2004a. *Cosmos and Community: The Ethical Dimension of Daoism*. Cambridge, Mass.: Three Pines Press.

_____. 2004b. *Supplement to Cosmos and Community: The Ethical Dimension of Daoism*. Cambridge, Mass.: Three Pines Press, E-Dao series.

_____. 2004c. *The Daoist Monastic Manual: A Translation of the Fengdao kejie*. New York: Oxford University Press.

_____. 2005. *Health and Long Life: The Chinese Way*. Cambridge, Mass.: Three Pines Press.

_____, ed. 2006. *Daoist Body Cultivation: Traditional Models and Contemporary Practices*. Magdalena, NM: Three Pines Press.

_____. 2007. *Daoist Mystical Philosophy: The Scripture of Western Ascension*. Magdalena, NM: Three Pines Press.

_____. 2008. *Chinese Healing Exercises: The Tradition of Daoyin*. Honolulu: University of Hawai'i Press.

_____. 2009. "Body and Identity." In *New Studies of the Liezi*, edited by Ronnie Littlejohn. Albany: State University of New York Press.

_____. 2010a. *Daoist Dietetics: Food for Immortality*. Dunedin, Fla.: Three Pines Press.

_____. 2010b. *Sitting in Oblivion: The Heart of Daoist Meditation*. Dunedin, Fla.: Three Pines Press.

_____. 2011. *Chuang-tzu: The Tao of Perfect Happiness. Selections Annotated and Explained*. Woodstock, VT: Skylight Paths Press.

_____, and Robin R. Wang, eds. 2009. *Internal Alchemy: Self, Society, and the Quest for Immortality*. Magdalena, NM: Three Pines Press.

_____, and Russell Kirkland. 2000. "Daoism in the Tang (618-907)." In *Daoism Handbook*, edited by Livia Kohn, 339-83. Leiden: E. Brill.

Komjathy, Louis. 2002. *Title Index to Daoist Collections*. Cambridge, Mass.: Three Pines Press.

_____. 2007. *Cultivating Perfection: Mysticism and Self-Transformation in Quanzhen Daoism*. Leiden: E. Brill.

_____. 2008. *Handbooks for Daoist Practice*. Hong Kong: Yuen Yuen Institute.

Kroll, Paul W. 1985. "In the Halls of the Azure Lad." *Journal of the American Oriental Society* 105: 75-94.

_____. 1996. "Body Gods and Inner Vision: *The Scripture of the Yellow Court.* In *Religions of China in Practice*, edited by Donald S. Lopez Jr., 149-55. Princeton: Princeton University Press.

Lagerwey, John. 2004. "Deux écrits taoïstes anciens." *Cahiers d'Extrême-Asie* 14:131-72.

Lam, Michael, Maria Sulindro, and Dorine Tan. 2002. *How to Stay Young and Live Longer: The Definite Guide to Anti-Aging.* Pasadena, Calif.: Academy of Anti-Aging Research.

Larre, Claude, J. Schatz, E. Rochat, and S. Stang. 1986. *Survey of Traditional Chinese Medicine.* Paris: Institut Ricci.

Li Ling 李零. 1993. *Zhongguo fangshu kao* 中國方術考. Beijing: Renmin Zhongguo chubashe.

Liu, Xun. 2009. "Numinous Father and Holy Mother: Late-Ming Duo-Cultivation Practice." In *Internal Alchemy: Self, Society, and the Quest for Immortality*, edited by Livia Kohn and Robin R. Wang, 122-41. Magdalena, NM: Three Pines Press.

Liu, Yanzhi. 1988. *The Essential Book of Traditional Chinese Medicine.* 2 Vols. New York: Columbia University Press.

Liu, Zhengcai. 1990. *The Mystery of Longevity.* Beijing: Foreign Languages Press.

Lo, Vivienne. 2000. "Crossing the *Neiguan*, "Inner Pass": A *Nei/Wai* "Inner/Outer" Distinction in Early Chinese Medicine." *East Asian Science, Technology, and Medicine* 17: 15-65.

_____. 2001a. "*Huangdi Hama jing* (Yellow Emperor's Toad Canon)." *Asia Major* 14.2:61-99.

_____. 2001b. "The Influence of Nurturing Life Culture on the Development of Western Han Acumoxa Therapy." In *Innovation in Chinese Medicine*, edited by Elisabeth Hsu, 19-50. Cambridge: Cambridge University Press.

_____. 2005. "Pleasure, Prohibition, and Pain: Food and Medicine in Traditional China." In *Of Tripod and Palate: Food, Politics and Religion in Traditional China*, edited by Roel Sterckx, 163-85. New York: Palgrave MacMillan.

Loon, Piet van der. 1984. *Taoist Books in the Libraries of the Sung Period.* London: Oxford Oriental Institute.

Lu, Henry C. 1986. *Chinese System of Food Cures: Prevention and Remedies.* New York: Sterling Publishing.

_____. 1996. *Chinese Foods for Longevity: The Art of Long Life.* Selanger, Malaysia: Pelanduk Publications.

Lu, Xichen. 2009. "The Southern School: Cultivating Mind and Inner Nature." In *Internal Alchemy: Self, Society, and the Quest for Immortality*, edited by Livia Kohn and Robin R. Wang, 73-86. Magdalena, NM: Three Pines Press.

Ma Daozong 马道宗, ed. 1999. *Zhongguo daojiao yangsheng mijue* 中国道教养生秘诀. Beijing: Zongjiao wenhua chubanshe.

Maher Derek, and Calvin Mercer, eds. 2009. *Religious Implications of Radical Life Extension*. New York: Palgrave MacMillan.

Mair, Victor H. 1994. *Wandering on the Way: Early Taoist Tales and Parables of Chuang Tzu*. New York: Bantam.

_____., ed. 2010 [1983]. *Experimental Essays on Chuang-tzu*. Dunedin, Fla.: Three Pines Press.

Maspero, Henri. 1981. *Taoism and Chinese Religion*. Translated by Frank Kierman. Amherst: University of Massachusetts Press.

Mather, Richard. 1976. *A New Account of Tales of the World*. Minneapolis: University of Minnesota Press.

Miles, Elisabeth. 1998. *The Feng Shui Cookbook: Creating Health and Harmony in Your Kitchen*. Secaucus, NJ: Carol Publishing Company.

Miller, James. 2008. *The Way of Highest Clarity: Nature, Vision and Revelation in Medieval Daoism*. Magdalena, NM: Three Pines Press.

Mori, Yuria. 2002. "Identity and Lineage: The *Taiyi jinhua zongzhi* and the Spirit-Writing Cult to Patriarch Lü in Qing China." In *Daoist Identity: History, Lineage, and Ritual*, edited by Livia Kohn and Harold D. Roth, 165-84. Honolulu: University of Hawaii Press.

Needham, Joseph, et al. 1983. *Science and Civilisation in China*, vol. V.5: *Spagyrical Discovery and Invention—Physiological Alchemy*. Cambridge: Cambridge University Press.

Neswald, Sara Elaine. 2009. "Internal Landscapes." In *Internal Alchemy: Self, Society, and the Quest for Immortality*, edited by Livia Kohn and Robin R. Wang, 27-53. Magdalena, NM: Three Pines Press.

Ngo, Van Xuyet. 1976. *Divination, magie et politique dans la Chine ancienne*. Paris: Presses Universitaires de France.

Ni, Hua-ching. 1989. *Attune Your Body with Dao-In: Taoist Exercises for a Long and Happy Life*. Malibu, Calif.: Shrine of the Eternal Breath of Tao.

Ni, Maoshing. 1995. *The Yellow Emperor's Classic of Medicine*. Boston: Shambhala.

_____. 2006. *Secrets of Longevity: Hundreds of Ways to Live to Be a 100*. San Francisco: Chronicle Books.

Olshansky, S. Jay, and Bruce A. Carnes. 2001. *The Quest for Immortality: Science at the Frontiers of Aging*. New York: W. W. Norton.

Oschman, James. 2000. *Energy Medicine: The Scientific Basis*. New York: Churchill Livingstone.

Palmer, David. 2007. *Qigong Fever: Body, Science, and Utopia in China*. New York: Columbia University Press.

Pas, Julian F., ed. 1989. *The Turning of the Tide: Religion in China Today*. Hong Kong: Oxford University Press.

Plasker, Eric. 2007. *The 100-Year Lifestyle*. Avon, Mass.: Adams Media.

Porkert, Manfred. 1974. *The Theoretical Foundations of Chinese Medicine*. Cambridge, Mass.: MIT Press.

Pregadio, Fabrizio. 2000. "Elixirs and Alchemy." In *Daoism Handbook*, edited by Livia Kohn, 165-95. Leiden: E. Brill.

_____. 2006. *Great Clarity: Daoism and Alchemy in Early Medieval China*. Stanford: Stanford University Press.

_____, ed. 2008. *The Encyclopedia of Taoism*. London: Routledge.

Reid, Daniel P. 1989. *The Tao of Health, Sex, and Longevity*. New York: Simon & Schuster.

_____. 2003. *The Tao of Detox: The Secrets of Yang-Sheng Dao*. Rochester, Vt.: Healing Arts Press.

Reiter, Florian C. 1990. *Der Perlenbeutel aus den drei Höhlen: Arbeitsmaterialien zum Taoismus der frühen T'ang-Zeit*. Asiatische Forschungen, vol. 12. Wiesbaden: Otto Harrassowitz.

Réquéna, Yves. 2010. *Le Qi Gong Anti-age*. Paris: Guy Trédaniel.

_____. 2012. "The Biochemistry of Internal Alchemy: Decapitating the Red Dragon." *Journal of Daoist Studies* 5:141-52.

Robbins, John. 2006. *Healthy at 100*. New York: Ballentine.

Robinet, Isabelle. 1977. *Les commentaires du Tao to king jusqu'au VIIe siècle*. Paris: Mémoirs de l'Institute des Hautes Etudes Chinoises 5.

_____. 1979. "Metamorphosis and Deliverance of the Corpse in Taoism." *History of Religions* 19: 37-70.

_____. 1983. "Kouo Siang ou le monde comme absolu." *T'oung Pao* 69: 87-112.

_____. 1984. *La révélation du Shangqing dans l'histoire du taoïsme*. 2 vols. Paris: Publications de l'Ecole Française d'Extrême-Orient.

_____. 1989. "Visualization and Ecstatic Flight in Shangqing Taoism." In *Taoist Meditation and Longevity Techniques*, edited by Livia Kohn, 157-90. Ann Arbor: University of Michigan, Center for Chinese Studies Publications.

_____. 1993. *Taoist Meditation*. Translated by Norman Girardot and Julian Pas. Albany: State University of New York Press.

_____. 1998. "Later Commentaries: Textual Polysemy and Syncretistic Interpretations." In *Lao-tzu and the Tao-te-ching*, edited by Livia Kohn and Michael LaFargue, 119-42. Albany: State University of New York Press.

_____. 2000. "Shangqing—Highest Clarity." In *Daoism Handbook*, edited by Livia Kohn, 196-224. Leiden: E. Brill.

Robson, James 2009. *Power of Place: The Religious Landscape of the Southern Sacred Peak in Medieval China*. Cambridge, Mass: Harvard University Asia Center.

Roizen, Michael F., and Mehmet C. Oz. 2007. *You Staying Young*. New York: Free Press.

Roth, Harold D. 1999. *Original Tao: Inward Training and the Foundations of Taoist Mysticism*. New York: Columbia University Press.

Russell, Terence C. 1990. "Chen Tuan's Veneration of the Dharma: A Study in Hagiographic Modification." *Taoist Resources* 2.1: 54-72.

Sabban, Françoise. 1996. "Follow the Seasons of the Heavens: Household Economy and the Absorption of Time in Sixth-century China." *Food and Foodways* 6.3/4:329-49.

Sakade Yoshinobu 坂川祥仲. 1986. "Chō Tan 'Yōsei yōshu' itsubun to sono shisō" 張湛養生要集逸文とその思想. *Tōhōshukyō* 東方宗教 68: 1-24.

_____, ed. 1988. *Chūgoku kodai yōsei shisō no sōgōteki kenkyū*. Tokyo: Hirakawa.

_____. 1989. "Longevity Techniques in Japan: Ancient Sources and Contemporary Studies." In *Taoist Meditation and Longevity Techniques*, edited by Livia Kohn, 1-40. Ann Arbor: University of Michigan, Center for Chinese Studies Publications.

_____. 1992. "Sun Simiao et le Bouddhisme." *Kansai daigaku bungaku ronshu* 42: 81-98.

_____. 2007a. *Taoism, Medicine, and Qi in China and Japan*. Osaka: Kansai University Press.

_____. 2007b. "The View of the Body in the *Laozi Heshang gong zhu*." In *Taoism, Medicine, and Qi in China and Japan*, edited by Yoshinobu Sakade, 29-36. Suita: Kansai University Press.

Santee, Robert. 2008. "Stress Management and the *Zhuangzi*." *Journal of Daoist Studies* 1:93-123.

Saso, Michael. 1978. "What is the *Ho-t'u?*" *History of Religions* 17: 399-416.

_____. 1995. *The Gold Pavilion: Taoist Ways to Peace, Healing, and Long Life*. Boston: Charles E. Tuttle.

_____. 2010 [1983]. "The *Zhuangzi neipian*: A Daoist Meditation." In *Experimental Essays on Zhuangzi*, edited by Victor H. Mair, 137-53. Dunedin, Fla.: Three Pines Press.

Schafer, Edward H. 1977. "The Restoration of the Shrine of Wei Hua-ts'un at Lin-ch'uan in the Eighth Century." *Journal of Oriental Studies* 15: 124-38.

Schipper, Kristofer M. 1965. *L'Empereur Wou des Han dans la legende taoïste*. Paris: Publications de l'Ecole Française d'Extrême-Orient 58.

_____. 1979. "Le Calendrier de Jade: Note sur le *Laozi zhongjing*." *Nachrichten der deutschen Gesellschaft für Natur- und Völkerkunde Ostasiens* 125: 75-80.

_____, and Franciscus Verellen, eds. 2004. *The Taoist Canon: A Historical Companion to the Daozang*. 3 vols. Chicago: University of Chicago Press.

Schwartz, Benjamin. 1985. *The World of Thought in Ancient China*. Cambridge, Mass: Harvard University Press.

Shahar, Meir, and Robert P. Weller, eds. 1996. *Unruly Gods: Divinity and Society in China*. Honolulu: University of Hawaii Press.

Shealy, C. Norman. 2011. *Energy Medicine: Practical Applications and Scientific Proof*. Virginia Beach: 4th Dimension Press.

Shostak, Stanley. 2002. *Becoming Immortal: Combining Cloning and Stem-Cell Therapy*. Albany: State University of New York Press.

Sivin, Nathan. 1967. "A Seventh-Century Chinese Medical Case History." *Bulletin of the History of Medicine* 41: 267-73.

_____. 1968. *Chinese Alchemy: Preliminary Studies*. Cambridge, Mass.: Harvard University Press.

_____. 1988. *Traditional Medicine in Contemporary China*. Ann Arbor: University of Michigan, Center for Chinese Studies.

Skar, Lowell, and Fabrizio Pregadio. 2000. "Inner Alchemy (*Neidan*)." In *Daoism Handbook*, edited by Livia Kohn, 464-97. Leiden: E. Brill.

Smith, Thomas E. 1992. "Ritual and the Shaping of Narrative: The Legend of the Han Emperor Wu." Ph.D. Diss., University of Michigan, Ann Arbor.

Stein, Rolf A. 1963. "Remarques sur les mouvements du taoïsme politico-religieux au IIe siecle ap. J.-C." *T'oung Pao* 50: 1-78.

Stein, Stephan. 1999. *Zwischen Heil und Heilung: Zur frühen Tradition des Yangsheng in China*. Uelzen: Medizinisch-Literarische Verlagsgesellschaft.

Strickmann, Michel. 1978. "The Mao-shan Revelations: Taoism and the Aristocracy." *T'oung Pao* 63: 1-63.

_____. 1981. *Le taoïsme du Mao chan; chronique d'une révélation*. Paris: Collège du France, Institut des Hautes Etudes Chinoises.

Tao Bingfu 陶秉福, ed. 1989. *Nüdan jicui* 女丹集萃. Beijing: Beijing shifan daxue chubanshe.

Teiser, Stephen F. 1988. "Having Once Died and Returned to Life: Representations of Hell in Medieval China." *Harvard Journal of Asiatic Studies* 48.2: 433-64.

_____. 1994. *The Scripture of the Ten Kings: And the Making of Purgatory in Medieval Chinese Buddhism*. Honolulu: University of Hawai'i Press.

Tsuchiya, Masaaki. 2002. "Confession of Sins and Awareness of Self in the *Taiping jing*." In *Daoist Identity: History, Lineage, and Ritual*, edited by Livia Kohn and Harold D. Roth, 39-57. Honolulu: University of Hawaii Press.

Valussi, Elena. 2003. "Beheading the Red Dragon: A History of Female Inner Alchemy in China." Ph. D. Diss., School of Oriental and African Studies, University of London, London.

_____. 2008. "Men and Women in He Longxiang's *Nüdan hebian* (*Collection of Female Alchemy*)." *Nannü: Men, Women and Gender in Early and Imperial China* 10:242-78.

_____. 2009. "Female Alchemy: An Introduction." In *Internal Alchemy: Self, Society, and the Quest for Immortality*, edited by Livia Kohn and Robin R. Wang, 142-64. Magdalena, NM: Three Pines Press.

Veith, Ilza. 1972. *The Yellow Emperor's Classic of Internal Medicine*. Berkeley: University of California Press.

Wagner, Rudolf G. 1973. "Lebensstil und Drogen im chinesischen Mittelalter." *T'oung Pao* 59: 79-178.

Wang, Shumin, and Penelope Barrett. 2006. "Profile of a *Daoyin* Tradition: The 'Five Animal Mimes'." *Asian Medicine: Tradition and Modernity* 2.2: 225-53.

Wang Zongyu 王宗昱. 2001. *Daojiao yishu yanjiu* 道教義樞研究. Shanghai: Shanghai wenhua chubanshe.

Ware, James R. 1966. *Alchemy, Medicine and Religion in the China of AD 320.* Cambridge, Mass.: MIT Press.

Watson, Burton. 1968a. *The Complete Works of Chuang-tzu.* New York: Columbia University Press.

_____. 1968b. *Records of the Grand Historian of China.* 2 vols. New York: Columbia University Press.

Weil, Andrew. 2005. *Healthy Aging: A Lifelong Guide to Your Well-Being.* New York: Anchor Books.

Weiss, Lucas. 2012. "Rectifying the Deep Structures of the Earth: Sima Chengzhen and the Standardization of Daoist Sacred Geography in the Tang." *Journal of Daoist Studies* 5:31-60.

Wells, Matthew. 2009. *To Die and Not Decay: Autobiography and the Pursuit of Immortality in Early China.* Ann Arbor: Association for Asian Studies.

Wenwu 文物. 1990. "Zhangjia shan Hanjian Yinshu shiwen" 張家山漢簡引書釋文. *Wenwu* 文物 1990/10: 82-86.

Wile, Douglas. 1992. *Art of the Bedchamber: The Chinese Sexual Yoga Classics Including Women's Solo Meditation Texts.* Albany: State University of New York Press.

Wilhelm, Hellmut. 1948. "Eine Zhou-Inschrift über Atemtechnik." *Monumenta Serica* 13: 385-88.

Winn, Michael. 2006. "Transforming Sexual Energy with Water-and-Fire Alchemy." In *Daoist Body Cultivation*, edited by Livia Kohn, 151-78. Magdalena, NM: Three Pines Press.

Wu, Baolin, with Michael McBride and Vincent Wu. 2011. *The Eight Immortals' Revolving Sword of Pure Yang.* Dunedin, Fla.: Three Pines Press.

Yang, Jwing-ming. 1988. *The Eight Pieces of Brocade: Improving and Maintaining Health.* Jamaica Plain, Mass.: Yang's Martial Arts Association.

Yao, Ted. 2000. "Quanzhen—Complete Perfection." In *Daoism Handbook*, edited by Livia Kohn, 567-93. Leiden: E. Brill.

Yoshioka, Yoshitoyo. 1979. "Taoist Monastic Life." In *Facets of Taoism*, edited by Holmes Welch and Anna Seidel, 220-52. New Haven, Conn.: Yale University Press.

Yü, Ying-shih. 1987. "O Soul, Come Back: A Study of the Changing Conceptions of the Soul and Afterlife in Pre-Buddhist China." *Harvard Journal of Asiatic Studies* 47: 363-95.

Zhu Yueli 朱越利. 1986. "*Yangxing yanming lu* kao" 養性延命錄考. *Shijie zongjiao yanjiu* 世界宗教研究 1986/1: 101-15.

Zukav, Gary. 1979. *The Dancing Wuli Masters: An Overview of the New Physics*. New York: Bantam.

Index

activities: and long life, 38-39, 44, 174; laugh, 36, 38, 43, 92, 170, 191, 222, 224; run, 38-39, 42, 93; sleep, 25, 33, 38-39, 42, 60, 71, 94, 111, 114, 124, 148, 151, 172, 178, 183-84, 187-89, 199, 237, 243; talk, 35, 38, 43, 161, 172-174, 222, 271; wake, 52-53; walk, 22, 37, 39, 41, 44, 93-94, 110, 130, 132, 148, 174-75, 177-78, 182-83, 185-88, 215, 241; wash, 25, 39, 69-70, 125, 148, 179-80, 184, 187, 195-97, 249; *see also* food

alchemy: internal, 11, 16, 141, 251-62; operative 10, 31-32, 34, 37, 46-47, 50-51, 74, 95, 119, 138; women's 11, 263-74; *see also* elixir

alcohol: abstention from, 9, 151, 185; harm of, 22, 38, 92, 107, 112, 116, 171-72, 176; in supplements, 121, 128-29; use of, 9, 120, 123, 136, 177, 183-84; and visions, 31

animals: bear, 181, 197-98; bird, 181, 197-98; cattle, 61; deer, 181, 197-98; in diet, 44, 123, 151, 153, 246; dragon, 61, 65, 91, 97, 105, 114, 227, 253, 256, 262; in exercise, 26-27, 95-97, 181; Five, 9, 11, 97, 181, 197-98, 218; frog, 101-03; goose, 105; monkey, 181, 197-98; owl, 180; ox, 163; rhino, 22; tiger, 27, 29, 61, 65, 86, 91, 123, 156, 169, 180, 181, 197-98, 227, 240, 253, 256, 262; toad, 97; turtle, 103-04, 106; wolf, 156, 169, 180, 240; worms, 49, 126, 145, 151, 184; zodiac, 75, 253

blood: in body, 5, 21, 35-36, 56-57, 193, 207, 218, 224, 246; harm to, 94, 123, 174, 185, 201, 239; and joints, 56; letting, 191; looking at, 124, 151, 154; menstrual, 267-74; opening of, 100, 104, 106, 125, 136, 155, 190, 197, 223, 246; Prime, 268, 273-74; and pulse, 83, 192; and *qi*, 171, 173, 176, 183, 195, 203, 229, 259; stagnation, 19, 58, 115, 126; as symptom, 44, 88, 184, 187; in women, 181, 261, 267

body care: bathing, 25, 30, 35, 39, 42, 69-71, 109, 119, 123-27, 150, 152-54, 178, 186, 190; hunger, 37, 39, 79-82, 132; sweat, 6, 27, 39, 42, 82, 121, 127, 186-91, 195, 198, 224, 226, 240-41, 271

body terms: Flowery Canopy, 156, 192, 208, 212; Flowery Pond, 113; 171, 244; Hall of Light, 61-62, 84, 158-59, 226; Mountain Spring, 51, 54, 61-62; Niwan Palace, 51, 58-59, 67, 76, 84, 104, 106, 232, 238, 249, 261; Numinous Root, 62, 77, 81, 171, 244, 261; Yellow Court, 77, 82

body: and administration, 35, 53; Chinese, 3-4, 35-36; joints in, 56, 58; meridians in, 6, 28, 37, 82; navel, 60; orifices, 52-54, 58, 60; palaces in, 67, 76, 80, 84;